ATLAS OF
ELECTROPHYSIOLOGY
IN HEART FAILURE

ATLAS OF ELECTROPHYSIOLOGY IN HEART FAILURE

Editors

Kalyanam Shivkumar, MD, PhD

Director, UCLA Cardiac Arrhythmia Center and Electrophysiology Program
Division of Cardiology
Department of Medicine
David Geffen School of Medicine at UCLA
Los Angeles, California

James N. Weiss, MD

Professor
Department of Medicine
Chief, Division of Cardiology
David Geffen School of Medicine at UCLA
Los Angeles, California

Gregg C. Fonarow, MD

Professor of Medicine
Department of Cardiology
David Geffen School of Medicine at UCLA
Director, Ahmanson-UCLA Cardiomyopathy Center
Los Angeles, California

Jagat Narula, MD, DM, PhD

Professor of Medicine
Chief, Division of Cardiology
Associate Dean
University of California, Irvine School of Medicine
Irvine, California

Series Editor

Eugene Braunwald, MD, MD (Hon), ScD (Hon)

Distinguished Hersey Professor of Medicine
Harvard Medical School
Chairman, TIMI Study Group
Brigham and Women's Hospital
Boston, Massachusetts

With 26 Contributors

Developed by Current Medicine LLC
Philadelphia

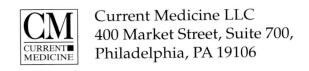

Current Medicine LLC
400 Market Street, Suite 700,
Philadelphia, PA 19106

Director of Editorial, Design, Production . . . . Wendy Vetter
Senior Developmental Editor . . . . Elizabeth Rexon
Commissioning Supervisor Books . . . . Annmarie D'Ortona
Cover Design . . . . Christine Keller-Quirk
Design and Layout . . . . William C. Whitman, Jr. and Christine Keller-Quirk
Illustrators . . . . Wieslawa Langenfeld, Maureen Looney,
                                                                                Kim Broadbent, Theresa Englehart,
                                                                                John McCullough, and William C. Whitman, Jr.
Assistant Production Manager . . . . Margaret La Mare
Indexer . . . . Holly Lukens

Left and *right* cover photos courtesy of Dr. Kalyanam Shivkumar; *middle* cover photo is
Figure 10-7B from Chapter 10.

Library of Congress Cataloging-in-Publication Data

Atlas of electrophysiology in heart failure / editors, Kalyanam Shivkumar ... [et al.] ; with 26 contributors.
    p. ; cm.
  Includes bibliographical references and index.
  ISBN 1-57340-225-7 (hardcover)
  1. Heart failure—Atlases. 2. Heart—Electric properties—Atlases. 3. Electrophysiology—Atlases.
  [DNLM: 1. Heart Failure, Congestive—physiopathology—Atlases. 2. Arrhythmia—diagnosis—Atlases. 3. Electrocardiography—
Atlases. 4. Heart Failure, Congestive—therapy—Atlases. WG 17 A88159 2005] I. Shivkumar, Kalyanam.
  RC685.C53A835 2005
  616.1'29'0222—dc22
                        2005045496

ISBN 1-57340-225-7

For more information, please call 1-800-427-1796 or email us at inquiry@phl.cursci.com
www.current-science-group.com

Although every effort has been made to ensure that drug doses and other information are presented accurately
in this publication, the ultimate responsibility rests with the prescribing physician. Neither the publishers nor
the authors can be held responsible for errors or for any consequences arising from the use of information
contained herein. Products mentioned in this publication should be used in accordance with the prescribing
information prepared by the manufacturers. No claims or endorsements are made for any drug or compound
at present under clinical investigation.

Printed by Phoenix Asia in China

10 9 8 7 6 5 4 3 2 1

Heart failure has emerged as a major cardiovascular health problem. Over the past several decades, it has become apparent that one of the most important causes of morbidity and mortality in patients with congestive heart failure relates to cardiac arrhythmias. Cardiac arrhythmias are thought to be directly responsible for sudden cardiac death in these patients. In addition, associated cardiac rhythm disturbances are important causes of morbidity, such as cerebral vascular accidents and increased propensity for tachyarrhythmias in the setting of heart failure. Over the past decade increasing data have accumulated defining the pathogenesis of these problems at cellular and molecular levels, in addition to the clinical setting.

Clinical cardiology has become progressively subdivided into more highly specialized domains, yet the modern management of the heart failure patient crosses these boundaries. Heart failure/cardiac transplantation training fellowships have emerged as a vital new subspecialty to train subspecialists in this area, but even heart failure subspecialists depend heavily on their clinical electrophysiology colleagues to optimize management of their heart failure patients, driven by the expanding roles of implantable cardioverter-defibrillators (ICDs) and cardiac resynchronization therapy.

Given the cross-disciplinary nature of heart failure management, we believe that this Atlas, which explores current concepts in the interface between heart failure and electrophysiology, comes at a timely juncture.

The first chapter, by Irmina Gradus-Pizlo and Douglas Zipes reviews the epidemiology of heart failure and the presents the rationale for the emergence of specialized heart failure training programs. The next two chapters explore the current state of knowledge about pathophysiology of arrhythmias in heart failure. Peng-Sheng Chen and Michael Fishbein provide an overview of structural remodeling in heart disease at the gross anatomical and microarchitectural levels, which, along with electrical remodeling, define the substrate promoting arrhythmogenesis. Neural remodeling, such as sympathetic nerve sprouting, is also discussed as a key factor that dynamically modulates the arrhythmogenic substrate. Next, James Weiss and Zhilin Qu review the electrophysiological mechanisms causing arrhythmias, focusing on the triggers and dynamic factors promoting wavebreaks that initiate reentry and ultimately lead to sudden cardiac death. The fourth chapter by Hein Wellens and Subramaniam Krishnan focuses on the electrocardiogram in heart failure. The fifth chapter by Gregg Fonarow focuses on the nuances of medical management and the impact of heart failure therapy on arrhythmias, and vice versa. The sixth chapter by David Kass deals with dyssynchronous ventricular contraction that forms the basis for therapies such as biventricular pacing in heart failure. The seventh chapter by William Dec, Rakesh Pai, Kalyanam Shivkumar, and Isaac Wiener takes a close look at the principles and practice of cardiac resynchronization therapy. They present the rationale supporting biventricular pacing and biventricular pacing with ICD therapy in heart failure patients, including discussion of recently concluded clinical trials. The eighth chapter by William Sauer, Hemal Nayak, and Francis Marchlinski deals with risk stratification for sudden death in heart failure patients, a topic of central importance to this Atlas. Criteria for patient selection for various therapeutic modalities are reviewed, based on a series of important multicenter trials appearing in the literature over the past several years. The ninth chapter by Samuel Asirvatham and Paul Friedman addresses supraventricular arrhythmias in heart failure, including their mechanistic basis, diagnosis, and management strategy, including trans-catheter and surgical interventions. The tenth and eleventh chapters deal with ventricular arrhythmias associated with ischemic and nonischemic cardiomyopathy, respectively. Bruce Koplan and William Stevenson discuss the diagnostic algorithms and management strategies for ischemic cardiomyopathy. Kalyanam Shivkumar, Miguel Valderrabano, and Jagat Narula review the same topics for nonischemic cardiomyopathy. Both chapters emphasize the appropriate usage of ICDs in heart failure and discuss at length the available clinical trials. The twelfth chapter by David Cesario, Dwight Reynolds, and Charles Swerdlow discusses novel implantable monitoring devices in heart failure, highlighting the use of devices such as implanted hemodynamic monitors, inotropic pacemakers, and integrated device platforms.

The intent of this Atlas is to provide the "bird's eye view" of the field of arrhythmias in heart failure, to define where we are in 2005, and hopefully to help us see where we are headed in the future. We are greatly indebted to all of the contributors to this Atlas, who, consistent with the old adage that "a picture is worth a thousand words," have culled through their personal collections of slides and figures to pick the most illustrative and informative.

Kalyanam Shivkumar, MD, PhD
James N. Weiss, MD
Gregg C. Fonarow, MD
Jagat Narula, MD, PhD

CONTRIBUTORS

Samuel J. Asirvatham, MD
Assistant Professor of Medicine
Department of Cardiovascular Diseases
Mayo Clinic College of Medicine
Rochester, Minnesota

David A. Cesario, MD
Cedars-Sinai Medical Center
Los Angeles, California

Peng-Sheng Chen, MD
Division of Cardiology
Cedars-Sinai Medical Center
Los Angeles, California

G. William Dec, MD
Chief, Cardiology Division
Massachusetts General Hospital
Boston, Massachusetts

Michael C. Fishbein, MD
Department of Pathology and
  Laboratory Medicine
David Geffen School of Medicine
  at UCLA
Los Angeles, California

Gregg C. Fonarow, MD
Professor of Medicine
Department of Cardiology
David Geffen School of Medicine
  at UCLA
Director, Ahmanson-UCLA
  Cardiomyopathy Center
Los Angeles, California

Paul A. Friedman, MD
Associate Professor of Medicine
Department of Cardiovascular Diseases
Mayo Clinic College of Medicine
Rochester, Minnesota

David A. Kass, MD
Department of Medicine
Division of Cardiology
The Johns Hopkins University
Baltimore, Maryland

Bruce A. Koplan, MD
Cardiovascular Division
Brigham and Women's Hospital
Boston, Massachusetts

Subramaniam C. Krishnan, MD
Henry Ford Heart and Vascular Institute
Detroit, Michigan

Francis E. Marchlinski, MD
Director, Cardiac Electrophysiology
University of Pennsylvania
  Health System
Department of Medicine/Cardiology
University of Pennsylvania School
  of Medicine
Philadelphia, Pennsylvania

Jagat Narula, MD, DM, PhD
Professor of Medicine
Chief, Division of Cardiology
Associate Dean
University of California, Irvine School
  of Medicine
Irvine, California

Hemal M. Nayak, MD
University of Pennsylvania
  Medical Center
Philadelphia, Pennsylvania

Rakesh K. Pai, MD
UCLA Cardiac Arrhythmia Center
Los Angeles, California

Irmina Gradus-Pizlo, MD
Director, Heart Failure Program
Krannert Institute of Cardiology
Indiana University School of Medicine
Indianapolis, Indiana

Zhilin Qu, PhD
David Geffen School of Medicine
  at UCLA
Los Angeles, California

Dwight W. Reynolds, MD
University of Oklahoma Health
  Sciences Center
Oklahoma City, Oklahoma

William H. Sauer, MD
University of Pennsylvania
  Medical Center
Philadelphia, Pennsylvania

Kalyanam Shivkumar, MD, PhD
Director, UCLA Cardiac Arrhythmia
  Center and Electrophysiology
  Program
Division of Cardiology
Department of Medicine
David Geffen School of Medicine
  at UCLA
Los Angeles, California

William G. Stevenson, MD
Director, Clinical Cardiac
  Electrophysiology Program
Brigham and Women's Hospital
Cardiovascular Division
Harvard Medical School
Boston, Massachusetts

Charles D. Swerdlow, MD
Cardiac Electrophysiology
Clinical Professor of Medicine, UCLA
Cedars Sinai Medical Center
Los Angeles, California

Miguel Valderrabano, MD
UCLA Cardiac Arrhythmia Center
Los Angeles, California

James N. Weiss, MD
Professor
Department of Medicine
Chief, Division of Cardiology
David Geffen School of Medicine at
  UCLA
Los Angeles, California

Hein J. Wellens, MD
Emeritus Professor of Cardiology
University of Maastricht
Maastricht, The Netherlands

Isaac Wiener, MD
UCLA Cardiac Arrhythmia Center
Los Angeles, California

Douglas P. Zipes, MD
Distinguished Professor of Medicine,
  Pharmacology, and Toxicology
Director, Division of Cardiology
Krannert Institute of Cardiology
Indiana University School of Medicine
Indianapolis, Indiana

CONTENTS

EPIDEMIOLOGY OF THE PROBLEM AND EMERGENCE OF A NEW SPECIALTY

Irmina Gradus-Pizlo and Douglas P. Zipes

Heart failure is a major health problem in the United States, with 5 million patients affected, 550,000 new cases diagnosed each year, and an increasing number of hospitalizations and death attributed to this disease [1]. Even though the complexity of management of heart failure is increasing, only 17% of patients with heart failure ever see a cardiologist. Primary care physicians deliver the majority of care to patients with heart failure [2]. To assist physicians taking care of heart failure patients, the American College of Cardiology/American Heart Association and the Heart Failure Society of America frequently revise heart failure treatment guidelines to include a position on data coming from new trials. However, guidelines have delayed penetration into the market, and despite the overwhelming evidence that patients with left ventricular systolic dysfunction should be treated with ACE inhibitors, their use in patients before referral to heart failure centers varies from 35% to 75%, depending on the geographic region and the background of the referring physician [3].

For the cardiology community to increase its role in the management of patients with heart failure, we have to address restructuring cardiology training programs to accommodate the emergence of the new specialty. As a spontaneous response to this need, multiple forms of heart failure training have emerged over the past several years. Some programs offer 1-year training to graduates from internal medicine programs, and some offer training as an additional year after cardiology fellowship. This additional year may or may not be combined with training in heart transplantation. At this time, no established guidelines exist regarding the curriculum of these programs or requirements that need to be fulfilled by trainees and by training programs.

One year of training for internal medicine physicians represents a practical approach, which should be considered in view of the enormous needs of the heart failure population. This training may result in the relatively quick emergence of internal medicine subspecialists who will play a leadership role in the primary care environment by providing quality, evidence-based care to heart failure patients and who will bridge the gap between primary and cardiologic subspecialty care for patients with more complex disease. The presence of primary care physicians with special interest in heart failure may increase interactions between primary care physicians and cardiologists, with potentially significant benefits to the patients. Even more important, this group of primary care physicians will be exceptionally positioned to champion heart failure prevention issues—an important aspect of heart failure. In view of the huge societal need, this opportunity has to be attractive to young physicians. It may require the creation of a heart failure training "track" in the selected internal medicine residency training programs, with a third year of residency devoted to training in heart failure, possibly with elements of geriatrics, followed by a special certification examination.

Heart failure fellowship for cardiology fellows should be planned for 2 years and should start after completion of the first 2 years of general cardiology training. Heart failure specialists should be able to deliver comprehensive care to their patients, assure optimal utilization of resources, and reduce the cost of follow-up. After completion of this training, heart failure fellows should be experts in the treatment of patients with heart failure, heart transplant, implanted devices such as biventricular pacemakers, and defibrillators. There is also a dynamically emerging surgical treatment of heart failure with ventricular assist devices (VADs). Adequate exposure to management of these patients should be a part of this fellowship because long-term follow-up of these patients will be best accomplished by a team comprising a heart failure specialist and a cardiovascular surgeon. The 2-year heart failure fellowship training period should be divided among clinical inpatient and outpatient experience, training in diagnosis and treatment of arrhythmias, training in device implantation and follow-up, and in-depth training in hemodynamics of the failing heart and performance of endomyocardial biopsy.

The future of this subspecialty may be even more exciting with the emergence of cardiovascular cell therapy. This therapy is based on delivering pluripotent stem cells or progenitor cells to the failing myocardium. Determining the exact mechanisms underlying the effects of cell therapy on the myocardium is currently an active area of research. A number of recent early human studies of cell therapy have demonstrated safety and feasibility as well as some degree of improvement in left ventricular function when compared with standard therapy. Confirmation of the beneficial effects of cell therapy in large-scale trials, assessment of long-term safety and benefits, and optimization of the cell delivery methods and types of cells delivered are all necessary before cell therapy becomes a mainstay in the treatment of cardiomyopathy; however, it is possible that it will open new opportunities for the treatment of the failing heart. Heart failure fellowship should include involvement in the research of this therapy and of other areas of this discipline.

The specific training requirements for the heart failure fellowship remain to be established, but there is an urgent need for a discussion to facilitate the emergence of this new subspecialty. The Subspecialty Board for Cardiovascular Disease of the American Board of Internal Medicine should formalize the training and procedural requirements for this subspecialty and develop a heart failure subspecialty board examination modeled on the Clinical Cardiac Electrophysiology and Interventional Cardiology examinations. This process will assure the highest quality of emerging training programs, will give this new subspecialty credentials, and will increase its attractiveness to the best cardiology fellowship candidates.

INCIDENCE OF HEART FAILURE

TEMPORAL TRENDS IN THE AGE-ADJUSTED INCIDENCE OF HEART FAILURE*

PERIOD	MEN		WOMEN	
	INCIDENCE OF HEART FAILURE	RATE RATIO	INCIDENCE OF HEART FAILURE	RATE RATIO
	RATE/100,000 PERSON-YEARS		RATE/100,000 PERSON-YEARS	
1950–1969[†]	627 (475–779)	1.00	420 (336–504)	1.00
1970–1979	563 (437–689)	0.87 (0.67–1.14)	311 (249–373)	0.63 (0.47–0.84)
1980–1989	536 (448–623)	0.87 (0.67–1.23)	298 (247–350)	0.60 (0.45–0.79)
1990–1999	564 (463–665)	0.93 (0.71–1.23)	327 (266–388)	0.69 (0.51–0.93)

*All values were adjusted for age (<55, 55 to 64, 65 to 74, 75 to 84, and >85 years). Values in parentheses are 95% confidence intervals.
[†]This period served as the reference period.

FIGURE 1-1. Temporal trends in the age-adjusted incidence of heart failure among subjects in the Framingham Heart Study during a 50-year interval from the 1950s through the 1990s [4]. The Framingham data show that the true, age-adjusted incidence of heart failure over time is not increasing. This study analyzed heart failure rates over the past 50 years. The incidence of heart failure has declined among women and remained unchanged among men. The data indicate that the decline in incidence occurred in the 1970s and that the incidence subsequently remained stable. There is no obvious explanation for this observation. Improvement in the treatment of hypertension may be a possible contributing factor to the noted decline in incidence in the 1970s. It is disap- pointing that more significant reduction in the incidence of heart failure was not observed. However, the fact that the age-adjusted incidence is not increasing is important because there are studies describing the increasing number of hospitalizations and deaths assigned a billing code for heart failure. Data based on billing codes have limitations because billing codes have not been constant over time and are not validated against standardized diagnostic criteria [5]. The strength of the Framingham study is that it used unified criteria for the diagnosis of heart failure. The potential weakness may be in the relatively small sample size of 1075 patients with heart failure to detect trends in incidence over time. (*Adapted from* Levy *et al.* [4].)

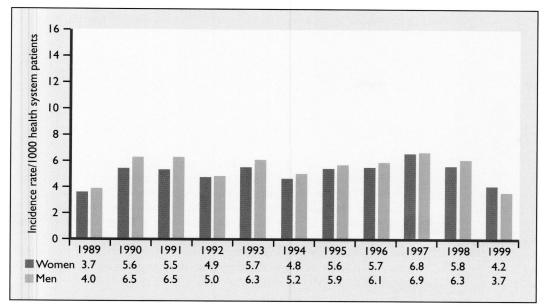

	1989	1990	1991	1992	1993	1994	1995	1996	1997	1998	1999
■ Women	3.7	5.6	5.5	4.9	5.7	4.8	5.6	5.7	6.8	5.8	4.2
▦ Men	4.0	6.5	6.5	5.0	6.3	5.2	5.9	6.1	6.9	6.3	3.7

FIGURE 1-2. Age- and gender-adjusted incidence of congestive heart failure in an integrated health system from 1989 to 1999; *P* > 0.05 for linear trend in both groups. Because the Framingham data set sample size was limited, it is reassuring that data from an integrated health care system serving more than 5 million people with 30,000 cases of heart failure also reported that the age- and gender-adjusted incidence of heart failure was stable from 1989 to 1999 [6]. Men predominated in almost all incident groups. The Resource Utilization Among Congestive Heart Failure (REACH) study included inpatients and outpatients with the diagnosis of heart failure. Patients with both systolic and diastolic heart failure were included. The population also represented a mix of people of all ages and ethnically diverse backgrounds with a variety of insurance plans. Fee-for-service, managed care, Medicaid, and underinsured patients were represented, which was not seen in other epidemiologic studies. The REACH study used ICD-9-CM billing codes as the basis for the definition of heart failure, which represents a significant limitation; however, in this study, a significant effort was made to verify diagnosis. (*Adapted from* McCullough *et al.* [6].)

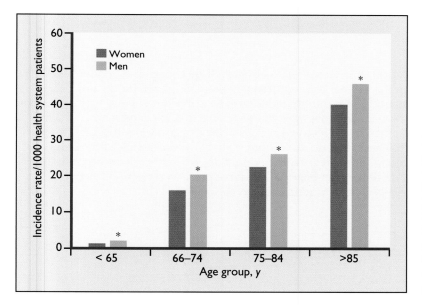

FIGURE 1-3. Incident cases of heart failure in men and women by age group in the Resource Utilization Among Congestive Heart Failure (REACH) study. Men predominated in all incident age groups. Again, cases of both systolic and diastolic heart failure patients are included in these data. These data show the stepwise rising of incidence of heart failure in different age groups for both men and women. The increasing incidence of heart failure with age, together with the increasing population of people 65 years and older, is responsible for the increasing number of patients with heart failure. *P < 0.0000001 for all pairwise comparisons. (*Adapted from* McCullough *et al.* [6].)

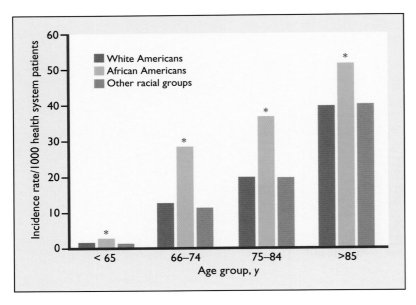

FIGURE 1-4. Incident cases of heart failure in racial groups by age group in the Resource Utilization Among Congestive Heart Failure (REACH) study. African Americans comprised 44.6% of the study sample. The rates of new cases of heart failure were consistently higher among African American patients than they were for whites or other racial groups in all age groups; *$P < 0.0000001$. The "other" racial group, comprising mainly those with "unknown or unstated" race, was relatively equally distributed among the age groupings. (*Adapted from* McCullough *et al.* [6].)

PREVALENCE OF HEART FAILURE BY AGE AND GENDER

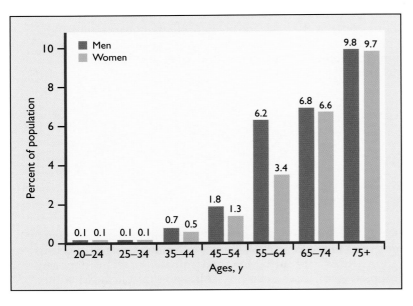

FIGURE 1-5. Prevalence of heart failure by age and gender based on the 44-year follow-up in the National Heart, Blood and Lung Institute's Framingham Heart Study. The prevalence increases from 1% to 2% in those ages 25 to 54 years to 6.2% in men and 3.4% in women in the 55-to-64 age group and approaches 10% after age 75. These data do not differentiate between systolic and diastolic heart failure. It is estimated that approximately half the patients with new-onset heart failure have preserved ejection fraction [7]. (*Adapted from* American Heart Association [1].)

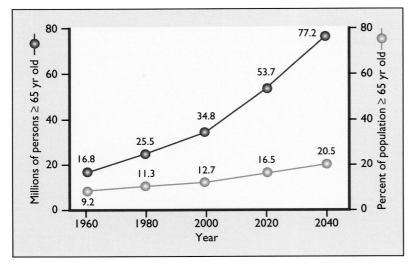

FIGURE 1-6. Projected increase in the US population 65 years of age and older. The rapid increase in the US population of people 65 years and older, together with the increasing incidence of heart failure in this age group, is responsible for the increasing number of patients with heart failure. In 2020, the population of people 65 years of age and older will increase by 54% as compared with 2000. This projection underscores the seriousness and scope of an emerging problem for the health care system. (*Data from* US Census Bureau [8].)

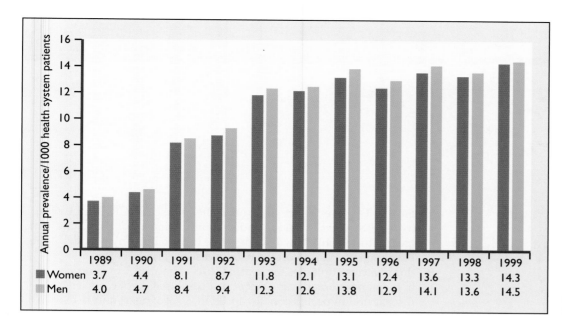

	1989	1990	1991	1992	1993	1994	1995	1996	1997	1998	1999
Women	3.7	4.4	8.1	8.7	11.8	12.1	13.1	12.4	13.6	13.3	14.3
Men	4.0	4.7	8.4	9.4	12.3	12.6	13.8	12.9	14.1	13.6	14.5

FIGURE 1-7. Age- and gender-adjusted prevalence of congestive heart failure in an integrated health system from 1989 to 1999. For both men and women, the prevalence of congestive heart failure has almost tripled over the decade of the 1990s; $P < 0.0001$ for linear trend in women and men. (*Adapted from* McCullough *et al.* [6].)

LIFETIME RISK

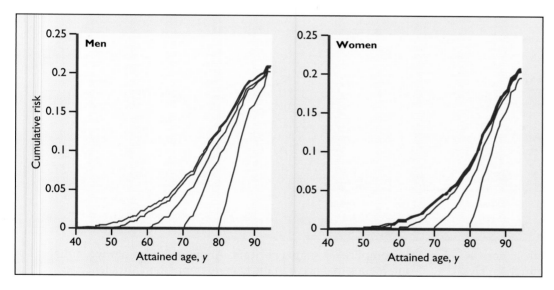

FIGURE 1-8. Cumulative risk for congestive heart failure at selected index ages for men and women. Based on 1972 to 1996 data from the National Heart, Lung and Blood Institute's Framingham Heart Study, the lifetime risk of developing heart failure for both men and women is one in five. At age 40, the lifetime risk of heart failure occurring without antecedent myocardial infarction is one in nine for men and one in six for women. The lifetime risk doubles for people with blood pressure greater than 160/90 mm Hg versus those with pressure less than 140/90 mm Hg. (*Adapted from* Lloyd-Jones *et al.* [9].)

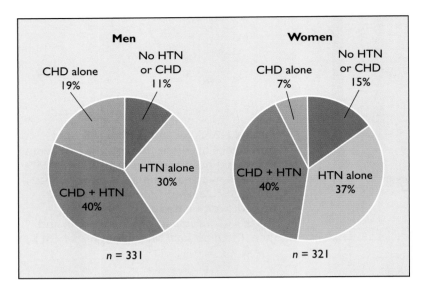

FIGURE 1-9. Prevalence of coronary heart disease (CHD) and hypertension (HTN) alone and in combination among Framingham Heart Study subjects with congestive heart failure, by gender. In the Framingham Study, coronary heart disease and hypertension predominate as etiologies for heart failure. About 40% of heart failure in men and women was a result of a combination of coronary disease and hypertension. In addition, 19% of heart failure in men and 7% in women was caused by coronary disease in isolation. This means that more than half the heart failure patients had coronary disease as a major contributing factor. (*Adapted from* Kannel [10].)

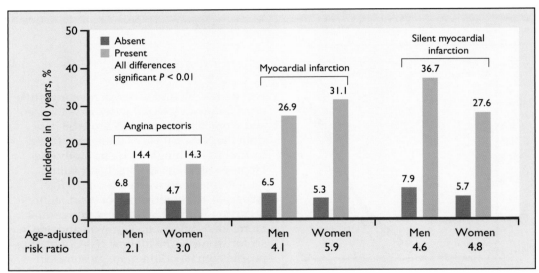

FIGURE 1-10. Risk of heart failure by clinical manifestations of coronary heart disease: 30-year follow-up of Framingham Heart Study subjects, 35 to 94 years of age [11]. People in the Framingham Heart Study with uncomplicated angina pectoris have about a twofold increased risk of congestive heart failure compared with people the same age in the general population. People who have documented myocardial infarction have twice the risk of those with uncomplicated angina pectoris. About one-third of myocardial infarctions that occur in the general population are silent and unrecognized. It is of interest that the occurrence of cardiac failure in people with such infarctions is just as great as in those with symptomatic recognized infarctions. Non–Q wave infarctions carry half the short- and long-term risk of Q wave infarction for development of heart failure. (*Adapted from* Kannel *et al.* [11].)

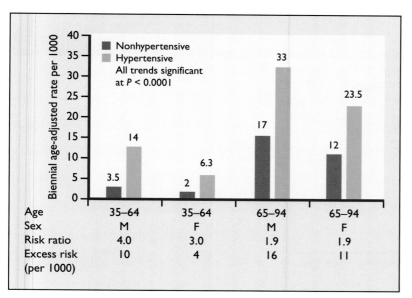

FIGURE 1-11. Cardiac failure by hypertensive status: 36-year follow-up of the Framingham Heart Study [11]. About 75% of heart failure is associated with hypertension with or without other conditions associated with it. Overall, hypertension increases the risk of heart failure by threefold. The risk of hypertension-induced cardiac failure increases with the degree to which the blood pressure is elevated. The isolated systolic hypertension is a powerful contributor to heart failure. In women, the systolic pressure appears to be most important; in men, pulse pressure appears to rival the impact of systolic blood pressure.

Left ventricular hypertrophy, whether diagnosed by roentgenogram, ECG, or echocardiogram, is associated with a greatly increased risk of heart failure. ECG evidence of left ventricular hypertrophy increased the risk of cardiac failure 15-fold. F—female; M—male. (*Adapted from* Kannel *et al.* [11].)

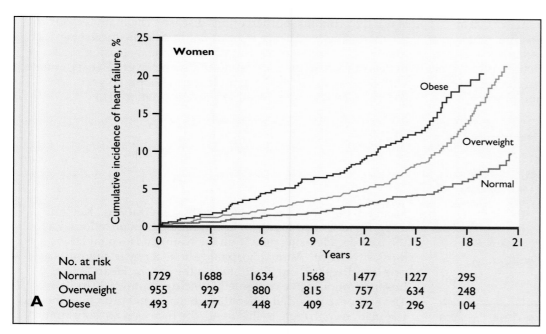

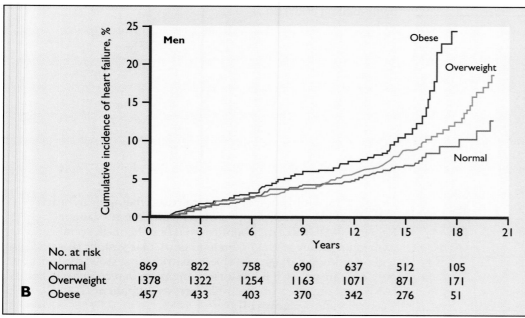

FIGURE 1-12. The role of obesity as a risk factor in the development of heart failure. The role of obesity as a risk factor in the development of heart failure was analyzed in participants in the Framingham Heart Study [12]. The figure shows cumulative incidence of heart failure according to category of body mass index at the baseline examination. The body mass index (defined as weight in kilograms divided by the square of the height in meters) is 18.5 to 24.9 in normal subjects, 25.0 to 29.9 in overweight subjects, and 30.0 or more in obese subjects. After adjustments for established risk factors, there was an increase in the risk of heart failure of 5% for men (**A**) and 7% for women (**B**) for each increment of 1 in body mass index, with no apparent threshold. Compared with subjects with normal body mass index, obese subjects had a doubling of the risk of heart failure. Although obesity is frequently associated with other risk factors for heart failure, such as coronary artery disease and hypertension, this study conclusion was that the risk of heart failure in obese subjects is at least partially independent of other factors associated with excessive body weight. Obesity alone was estimated to account for 11% of cases of heart failure in men and 14% of heart failure in women. These results are particularly important in view of the alarming increase in the incidence of obesity in the United States. (*Adapted from* Kenchaiah *et al.* [12].)

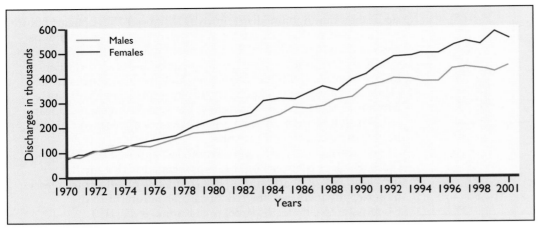

FIGURE 1-13. Hospital discharges for congestive heart failure by sex. Hospital discharges for heart failure rose from 377,000 in 1979 to 995,000 in 2001 for both men and women. This represents an increase of 164%. The increase in hospital discharges does not equal increasing incidence. The number of discharges is based on billing codes, which are not validated and tend to change over time because of changing economic incentives and practice patterns. However, these data provide important information about the economic burden of this disease. The main reason for the increasing prevalence of heart failure and the increasing number of hospitalizations and deaths is the increasing incidence of heart failure in the population of patients over 65 years, coupled with the increase in the US population of people 65 years and older. (*Adapted from* American Heart Association [1].)

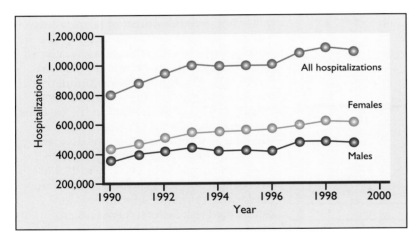

FIGURE 1-14. Trends in heart failure hospitalizations. Koelling *et al.* [13] described trends in heart failure hospitalizations over the past decade using data from the National Hospital Discharge Survey (NHDS). Annual hospitalizations for heart failure as a primary diagnosis are illustrated on the graph. Heart failure hospitalizations have continued to increase from 1990 to 1999. The authors concluded that although aging and growth of the US population contribute to this trend, the increases are substantially influenced by changes in hospitalization rates in women. (*Adapted from* Koelling *et al.* [13].)

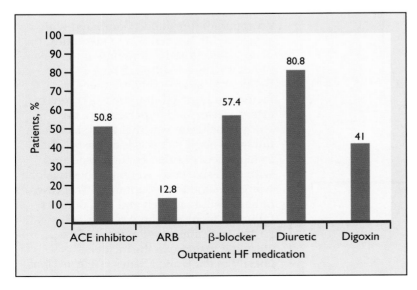

FIGURE 1-15. Utilization of evidence-based therapies in heart failure (HF). Acute Decompensated Heart Failure National Registry (ADHERE) data confirm that of patients hospitalized with heart failure with known left ventricular systolic dysfunction and prior known diagnosis of left ventricular systolic dysfunction, only 64% are on ACE inhibitors or angiotensin receptor blockers (ARB) and only 57% are on β-blockers as outpatients [14]. (*Adapted from* Fonarow [14].)

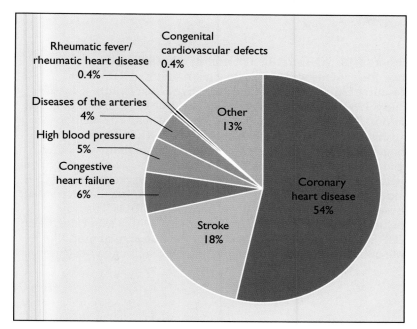

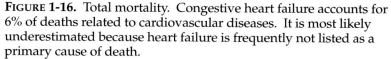

FIGURE 1-16. Total mortality. Congestive heart failure accounts for 6% of deaths related to cardiovascular diseases. It is most likely underestimated because heart failure is frequently not listed as a primary cause of death.

According to a 44-year follow-up of the National Heart, Lung and Blood Institute's Framingham Heart Study, 80% of men and 70% of women under age 65 who have heart failure will die within 8 years. After heart failure is diagnosed, survival is poorer in men than in women, but fewer than 15% of women survive more than 8 to 12 years. The 1-year mortality rate is high, with one in five patients dying. In people diagnosed with heart failure, sudden cardiac death occurs at six to nine times the rate it occurs in the general population. (*Adapted from* American Heart Association [1].)

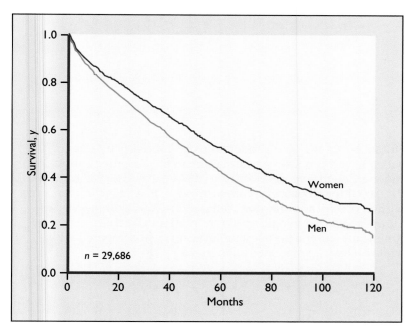

FIGURE 1-17. Age- and race-adjusted survival for men and women with congestive heart failure (CHF) in the Resource Utilization Among Congestive Heart Failure (REACH) study, 1989 to 1999 ($P < 0.0001$). The overall median survival for CHF in the REACH study was 4.5 years for women versus 3.7 years for men. These survival times are longer than previously reported—3.2 years for women and 1.7 years for men—from the combined Framingham Heart and Offspring study cohorts [11]. These differences should be noted in light of the similar mean ages at diagnosis in REACH (69.5 ± 14.5 years) and Framingham (70.0 ± 10.8 years) [6,11]. (*Adapted from* McCullough *et al.* [6].)

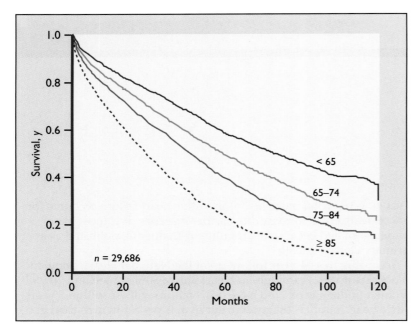

FIGURE 1-18. Age-stratified mortality, adjusted for gender and race, for patients with congestive heart failure (CHF) in the Resource Utilization Among Congestive Heart Failure (REACH) study, 1989 to 1999. Age is taken at the time of diagnosis of heart failure; $P < 0.0001$ for all pairwise comparisons. The median survival for those younger than 65 years in REACH was 6 years, longer than that previously reported in Framingham and other epidemiologic studies [11]. It is supporting the case that improved therapies for myocardial infarction are creating more cases of CHF and that improved treatment of CHF is prolonging the survival of these patients. This is also likely because the REACH study included patients identified as outpatients, with a lesser degree of CHF and, hence, is more reflective of the true annual mortality rate of this condition [6]. (*Adapted from* McCullough *et al.* [6].)

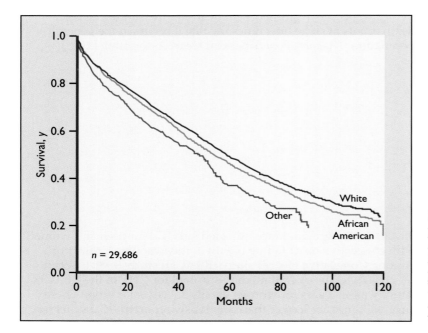

FIGURE 1-19. Age- and gender-adjusted mortality by race for patients with congestive heart failure in the Resource Utilization Among Congestive Heart Failure (REACH) study, 1989 to 1999; $P < 0.0001$ for all pairwise comparisons. REACH included a large portion of African Americans not previously captured in US or European epidemiologic studies or randomized trials. African Americans suffer a poorer long-term survival compared with whites. (*Adapted from* McCullough *et al.* [6].)

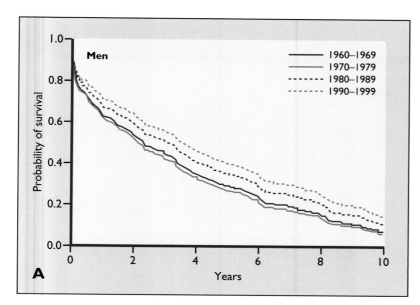

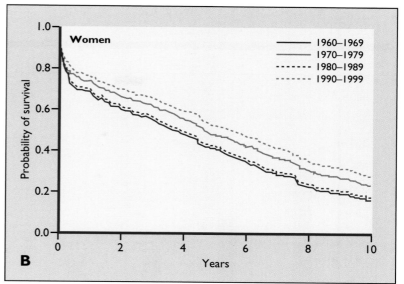

FIGURE 1-20. Temporal trends in age-adjusted survival after the onset of heart failure among men (**A**) and women (**B**) from the Framingham Heart Study. The study period included a 50-year interval from the 1950s through the 1990s [4]. Age-adjusted survival rates after the onset of heart failure improved over time.

The 5-year mortality rate among men declined from 70% in the period from 1950 through 1969 to 59% in the period from 1990 through 1999. The respective rates among women declined from 57% to 45%. The overall trend across time periods was a decline in the risk of death of 12% per decade. (*Adapted from* Levy *et al.* [4].)

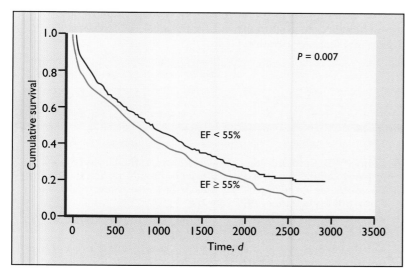

FIGURE 1-21. Survival of patients with congestive heart failure with normal and reduced left ventricular ejection fraction (LVEF) [15]. Approximately one-half of patients with a diagnosis of congestive heart failure have preserved LVEF [16]. Varadarajan and Pai [15] investigated the survival patterns of 2258 patients with a primary discharge diagnosis of congestive heart failure between 1990 and 1999. Mean duration of follow-up was 786 days. Ninety-seven percent of patients were male. Patients with normal LVEF were the same age (mean age 71 ± 11 years) as those with reduced LVEF but had lower prevalence of atrial fibrillation, left bundle branch block, significant mitral regurgitation, and ECG evidence of myocardial infarction. Despite lesser comorbidities, they had a higher mortality hazard, with a 5-year survival of 22% compared with 28% for those with systolic heart failure. It indicates that hospitalized patients with heart failure and normal ejection fraction (EF) have a very poor prognosis. (*Adapted from* Varadarajan and Pai [15].)

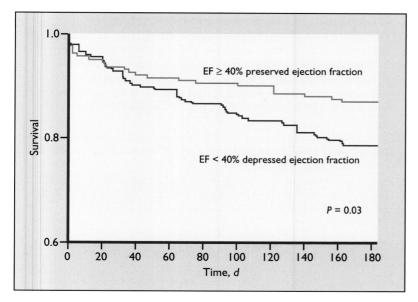

FIGURE 1-22. Clinical outcomes in patients hospitalized with congestive heart failure (CHF). Smith *et al.* [17] also investigated clinical outcomes in a prospective cohort of 413 patients (74% men) hospitalized with CHF. After 6 months, 13% of patients with preserved ejection fraction (EF) died compared with 21% of patients with depressed ejection fraction. The rates of functional decline were similar in both groups. Even though in this study mortality rates were lower in patients with CHF and preserved systolic function, the study confirms that these patients still experience substantial mortality. (*Adapted from* Smith *et al.* [17].)

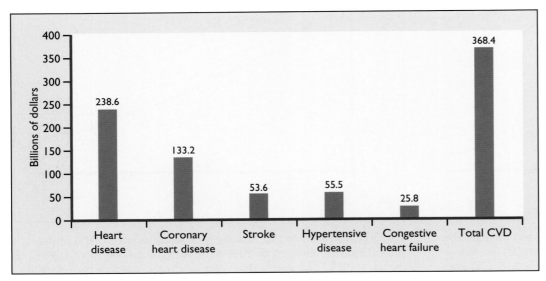

FIGURE 1-23. Estimated direct and indirect costs of cardiovascular diseases (CVD) and stroke. The economic burden of heart failure is substantial. In 2004, the estimated direct and indirect costs of heart failure in the United States is $25.8 billion. The cost is accounted for by hospital care, outpatient care, medications, laboratory tests, procedures, and transplantation. The expenditure dedicated to the treatment of heart failure can be expected only to escalate in the future. Development of a heart failure subspecialty and an increase in the cardiology community's role in the development of a cost-effective strategy for the comprehensive management of heart failure are ways to potentially reduce this cost. (*Adapted from American Heart Association [1].*)

REFERENCES

1. American Heart Association. *Heart Disease and Stroke Statistics—2004 Update.* Dallas, TX: American Heart Association, 2004.

2. O'Connell JB, Bristow MR: Economic impact of heart failure in the United States: time for a different approach. *J Heart Lung Transplant* 1994, 13:(Suppl):107–112.

3. Stevenson LW, Massie BM, Francis GS, *et al.*: Optimizing therapy for complex or refractory heart failure: a management algorithm. *Am Heart J* 1998, 135(6 Part 2):S293–S309.

4. Levy D, Kenchaiah S, Larson MG, *et al.*: Long-term trends in the incidence of and survival with heart failure. *N Engl J Med* 2002, 347:1397–1402.

5. Redfield MM: Heart failure—an epidemic of uncertain proportions. *N Engl J Med* 2002, 347:1442–1444.

6. McCullough PA, Philbin EF, Spertus JA, *et al.*: Confirmation of a heart failure epidemic: findings from the Resource Utilization Among Congestive Heart Failure (REACH) study. *J Am Coll Cardiol* 2002, 39:60–69.

7. Senni M, Tribouilloy CM, Rodeheffer RJ, *et al.*: Congestive heart failure in the community. A study of all incident cases in Olmsted County, Minnesota, in 1991. *Circulation* 1998, 98:2282–2289.

8. US Census Bureau: *National Population Projections.* Washington, DC: US Census Bureau, 2002. Accessible at http://www.census.gov/population/www/projections/natproj.html. Accessed October 10, 2002.

9. Lloyd-Jones DM, Larson MG, Leip EP, *et al.*: Lifetime risk for developing congestive heart failure. The Framingham Heart Study. *Circulation* 2002, 106:3068–3072.

10. Kannel WB: Epidemiology of heart failure in the United States. In *Heart Failure. Scientific Principles and Clinical Practice.* Edited by Poole-Wilson PA, Colucci WS, Massie BM, *et al.* New York: Churchill Livingstone; 1997:279–288.

11. Kannel WB, Ho K, Thom T: Changing epidemiological features of cardiac failure. *Br Heart J* 1994, 72(Suppl S):3–9.

12. Kenchaiah S, Evans JC, Levy D, *et al.*: Obesity and the risk of heart failure. *N Engl J Med* 2002, 347:305–313.

13. Koelling TM, Chen RS, Lubwama RN, *et al.*: The expanding national burden of heart failure in the United States: the influence of heart failure in women. *Am Heart J* 2004, 147:74–83.

14. Fonarow GC: ADHERE registry report Q1 2002 (4/01-3/02) of 180 US hospitals. Presented at the Heart Failure Society of America Satellite Symposium. Boca Raton, FL; September 23, 2002.

15. Varadarajan P, Pai RG: Prognosis of congestive heart failure in patients with normal versus reduced ejection fraction: results from a cohort of 2258 hospitalized patients. *J Cardiac Fail* 2003, 9:107–112.

16. Vasan R, Benjamin E, Levy D: Prevalence, clinical features and prognosis of diastolic heart failure: an epidemiologic perspective. *J Am Coll Cardiol* 1995, 26:1565–1574.

17. Smith GL, Masoudi FA, Vaccarino V, *et al.*: Outcomes in heart failure patients with preserved ejection fraction. Mortality, readmission and functional decline. *J Am Coll Cardiol* 2003, 41:1510–1518.

STRUCTURAL SUBSTRATES FOR ARRHYTHMIAS IN HEART FAILURE

Michael C. Fishbein and Peng-Sheng Chen

A large number of cardiac disorders result in heart failure and are associated with severe arrhythmias that may be fatal. Of the cases of cardiac arrhythmic death, more than 75% are associated with ventricular tachyarrhythmias [1]. The generally accepted paradigm is that there is a preexisting structural abnormality providing a substrate for foci or pathways of intermittent or sustained arrhythmias. Often, there is more than one structural abnormality that is associated with an increased risk of arrhythmia. Then, an acute trigger (*ie*, stress, exercise) or a modification of the environment (electrolyte disturbance), converts a stable situation into an unstable, life-threatening arrhythmic state [2–4].

Usually, it is difficult to recognize, and often impossible to prove, the triggering event. Knowledge of the diurnal variation of sudden death and some pathophysiologic states associated with increased demand on the heart or a decreased substrate supply may provide insights. Indeed, the increased risk of triggering a myocardial infarction by anger, heavy physical exertion, or sexual activity has been quantitated [5]. It is known that there is an increased incidence of cardiac death associated with bereavement and retirement [6], but the moment chosen for the fatal arrhythmias is enigmatic. Reich *et al.* [7] reported 25 patients who had "acute psychologic disturbances" within 24 hours of a ventricular arrhythmia; two-thirds of these were within 1 hour of the event. These and other authors suggest that sympathetic arousal is involved in the genesis of these arrhythmias [8,9]. Such studies are difficult to control and reproduce and depend on subjective interpretations on the part of patients and investigators. "Identifying" an emotional trigger may provide an explanation comforting to the physician and family of the decedent, be it related or not.

Acute ischemia is by far the most common trigger of a fatal arrhythmia. Alone, or superimposed on heart failure, ischemia results in a number of alterations that are proarrhythmic: 1) resting membrane depolarization, 2) a rise in extracellular potassium, 3) increased intracellular calcium, 4) intracellular accumulation of lysophosphoglycerides, 5) increased conduction, and 6) prolongation of the action potential duration. Changes in ischemia also increase tissue inosotropy, which favors re-reentrant arrhythmias [10].

Acute myocardial infarction also results in immediate nerve sprouting, which may lead to heterogeneous sympathetic hyperinnervation, arrhythmia, and sudden death during the convalescent or chronic phase of infarction [11,12]. Dogs with increased cardiac sympathetic nerve density have increased arrhythmias. The arrhythmias and sudden deaths show diurnal variations, with the highest incidence of arrhythmia occurring in the morning hours to early afternoon. These findings suggest that abnormally increased cardiac sympathetic innervation may play an important role in the increased incidence of arrhythmia and sudden death after myocardial infarction.

Ventricular fibrillation is a complex process. The exact mechanisms involved in the initiation, maintenance, and termination of ventricular fibrillation are not completely understood. Activation patterns within the myocardium and vulnerability to fibrillation vary in location and timing. Functional reentry can be demonstrated in myocardium with no structural abnormalities, with activation occurring in the form of meandering spiral-shaped waves [13,14], but the mechanisms by which spiral waves are spontaneously generated are unclear. The sequence of activation in the myocardium has a major impact on the sequence of repolarization. This relationship may be important in determining vulnerability to ventricular fibrillation. Myocardial fiber orientation also influences the timing of both depolarization and repolarization in subepicardial myocytes [15–17]. The spiral waves may also anchor to anatomic structures, such as the root of the papillary muscle [18]. Anchored spiral waves are more stationary and persistent than nonanchored ones. Rapid activation from these spiral waves could serve as a focus for rapid activation that sustains ventricular fibrillation.

There are structural substrates common to heart diseases associated with an increased risk of arrhythmia, regardless of the specific underlying disease. These include 1) ventricular dilatation, 2) myocardial hypertrophy, and 3) myocardial fibrosis.

One or more of these three contribute to decreased ejection fraction and heart failure, a pathophysiologic state that is clearly linked to increased risk of fatal arrhythmia.

Depressed cardiac function is a strong predictor of sudden death. In patients with New York Heart Association class III or IV heart failure, the 1-year mortality in some populations may be as high as 50%, with half of these deaths being sudden [17]. Holter monitor studies have shown that most sudden deaths under these circumstances are related to ventricular tachyarrhythmias. The preponderance of evidence indicates that these arrhythmias are based on reentry. Failed left ventricles are dilated and hypertrophied and have fibrosis and changes in fiber orientation. The myocytes may be subjected to stretch, increased wall tension, increased catecholamines, ischemia, and electrolyte/biochemical changes. It is not surprising that the basic electrophysiologic mechanisms causing arrhythmias in heart failure remain to be clarified.

Structural abnormalities also play an important role in atrial arrhythmogenesis. Recent clinical studies showed that the source of atrial fibrillation is sometimes in the thoracic veins, and radiofrequency ablation within the thoracic veins may lead to a cure of both acute and chronic atrial fibrillation [19]. The muscle sleeves within the pulmonary veins [20] and the muscle bundles in the ligament of Marshall [21,22] both participate in cardiac arrhythmogenesis. Anatomic complexities in these muscle sleeves might contribute to rapid discharges from these structures.

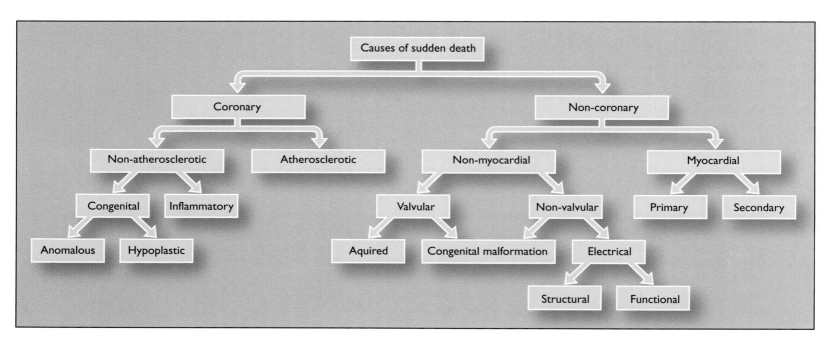

FIGURE 2-1. A categorization of the cardiac diseases in which there is an increased risk of arrhythmic death. In most of these, the substrate (dilatation, hypertrophy, fibrosis, decreased ejection fraction) is evident. In some diseases, such as anomalous coronary artery or myxomatous degeneration of the mitral valve, there may be none of the above substrates preceding an arrhythmic event.

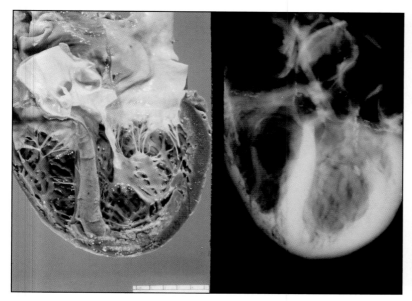

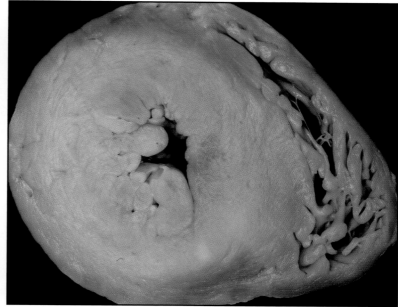

FIGURE 2-2. Ventricular dilatation: gross photograph and post-mortem radiograph of the heart in dilated cardiomyopathy. Independent of its cause, ventricular dilatation is associated with increased left- and, eventually, right-sided filling pressures and neurohumoral activation. Besides these physiologic changes, hypertrophy and some degree of fibrosis are usually present. Ventricular wall thickness may be normal in a dilated, hypertrophied heart, but heart weight will be increased (eccentric hypertrophy). The remodeling associated with dilatation may also result in increased stretch of fibers, which is also arrhythmogenic [17]. Agents such as ACE inhibitors, which prevent postinfarction scar expansion and dilatation, have been associated with improved survival after myocardial infarction [23]. In a rat model, captopril also decreased inducibility of ventricular arrhythmias [24].

FIGURE 2-3. Myocardial hypertrophy: cross-section of ventricles from a patient with long-standing systemic hypertension. Note the markedly thickened left ventricular wall. Regardless of the cause, hypertrophy is a risk factor for sudden death [25]. Studies of the electrophysiology of hypertrophied myocardium have yielded conflicting results. Some experimental studies of hypertrophied myocardium using different preparations and a variety of animals have shown a significant lengthening of action potential duration and a reduction in maximum polarization rate (dV/dtmax) and conduction velocity [17]. Action potential duration increases more in the subepicardial myocardial myocardium, increasing tissue anisotropy, which may contribute to reentrant arrhythmias. Some investigators have found no electrophysiologic changes associated with ventricular hypertrophy. Apparently, basic characteristics of the models being studied are responsible for these differences. Because hypertrophy is almost always associated with interstitial fibrosis, remodeling, and perfusion abnormalities [26,27], it is difficult to relate electrophysiologic abnormalities to the presence of hypertrophy alone, as opposed to hypertrophy plus dilatation, fibrosis, and/or ischemia. Systemic hypertension is the most common cause of left ventricular hypertrophy in humans [28]. Arrhythmias contribute to the increased mortality observed in this population. In addition to the pathophysiologic findings in hypertensive hearts, patients with hypertension may be treated with agents that cause hypokalemia and/or hypomagnesemia, further contributing to arrhythmogenesis.

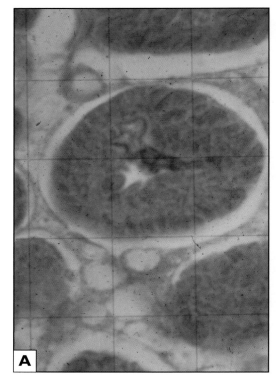 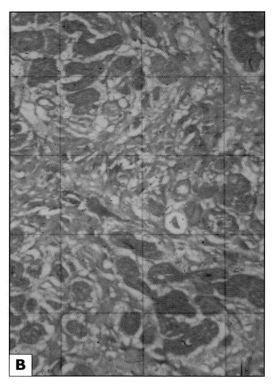

FIGURE 2-4. Quantitation of hypertrophy. **A**, Hypertrophied myocyte (21 μm in diameter by ocular micrometry, normal <15 μm; hematoxylin-eosin stain, ×250). **B**, Lower magnification view showing interstitial fibrosis (*blue staining*) often present in hypertrophied hearts (trichrome stain ×25). The best index of myocardial hypertrophy is increased heart weight. In most species of animals, normal heart weight is about 0.5% of lean body weight. Because there is so much obesity in our society, it is probably better to normalize heart weight to body length rather than body weight, and there are formulas for this purpose [29]. In men, normal heart weight equals 1.9 × height (in centimeters) – 2.1 ± 40 g. In women, normal heart weight equals 1.78 × height (in centimeters) – 21.6 ± 30 g. Wall thickness will be increased in concentric hypertrophy but may not be in eccentric hypertrophy. What about physiologic hypertrophy—so-called athlete's heart? Are athletic individuals at increased risk of arrhythmias and sudden death? In animal models, exercise training prolongs the action potential duration. In humans, increased QT and QTc intervals, heart block with prolongation of other ECG intervals, and complex ventricular ectopy have been described in trained athletes. Although sudden death in athletes is rare, in up to 15% of cases, the only morphologic abnormality is a hypertrophied heart [30]. How does one diagnose hypertrophy in large individuals who undergo intense physical activity and are expected to have large hearts? At what point does "physiologic" hypertrophy become "pathologic" hypertrophy?

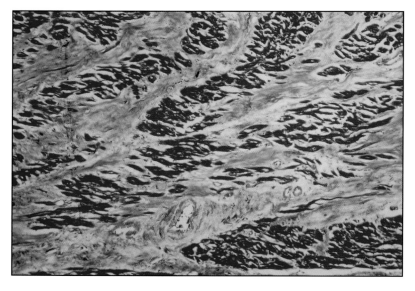

FIGURE 2-5. Fibrosis: photomicrograph of the left ventricle of a patient with idiopathic restrictive cardiomyopathy. Dilatation and hypertrophy are diffuse processes. Fibrosis, on the other hand, is focal or regional and because of its regional distribution, provides a basis for conduction block and reentrant arrhythmias. Large regions of replacement fibrosis may create an anatomic obstacle to conduction, contribute to dilatation and heart failure, and result in compensatory hypertrophy of residual myocardium. Interstitial fibrosis disturbs myocyte interconnections, which may result in unidirectional blocks and slowed conduction. Reentry may occur around fibrotic tissues during ventricular fibrillation [31].

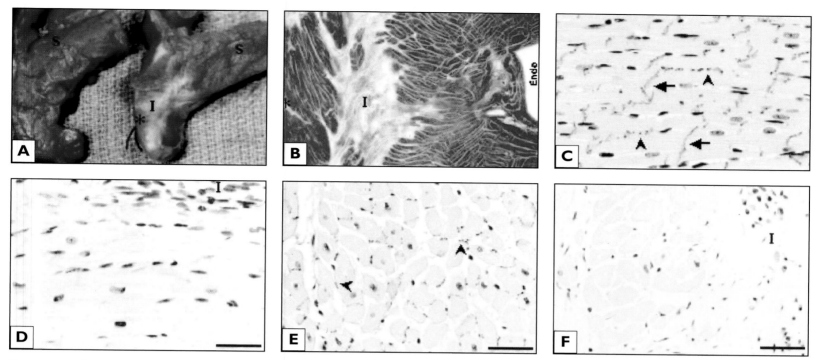

FIGURE 2-6. Gap junctions and arrhythmias. Immunohisto-chemical staining of gap junctions using antibodies to connexin 43 demonstrates end-to-end and side-to-side connections in normal myocardium (**C** and **E**). Around a healed infarct (*I* in **A** and **B**), these connections are absent (**D** and **F**) (bar = 30 μm). Loss of gap junctions has been implicated in arrhythmogenesis [32,33]. Luke and Saffitz [34] demonstrated that interstitial collagen is associated with disruption and remodeling of inter-cellular junctions that would disproportionately enhance axial resistivity in the transverse direction, potentially contributing to the development of reentry arrhythmias. Decreased connexin might play a role in decreased conduction velocity and wave break in the epicardial border zone [35] and facilitate the maintenance of ventricular fibrillation. Gap junctions now represent an entire field of investigation into arrhythmogenesis.

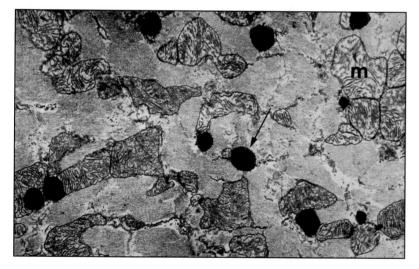

FIGURE 2-7. Acute ischemia: electron photomicrograph of canine myocardium with irreversible acute ischemic changes. Mito-chrondria (m) are swollen with disrupted cristae, and numerous lipid droplets (*arrow*) are present. Within minutes after the onset of myocardial ischemia, ultrastructural changes are apparent in the injured myocardium [36]. Although all "triggers" of ventricular arrhythmias probably have not been identified, the majority of arrhythmias are thought to be triggered by four interactive, not mutually exclusive mechanisms: 1) ischemia, 2) biochemical/metabolic changes, 3) neural/hormonal changes, and/or 4) toxic effects on myocytes [2,3,37]. Ischemia, an imbalance in oxygen supply and demand, results in substrate deprivation, generation of arrhythmogenic metabolites, and ionic shifts. The effects of neural/hormonal change on arrhyth-mogenesis may also be eventually mediated by changes in intra-cellular ions. (Uranyl acetate/lead citrate stain ×10,000.)

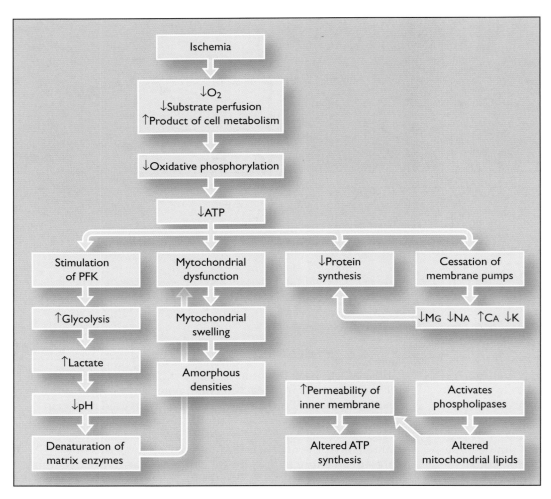

FIGURE 2-8. Biochemical, functional, and structural abnormalities early (minutes) after the onset of ischemia. Even before morphologic changes occur, there are profound metabolic changes, which have been shown to be arrhythmogenic. These include elevated extracellular potassium and intracellular accumulation of calcium, hydrogen ions, lactate, cyclic mono-phosphate, lysophospholipid, fatty acid esters, free fatty acids, and free radicals. Metabolic and ultrastructural changes persist in the reversibly injured fibers. These are usually most easily detected in adjacent surviving subendocardial and subepicardial myocytes [38–40]. PFK—phosphofructokinase.

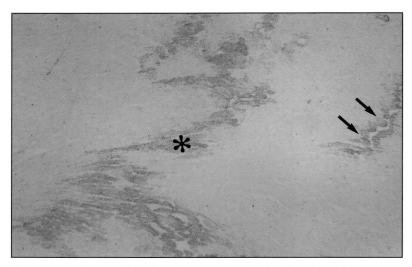

FIGURE 2-9. Lateral border of rat myocardial infarction 24 hours after coronary occlusion. Note the presence of abundant lipid at the edge of the infarct (*asterisk*) and within the infarct (*arrows*). Although a lateral border zone around an infarct is a disputed entity, metabolic derangements are demonstrable in these regions [40]. These metabolic changes contribute to an environment for reentry and probably automaticity-related arrhythmia as well. It has been shown that subendocardial Purkinje cells that survive an acute ischemic insult are necessary for the development of an endocardial-epicardial activation rate gradient that develops during ventricular fibrillation [41]. (Oil red O stain ×10.) (*From* Fishbein *et al.* [40]; with permission.)

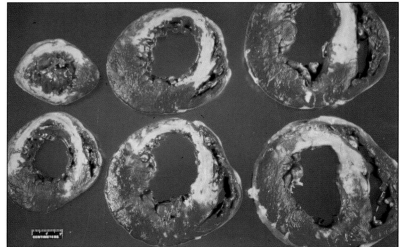

FIGURE 2-10. Serial transverse slices of ventricles, from apex to base, stained with triphenyltetrazolium chloride to identify regions of acute necrosis (*yellow color*). This patient had a massive anterolateral-septal myocardial infarction and died of congestive heart failure, never experiencing serious ventricular arrhythmias. Why some patients with large infarcts never suffer arrhythmias whereas others with ischemia but no infarcts die suddenly is not known.

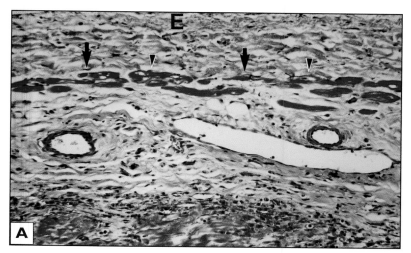

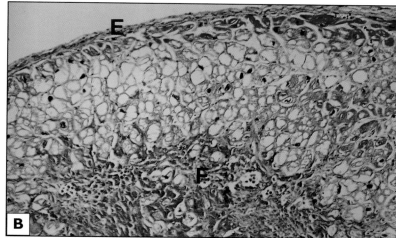

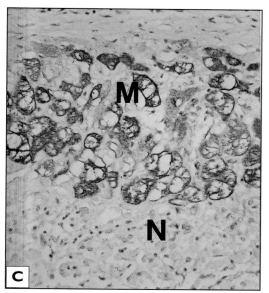

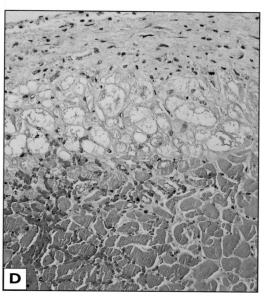

FIGURE 2-11. Residual myocardial fibers after myocardial infarction. **A**, Subendocardial fibers (*arrowheads*) are almost always present late after infarction, presumably because these regions get their blood supply from the ventricular cavity. **B**, Preserved subendocardial fibers between the endocardium (E) and old fibrous scar (F) showing extensive myocytolysis (vacuolar change). **C**, Immunohistochemical stain for myoglobin demonstrating the viability of cells with myocytolysis (M) as opposed to necrotic cells (N), which fail to stain. **D**, Hematoxylin-eosin–stained section of the same area (×50). The heart with established ischemic injury,

ie, healed myocardial infarction, has been the best-studied model of reentrant pathways in arrhythmogenesis. Witt *et al.* [42], using a canine model of myocardial infarction, was able to demonstrate an epicardial origin of reentry arrhythmias. Bolick *et al.* [43] studied human hearts from patients who had a history of ventricular tachycardia after myocardial infarction and found that these hearts had a thick ribbon of surviving subendocardial myocytes, with prominent myocytolysis (vacuolar change) present. Myocytolysis is thought to reflect chronic ischemic injury of fibers. Such fibers are viable and contain increased lipids, which are arrhythmogenic [39].

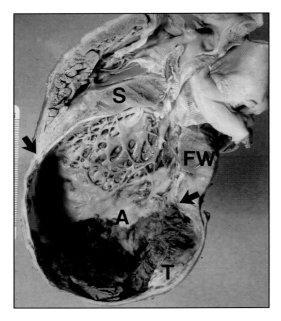

FIGURE 2-12. Sagittal section of the heart of a man who experienced excruciating chest pain after jogging. He continued to jog for about 1 week to try to get into better shape. About 2 months later, he developed severe, congestive heart failure with arrhythmias. Autopsy showed a massive apical aneurysm (A) with mural thrombus (T). The *arrows* indicate where the aneurysm begins. In a canine model of infarction, Garan *et al.* [44] demonstrated that sustained ventricular tachycardia could be related to the presence of epicardial, endocardial, and/or intramural reentry circuits. In the hearts of such patients, the surviving myocardium around regions of infarction is not normal. Such regions demonstrate acute and/or chronic ischemic changes, fibrosis, and/or hypertrophy [45–49]. FW—free wall; S—septum.

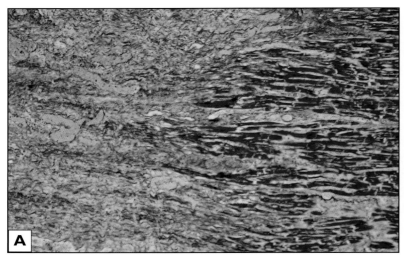

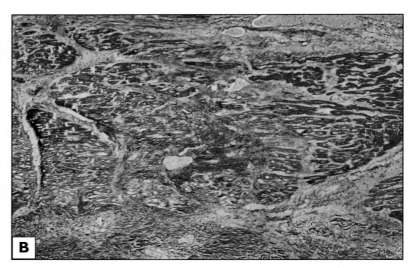

FIGURE 2-13. **A**, Junction of a circumscribed scar of an old, healed myocardial infarction with viable myocardium. **B**, A different infarct, at the edge of which is heterogeneous tissue composed of a mosaic of patchy fibrosis and residual viable myocardium (trichrome stain ×25). Although any heart with ischemic injury is susceptible to ventricular arrhythmias, those with large infarcts and/or aneurysms are at greatest risk [49], but infarct geometry also plays a role, as patchiness of fibrosis at the edge of an infarct may increase inducibility of arrhythmias. Evaluation of individual factors that might increase the risk of arrhythmias is complicated by the presence of other factors, such as compensatory hypertrophy, remodeling with dilatation of the ventricle, and decreased ejection fraction, which are independent predictors of ventricular tachyarrhythmias.

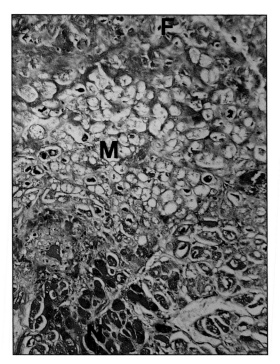

FIGURE 2-14. Section of heart from a patient with chronic, ischemic heart disease who died suddenly. Note the healed, fibrous scar (F), adjacent myocytolysis (M), and focal acute coagulation necrosis (N) (trichrome stain ×50). In a heart with chronic ischemic injury, arrhythmogenesis depends on 1) the size and geometry of the infarct, 2) surrounding extracellular matrix abnormalities, 3) altered connections between myocytes, and 4) changes in surviving myocytes, including hypertrophy, atrophy, and acute (coagulation necrosis) and/or chronic (myocytolysis) ischemic injury.

CONDITIONS ASSOCIATED WITH HYPERTROPHY

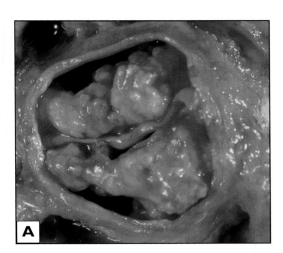
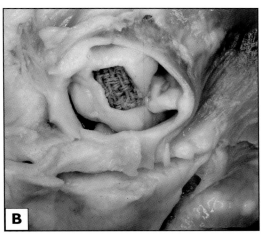

FIGURE 2-15. Aortic stenosis. **A,** Severely stenotic bicuspid aortic valve of an elderly man who presented with severe right-sided heart failure. No murmur was heard, presumably because cardiac output was so low. The patient did not have arrhythmias. **B,** Bicuspid valve of an 11-year-old boy who died suddenly, presumably of a ventricular tachyarrhythmia. The degree of stenosis is only moderate. Valvular heart disease may be associated with hypertrophy, dilatation, fibrosis, heart failure, and/or ischemia. The best example of the lethal combination of the above factors is aortic valve stenosis, in which sudden death is common. The valve shown in *panel B* is not nearly as stenotic as the valve shown in *panel A.* The 11-year-old boy would take daily walks with his father up a small hill. During one of these walks, the boy collapsed and died. These cases illustrate that there is not always a close correlation between the degree of valvular stenosis, sudden death, and heart failure. Furthermore, it demonstrates an inability to identify "triggers" to cardiac arrhythmias. Why did this young man choose this particular day to die? Nothing was different during this walk, as opposed to other walks this child had taken with his father on previous days.

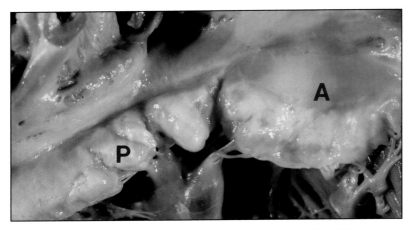

FIGURE 2-16. Mitral valve prolapse: mitral valve with slight thickening of the anterior leaflet (A) and more prominent thickening and scalloping of the posterior leaflet (P). Mitral valve prolapse is a valvular disease associated with sudden death in

which the pathogenesis of the arrhythmia is even less clear. Such hearts may be normal in size (no hypertrophy), without gross fibrosis, and free of ischemia. Some investigators have even reported an inverse relationship between the degree of valvular dysfunction and risk of sudden death in this entity [50]. Proposed mechanisms of sudden death in mitral valve prolapse include 1) coexisting myopathy, 2) increased "irritability" due to friction between abnormal chordae and left ventricular endocardium, 3) abnormal tension on the papillary muscles caused by the valvular abnormalities, 4) coexisting abnormal conduction pathways, and 5) intracoronary microemboli [51]. Sometimes microscopic fibrosis is present, particularly in the posterior wall of the left ventricle. The valve in the photograph is from a 16-year-old girl who participated in competitive track at her high school. She was at a movie theater with her sister, apparently completely well. Her sister went out for popcorn, and when she returned, she found her sister dead. At autopsy, the mitral valve showed myxomatous changes. There was focal fibrosis of the posterior wall of the left ventricle. There was no history of any cardiac abnormalities.

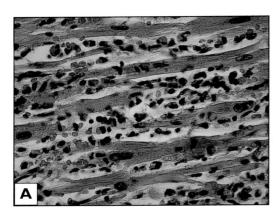
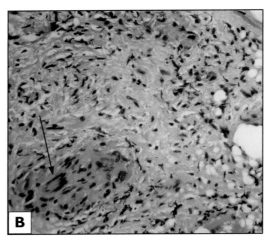

FIGURE 2-17. Infiltrative disorders. **A,** Histologic section of myocardium showing severe myocarditis (hematoxylin-eosin stain ×50). A number of inflammatory and neoplastic conditions may present with heart failure and/or ventricular arrhythmias or sudden death, presumed to be on the basis of ventricular tachyarrhythmias. Myocarditis accounts for about 10% of sudden death in young people who die during strenuous exercise. *Panel A* shows the histology of the heart of a college student who came home for the winter holidays

and died suddenly during Christmas dinner with her family. She was apparently asymptomatic in spite of the presence of severe myocarditis. Sudden death may be the first manifestation of cardiac sarcoidosis [52]. **B,** Endomyocardial biopsy of a young woman who was successfully resuscitated from an episode of sudden death. At the time of electrophysiologic studies, an endomyocardial biopsy was obtained that showed non-necrotizing granulomas (*arrow*), leading to the diagnosis of isolated cardiac sarcoidosis.

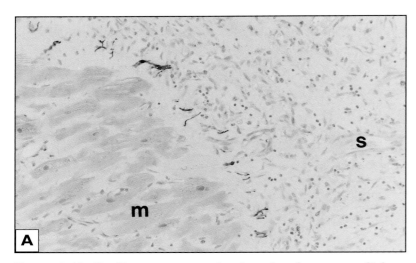
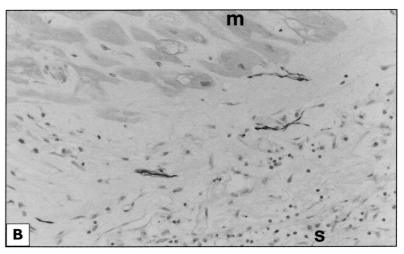

FIGURE 2-18. Cardiac nerve sprouting 2 weeks after myocardial infarction. **A,** Results of S100 staining. Brown nerve twigs are evident between surviving myocytes (m) and scar tissue (s).

B, Higher-power view of the same slide. Nerve sprouting occurs early after infarction. Experimental studies suggest that nerve sprouting plays a role in sudden death after infarction [53].

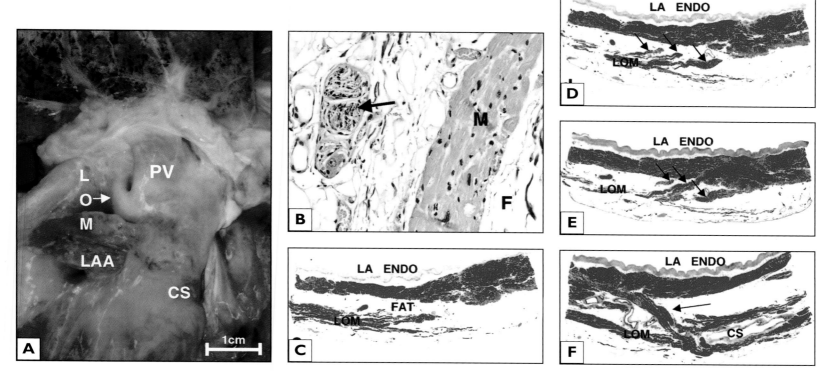

FIGURE 2-19. Ligament of Marshall (LOM) in a human patient.
A, Gross photograph showing location on the posterior surface of
the heart. **B,** Immunohistochemical staining for tyrosine hydroxylase showing positively in nerve (*brown staining—arrow*)
(avidin-biotin-peroxidase stain ×120). **C–E,** Subserial sections
showing the ligament of Marshall isolated from the left atrial wall
(*panel C*), with three tracts (*arrows*) emerging from it (*panel D*), and
eventually inserting into the atrial wall (*panel E*) (hematoxylin-
eosin [H & E] stain ×10). **F,** Section from the lower end of
ligament of Marshall showing the tract inserting into the left atrial
wall (*arrow*) and coronary sinus (CS) (H & E stain ×10). F—fat;
LAA—left atrial appendage; M—myocardium; PV—left superior
pulmonary vein. (*From* Kim *et al.* [22]; with permission.)

Acknowledgments

This work was supported by a generous endowment from the
Piansky Family Trust (MCF), by a Pauline and Harold Price
Endowment (PSC), and by National Institutes of Health grants
P50HL52319, R01HL66389, and R01HL71140.

References

1. Myerburg RJ, Kessler KM, Zaman L, et al.: Survivors of pre-
hospital cardiac arrest. *JAMA* 1982, 247:1485–1490.

2. Myerburg RJ, Kessler KM, Bassett AL, Castellanos A: A biological
approach to sudden cardiac death: structure, functions, and cause.
Am J Cardiol 1989, 63:1512–1516.

3. Myerburg RJ, Kessler KM, Castellanos A: Pathophysiology of
sudden cardiac death. *Pacing Clin Electrophysiol* 1991, 14:935–943.

4. Jimenez RA, Myerburg RJ: Sudden cardiac death: magnitude of
the problem, substrate/trigger interaction and populations at high
risk. *Cardiol Clin* 1993, 11:108.

5. Muller JE, Mittleman MA, Maclure M, *et al.*: Triggering myocardial
infarction by sexual activity. Low absolute risk and prevention by
regular physical exertion. *JAMA* 1996, 275:1405–1409.

6. Greene WA, Goldstein S, Moss AJ: Psychosocial aspects of sudden
death. *Arch Intern Med* 1972; 129:725–731.

7. Reich P, DeSilva RA, Lown B, Murawski BJ: Acute psychological
disturbances preceding life-threatening ventricular arrhythmias.
JAMA 1981, 246:233–235.

8. Lown B, Temte JV, Reich P, *et al.*: Basis for recurring ventricular
fibrillation in the absence of coronary heart disease and its
management. *N Eng J Med* 1976, 294:623–629.

9. Meredith IT, Broughton A, Jennings GL, Esler MD: Evidence of a
selective increase in cardiac sympathetic activity in patients with
sustained ventricular arrhythmias. *N Eng J Med* 1991, 325:618–624.

10. Ehlert FA, Goldberger JJ: Cellular and pathophysiological
mechanisms of ventricular arrhythmias in acute ischemia and
infarction. *Pacing Clin Electrophysiol* 1997, 20:966–975.

11. Cao JM, Chen LS, Ken-Knight BH, *et al.*: Nerve sprouting and
sudden cardiac death. *Circ Res* 2000, 86:816–821.

12. Cao JM, Fishbein MC, Han JB, *et al.*: Relationship between regional
cardiac hyperinnervation and ventricular arrhythmia. *Circulation*
2000, 101:1960–1969.

13. Pertsov AM, Davidenko JM, Salomonsz R, *et al.*: Spiral waves of
excitation underlie reentrant activity in isolated cardiac muscle.
Circ Res 1993, 72:631–650.

14. Spach MS, Miller WT, Geselowitz DB, *et al.*: The discontinuous nature of propagation in normal canine cardiac muscle. Evidence for recurrent discontinuities of intracellular resistance that affect the membrane current. *Circ Res* 1981, 49:39–54.

15. Gotoh M, Uchida T, Fan W, *et al.*: Anisotropic repolarization in ventricular tissue. *Am J Physiol* 1997, 272:H107–H113.

16. Osaka T, Kodama I, Tuboi N, *et al.*: Effects of activation sequence and anisotropic cellular geometry on the repolarization phase of action potential of dog ventricular muscles. *Circulation* 1987, 76:226–236.

17. Pye MP, Cobbs SM: Mechanisms of ventricular arrhythmias in cardiac failure and hypertrophy. *Cardiovasc Res* 1992, 26:740–750.

18. Valderrabano M, Lee MH, Ohara T, *et al.*: Dynamics of intramural and transmural reentry during ventricular fibrillation in isolated swine ventricles. *Circ Res* 2001, 88:839–848.

19. Chen P-S, Wu TJ, Hwang C, *et al.*: Thoracic veins and the mechanisms of non-paroxysmal atrial fibrillation. *Cardiovas Res* 2002, 54:295–301.

20. Hamabe A, Okuyama Y, Miyauchi Y, *et al.*: Correlation between anatomy and electrical activation in canine pulmonary veins. *Circulation* 2003, 107:1550–1555.

21. Doshi RN, Wu TJ, Yashima M, *et al.*: Relation between ligament of Marshall and adrenergic atrial tachyarrhythmia. *Circulation* 1999, 100:876–883.

22. Kim DT, Lai AC, Hwang C, *et al.*: The ligament of Marshall: a structural analysis in human hearts with implications for atrial arrhythmias. *J Am Coll Cardiol* 2000, 36:1324–1327.

23. Pfeffer MA, Pfeffer JM, Steinberg CR, Finn P: Survival after an experimental myocardial infarction: beneficial effects of long-term therapy with captopril. *Circulation* 1985, 72:406–412.

24. Belichard P, Savard P, Cardoma R, *et al.*: Markedly different effects on ventricular remodeling result in a decrease in inducibility of ventricular arrhythmias. *J Am Coll Cardiol* 1994, 34:505–513.

25. Levy D, Garrison RJ, Savage DD, *et al.*: Prognostic implications of echocardiographically determined left ventricular mass in the Framingham Heart Study. *N Eng J Med* 1990, 322:1561–1566.

26. Murray PA, Baig H, Fishbein MC, Vatner SF: Effects of experimental right ventricular hypertrophy on myocardial blood flow in conscious dogs. *J Clin Invest* 1979, 64:421–427.

27. Marcus ML, Harrison DG, Chilian WM, *et al.*: Alterations in the coronary circulation in hypertrophied ventricles. *Circulation* 1987, 75(Suppl I):I19–I25.

28. Frohlich ED, Apstein C, Chobanian AV, *et al.*: The heart in hypertension. *N Eng J Med* 1992, 327:998–1008.

29. Zeek PM: The weight of the normal human heart. *Arch Pathol* 1942, 34:820–832.

30. Hart G: Exercise-induced cardiac hypertrophy: a substrate for sudden death in athletes. *Exp Physiol* 2003, 88:639–644.

31. Wu TJ, Ong JJ, Hwang C, *et al.*: Characteristics of wave fronts during ventricular fibrillation in human hearts with dilated cardiomyopathy: role of increased fibrosis in the generation of reentry. *J Am Coll Cardiol* 1998, 32:187–196.

32. Saffitz JE: Myocyte interconnections at gap junctions and the development of anatomic substrates of ventricular arrhythmias. *Cardiovasc Pathol* 1994, 3:87–91.

33. Ino T, Fishbein MC, Mandel WJ, *et al.*: Cellular mechanisms of ventricular bipolar electrograms showing double and fractionated potentials. *J Am Coll Cardiol* 1995, 26:1080–1089.

34. Luke RA, Saffitz JE: Remodeling of ventricular conduction pathways in healed canine infarct border zones. *J Clin Invest* 1991, 87:1594–1602.

35. Ohara T, Ohara K, Cao JM, *et al.*: Increased wavebreak during ventricular fibrillation in the epicardial border zone of hearts with healed myocardial infarction. *Circulation* 2001, 103:1465–1472.

36. Kloner RA, Fishbein MC, Hare CM, Maroko PR: Early ischemic ultrastructural and histochemical alterations in the myocardium of the rat following coronary artery occlusion. *Exp Mol Pathol* 1979, 30:129–143.

37. Opie LH, Nathan D, Lubbe WF: Biochemical aspects of arrhythmogenesis and ventricular fibrillation. *Am J Cardiol* 1979, 43:131–148.

38. Friedman PL, Fenoglio JJ Jr, Wit AL: Time course for reversal of electrophysiological and ultrastructural abnormalities in subendocardial Purkinje fibers surviving extensive myocardial infarction in dogs. *Circ Res* 1975, 36:127–144.

39. Edwalds GM, Said JW, Block MI, *et al.*: Myocytolysis (vacuolar degeneration) of myocardium. *Hum Pathol* 1984, 15:753–756.

40. Fishbein MC, Hare CA, Gissen SA, *et al.*: Identification and quantification of histochemical border zones during the evolution of myocardial infarction in the rat. *Cardiovasc Res* 1980, 19:41–49.

41. Cha YM, Uchida T, Wolf PL, *et al.*: Effects of chemical subendocardial ablation on activation rate gradient during ventricular fibrillation. *Am J Physiol* 1995, 269:H1998–H2009.

42. Witt AL, Allessie MA, Bonke FIM, *et al.*: Electrophysiologic mapping to determine the mechanisms of experimental ventricular tachycardia initiated by premature impulses: experimental approach and initial results demonstrating re-entrant excitation. *Am J Cardiol* 1982, 49:166–185.

43. Bolick DR, Hackel DB, Reimer KA, Ideker RE: Quantitative analysis of myocardial infarct structure in patients with ventricular tachycardia. *Circulation* 1986, 74:1266–1279.

44. Garan H, Fallon JT, Rosenthal S, Ruskin JN: Endocardial, intramural and epicardial activation pattern during sustained monomorphic ventricular tachycardia in late canine myocardial infarction. *Circ Res* 1987, 60:879–896.

45. Rubin SA, Fishbein MC, Swan HJC: Compensatory hypertrophy in the heart after myocardial infarction in the rat. *J Am Coll Cardiol* 1983, 1435–1441.

46. De Bakker JMT, Coronel R, Tusseron S, *et al.*: Ventricular tachycardia in the infarcted, Langerdorff-perfused human heart: role of the arrangement of surviving cardiac fibers. *J Am Coll Cardiol* 1990, 15:1594–1607.

47. Sugi K, Karagueuzian HS, Fishbein MC, *et al.*: Cellular electrophysiologic characteristics of surviving subendocardial fibers in chronically infarcted right ventricular myocardium susceptible to inducible sustained ventricular tachycardia. *Am Heart J* 1987, 114:559–569.

48. Gang ES, Bigger JT Jr, Livelli FD Jr: A model of chronic ischemic arrhythmias: the relation between electrically inducible ventricular tachycardia, ventricular fibrillation threshold and myocardial infarct size. *Am J Cardiol* 1982, 50:469–477.

49. Karagueuzian HS, Sugi K, Ohta M, *et al.*: Inducible sustained ventricular tachycardia and ventricular fibrillation in conscious dogs with isolated right ventricular infarction: relation to infarct structure. *J Am Coll Cardiol* 1986, 7:850–858.

50. Dollar AL, Roberts WC: Morphologic comparison of patients with mitral valve prolapse who died suddenly with patients who died from severe valvular dysfunction or other conditions. *J Am Coll Cardiol* 1991, 17:921–931.

51. Chesler E, King RA, Edwards JE: The myxomatous mitral valve and sudden death. *Circulation* 1983, 67:632–639.

52. James TN: Clinicopathologic correlations. De subitaneis mortibus. XXV. Sarcoid heart disease. *Circulation* 1977, 56:320–326.

53. Chen PS, Chen LS, Cao JM, *et al.*: Sympathetic nerve sprouting, electrical remodeling and the mechanisms of sudden cardiac death. *Cardiovas Res* 2001, 50:409–416.

MOLECULAR AND CELLULAR BASIS OF ARRHYTHMIAS IN HEART FAILURE

James N. Weiss and Zhilin Qu

The goal of this chapter is to discuss the factors that promote a high incidence of ventricular arrhythmias and sudden cardiac death (SCD) in the setting of heart failure. First, some basics of cardiac electrophysiology are reviewed, including the ionic currents generating the ventricular action potential and the principles underlying propagation of the cardiac electrical wave. Second, the mechanisms of wave break that lead to cardiac reentry are described, emphasizing the roles of both preexisting tissue heterogeneity and dynamic wave instability. Third, the effects of structural and electrical remodeling in heart failure on induction of reentry are discussed, including the mechanisms underlying the increased incidence of triggering events. Finally, the roles of neural remodeling and autonomic dysfunction are addressed as factors that dynamically modulate the heterogeneous electrical substrate of heart failure to promote ventricular arrhythmias and SCD.

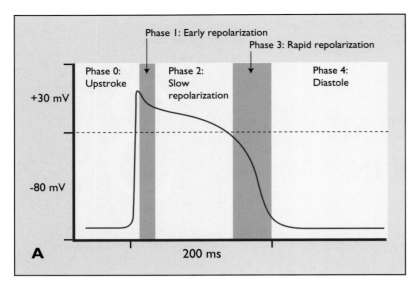

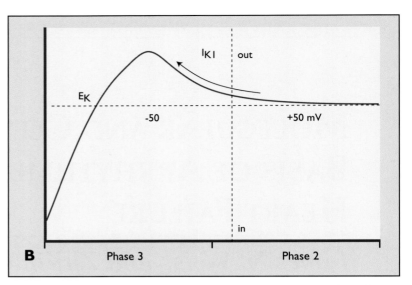

FIGURE 3-1. Basics of the cardiac action potential (AP). The cardiac AP is divided into five phases (**A**). *Phase 0* refers to the AP upstroke and is carried predominantly by the sodium (Na) current (SCN5A channels) in atrial, ventricular, and His-Purkinje muscle, and by the L-type calcium (Ca) current in the sinoatrial node and atrioventricular node. The AP upstroke plays a critical role in determining conduction velocity, with a faster rate of depolarization (dV/dt_{max}) corresponding to a faster conduction velocity.

Phase 1 refers to the early repolarization phase, or notch, and is more prominent in ventricular epicardium than endocardium. It is mediated primarily by the transient outward potassium (K) current (I_{to}), which is activated during the AP upstroke but then inactivates, causing a notch in the early portion of the AP plateau. The physiologic significance of this current, including why it is more prominent in epicardium versus endocardium, is uncertain; however, it may play a role in enhancing the efficiency of Ca_i release by increasing the driving force for Ca entry through L-type Ca channels during the early portion of the AP plateau.

Phase 2 refers to slow repolarization during the AP plateau and is the major determinant of AP duration (APD). Ionic currents arising from multiple ion channels and electrogenic transporters (such as Na-Ca exchanger) all influence phase 2. Physiologically, the L-type Ca current and time-dependent K currents, such as I_{Kr} (HERG channels) and I_{Ks} (KvLQT1 channels), are particularly important in regulating the duration of phase 2 and, hence, APD. The L-type Ca current is activated during the AP upstroke, peaks within 10 ms, and then begins to inactivate. Meanwhile, the time-dependent K currents activate more slowly, causing a progressive increase in outward K current. Thus, as the inward L-type Ca current turns off and the K currents turn on, net current becomes progressively more outward, causing gradual repolarization of the membrane potential during the AP plateau. Different expression levels of ion channels, particularly K channels, underlie transmural and base-to-apex gradients in APD, as well as the prolonged APD characteristic of the midmyocardial wall (the M cell layer). This normal AP heterogeneity becomes exaggerated in heart failure and has important implications for arrhythmias

(*see* Fig. 3-8). Physiologic regulation of the APD is critical: as heart rate increases, APD must shorten to preserve diastole for both ventricular filling and coronary flow. The relationship between APD and diastolic interval is referred to as APD restitution. As discussed later, APD restitution plays a key role in regulating the dynamic stability of electrical wave propagation.

Phase 3 refers to the rapid repolarization phase of the AP. Once the AP has triggered Ca_i release to generate contraction, heart cells must repolarize quickly and synchronously to allow for efficient refilling of the ventricles and coronary flow during diastole. Rapid repolarization is mediated primarily by the inward rectifier K current I_{K1} (Kir2 channels), with some initial contribution by I_{Kr} as well. Both currents have the interesting property of anomalous rectification, defined by a negative slope region in their current-voltage (I-V) relationships (**B**). Thus, as membrane voltage decreases gradually during the AP plateau, I_{Kr} and I_{K1} generate progressively more outward current, which facilitates more rapid repolarization, in a positive feedback cycle. Once the membrane potential during the AP approaches ~ 0 millivolts (mV), repolarization becomes progressively more rapid and regenerative, first via I_{Kr} and then via I_{K1}.

Phase 4 refers to diastole. In ventricular muscle, membrane potential during phase 4 is normally stable near –80 mV. In His-Purkinje tissue, however, spontaneous diastolic depolarization occurs, corresponding to an idioventricular escape rhythm of 20 to 30 bpm, which is normally overdriven by the faster sinus rate. The stable resting potential of ventricular muscle is mediated by the inward rectifier K current I_{K1}. These channels remain open when membrane potential is near the K equilibrium potential (EK; normally ~ –95 mV), ensuring a high K conductance during diastole. However, when membrane potential is driven away from EK by depolarization, I_{K1} shuts off as positively charged intracellular polyamines and magnesium are driven into the pore of the channel, blocking K permeation. This feature is nature's elegant solution to preventing excessive K loss during the long cardiac AP plateau, when the driving force for K efflux ($E_m – E_K$) increases by an order of magnitude. It also reduces the magnitude of inward current required to maintain the long AP plateau.

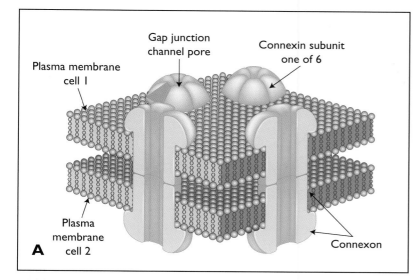

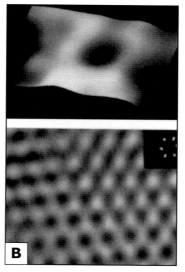

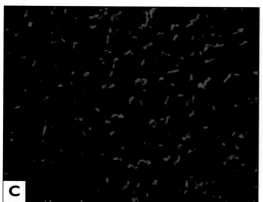

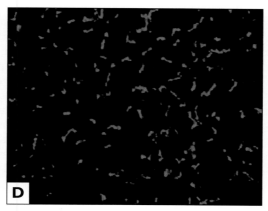

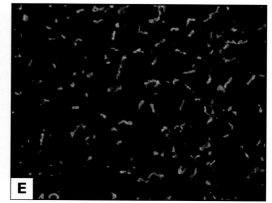

FIGURE 3-2. Basics of electrical wave propagation in the heart. Propagation of the action potential (AP) from myocyte to myocyte is mediated via intercellular ion channels formed by arrays of proteins known as connexins, concentrated in gap junctions. **A**, Six connexin subunits form a hemichannel (connexon) in the membrane of one myocyte and connect to a hemichannel from an adjacent myocyte to form an intercellular channel. **B**, High- (*top*) and low-resolution (*bottom*) images of a gap junction plaque using atomic force microscopy. The hexagonal symmetry of the hemichannels is apparent. **C–E**, The distribution of intercalated discs (*panel C*, using cadherin antibodies) and gap junction protein (*panel D*, using connexin 43 antibodies) in intact ventricular muscle, with the overlay (*yellow*) shown in *panel E* [1].

Gap junction plaques at the intercalated disks contain up to several hundred thousand intercellular channels. Each ventricular myocyte makes connections via gap junctions with about 11 other myocytes. The end-to-end gap connections are more prominent than side-to-side connections, which makes conduction velocity (CV) two- to threefold faster parallel than

perpendicular to fiber direction. This property is known as anisotropic conduction. Although CV is faster parallel to fiber direction, the safety factor for propagation is lower than in the perpendicular direction. This can lead to unidirectional conduction block parallel to fiber direction, potentially initiating reentry. In addition, the fiber angle twists by more than 180° from the ventricular epicardium to endocardium, which can also play a role in facilitating reentry [2,3].

Two major factors determine how rapidly the AP propagates. The first is a property of the cell—how quickly the voltage changes during the AP upstroke (dV/dt_{max}). In the atrial and ventricular myocardium, dV/dt_{max} is mainly determined by the amplitude of the sodium current. The second is a property of the tissue—the degree to which cells are interconnected by gap junctions. Gap junctional conductance determines how quickly the current generated by depolarized cells can flow into adjacent cells to bring them to their AP threshold. Together, these properties determine CV of the cardiac electrical wave. (*Panels C–E from* Gutstein *et al.* [1]; with permission.)

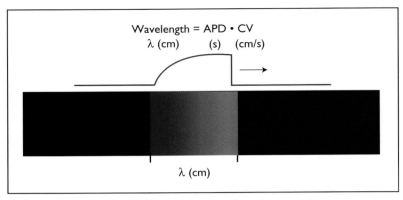

Wavelength = APD • CV
λ (cm)   (s)   (cm/s)

λ (cm)

FIGURE 3-3. Propagation of the action potential (AP). The cardiac impulse can be characterized as an electrical wave, with a wave front (*red*) corresponding to the AP upstroke (phase 0), and a wave back (*light blue*) corresponding to rapid repolarization (phase 3). The wavelength, *ie*, the distance between the wave front and wave back, is defined as the product of action potential duration (APD) and conduction velocity (CV). This concept is critically important for understanding arrhythmias, because reentry, the most common form of clinically important arrhythmias, is fundamentally related to wave break. Wave break occurs when wavelength goes to zero, *ie*, propagation fails, in a region of the ventricle. Normally, when a wave propagates through cardiac tissue, wave front and wave back never touch. If they do, their point of intersection (zero wavelength) defines a wave break. Under the right conditions, localized wave break can induce reentry.

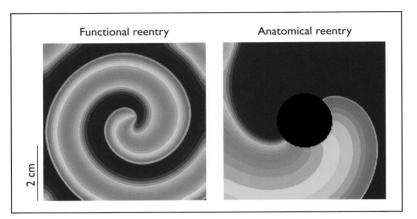

Functional reentry   Anatomical reentry

2 cm

FIGURE 3-4. Anatomic and functional reentry. Reentry begins at a localized wave break because the curvature of the wave front at that point is very high. The high curvature produces a source-sink mismatch that slows conduction of the propagating wave near this point, causing the wave to rotate around the wave break point. If this wave break rotates around an anatomically defined circuit, such as an infarct (*black circle, right panel*), it is called anatomic reentry. However, the wave break can also rotate without an anatomic circuit as functional reentry, called a rotor, which is equivalent to a spiral wave in two-dimensional or a scroll wave in three-dimensional tissue (*left panel*). The *panels* show voltage snapshots, with the most depolarized tissue in red, changing from yellow to green to most repolarized in blue.

Rotor formation as a possible cause of cardiac arrhythmias was first proposed by Krinsky [4], Gul'ko and Petrov [5], and Winfree [6]. Key experimental evidence was obtained by Allessie *et al.* [7–9], who in the 1970s showed that functional ("leading circle") reentry could occur in the absence of an anatomic obstacle. In 1992, Davidenko *et al.* [10] established the relationship conclusively by documenting spiral/scroll wave reentry in ventricular tissue, which they proposed as a mechanism of fibrillation [11].

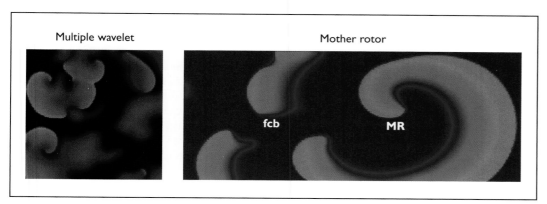

Multiple wavelet   Mother rotor

FIGURE 3-5. Fibrillation: multiple wavelet versus mother rotor (MR)? It is generally accepted that fibrillation requires an initial wave break to create the first rotor, although it is possible that focal activity underlies some types of fibrillation, especially in the atrium and thoracic veins [12,13]. However, a controversy exists over whether subsequent wave breaks are required to maintain fibrillation. In the multiple wavelet hypothesis [14–16], continual wave break is proposed to be the engine of fibrillation (*left panel*), whereas the mother rotor hypothesis [17,18] postulates that a relatively stable fast "mother rotor" caused by the initial wave break drives fibrillation (*right panel*). In the latter case, subsequent wave breaks occur as epiphenomena, related to fibrillatory con-duction block (fcb) in outlying regions that are unable to follow the mother rotor with one-to-one conduction. For both mechanisms of ventricular fibrillation, however, the initial wave break is critically important, and understanding its mechanism holds the key to developing effective preventive therapy for fibrillation.

Wave breaks may be caused by either preexisting or dynamically generated tissue heterogeneity. The mechanisms by which these types of heterogeneity promote wave break, as well as how they interact to make the heart susceptible to ventricular fibrillation and sudden cardiac death in the setting of heart failure, are discussed in the next series of figures.

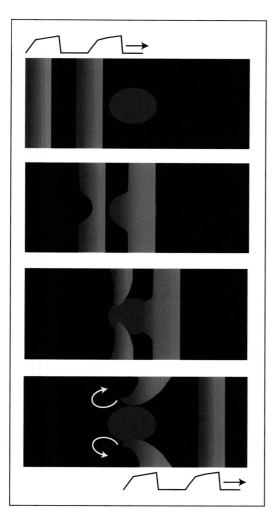

FIGURE 3-6. Causes of wave break: preexisting tissue heterogeneity. Wave break occurs when the diffusive current generated by the wave front (the source) is insufficient to sustain regenerative depolarization in the tissue beyond the wave front (the sink). This situation may arise as a result of either preexisting or dynamically generated tissue heterogeneity. Traditionally, preexisting tissue heterogeneities have been viewed as the major factor predisposing ventricular muscle to wave break, causing rotor formation and ventricular fibrillation. The illustration shows a wave propagating into a region with prolonged action potential duration (APD; *light blue oval*). If the wavelength, which is proportional to APD, lengthens sufficiently in this region, the excitable gap between the wave back and the advancing wave front of the next wave will be eliminated, resulting in localized wave break. A rotor begins to form, and if the rotor has enough excitable tissue, functional reentry results. Subsequently, reentry can either remain functional as a sustained rotor, or be converted to anatomic reentry by anchoring to a structural element, as shown in Figure 3-4. In addition, sustained reentry requires a critical tissue size such that the wave front can always find new excitable tissue. If wavelength is too long relative to tissue size, reentry is nonsustained. Thus, a critical mass of tissue, relative to wavelength, is required for reentry to sustain itself. The principle of type 3 anti-arrhythmic drug action is to prolong refractoriness so that the wavelength's exceeding the threshold above reentry can be sustained in normal cardiac tissue dimensions.

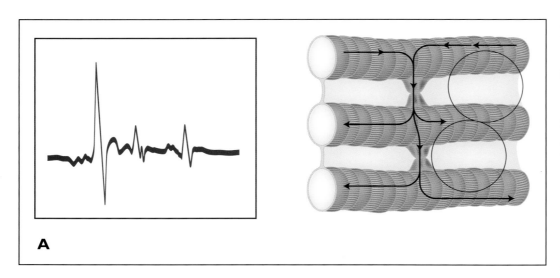

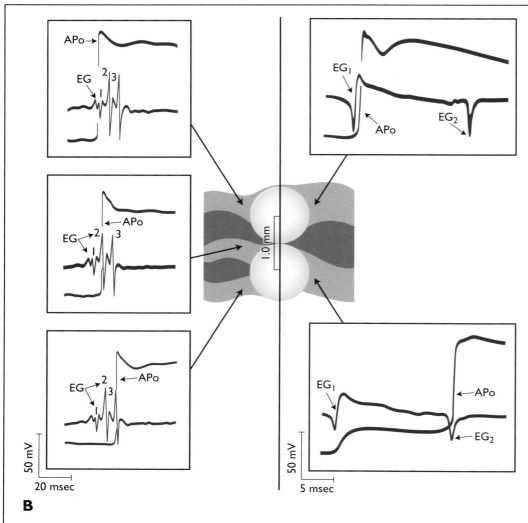

FIGURE 3-7. Effects of heart failure (HF) on preexisting tissue heterogeneity: structural remodeling. In ischemic HF, the border zone between nonischemic and ischemic tissue is characterized by strands of surviving ventricular myocardium fibers interlaced with collagen bundles (**A** [*right*]). The poor connectivity due to reduced gap junction connections between fibers creates nonuniform anisotropy with slow, even, discontinuous conduction in these areas (*arrows*) facilitating wave break and reentry. Such areas are often characterized by fractionated delayed electrograms (**A** [*left*]). Fractionated electrograms (EG) are composed of multiple spikes, each of which correspond to local action

potential activations in the complex anatomy of the muscle strands (**B**). Fractionated electrograms may be detected noninvasively as late potentials in the signal-averaged electrocardiogram, and are also often identified during intracardiac mapping studies in patients with ischemic HF. If implicated (by various pacing protocols) in the ventricular tachycardia (VT) reentry circuit, they may identify ablation sites to cure the arrhythmia.

Increased tissue heterogeneity such as that in an infarct border zone plays a key role in increasing the susceptibility of the failing heart to VF. Disease processes that increase tissue heterogeneity increase the likelihood that physiologic triggers, such as spontaneous premature extrasystoles, will succeed in causing a localized wave break, typically at the border between normal and diseased tissue. Once a localized wave break initiates reentry, a rotor may then either be unstable and break up into fibrillation or become anchored by a tissue heterogeneity to produce monomorphic tachycardia. A major component of increased tissue heterogeneities in HF is structural remodeling.

Structural remodeling in HF occurs over several scales. In HF due to ischemic heart disease, myocardial infarct scars often produce macroscopic heterogeneities. Macroscopic anatomic defects act not only as sites that promote the initial wave break–inducing reentry, but also may subsequently anchor the rotor to produce stable reentry around an anatomically defined circuit. This is thought to be the reason why monomorphic VT is more common in ischemic HF than in non-ischemic HF. In nonischemic HF, myocardial fibrosis is more diffuse and typically does not create macroscopic structural defects, despite global dilation and/or hypertrophy of the ventricles. Reduced connectivity still promotes wave break leading to rotor formation, but rotors are less likely to become anchored around an anatomically defined circuit. In non-ischemic HF, VT is typically polymorphic because of the changing electrical axis as the rotor meanders through the ventricles.

In addition to fibrosis that disrupts connectivity between myocardial fibers, gap junction remodeling also occurs at the myocyte level in HF. Overall, gap junction density is reduced, and the preferential end-to-end distribution of gap junctions is disrupted. In summary, structural remodeling in HF increases preexisting tissue heterogeneity at multiple levels, from macroscopic to microscopic.

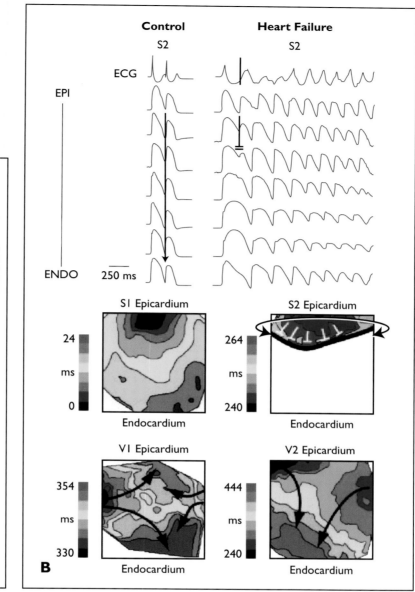

FIGURE 3-8. Effects of heart failure (HF) on preexisting tissue heterogeneity: electrical remodeling. HF also induces changes in the expression of a variety of ion channels and transporters that alter both the action potential (AP) and intracellular calcium (Ca) transient. Generally, HF prolongs the ventricular AP. The molecular alterations underlying these changes are complex, but prominent among them are down-regulation of time-dependent potassium (K) currents such as I_{Ks} and I_{to}, up-regulation of sodium-calcium exchange, and down-regulation of the sarcoplasmic reticulum Ca ATPase (SERCA pump). The K current changes lead to AP prolongation, producing modest QT interval prolongation. It has been speculated that increased arrhythmogenesis in HF may represent a form of acquired long QT syndrome [19]. **A,** In a canine HF model, normal transmural AP heterogeneity is markedly accentuated, with the AP duration prolongation greatest in the M cell layer compared with the epicardial (EPI) and endocardial (ENDO) layers. This increased transmural AP heterogeneity may be a major factor increasing susceptibility to wave break and reentry. **B,** A single premature extrastimulus (S2) failed to induce reentry in normal hearts but consistently induced ventricular tachycardia/fibrillation in the HF hearts. The mechanism is shown in the *lower right panel*: a focal extrastimulus delivered at the epicardium was initially blocked in the M cell layer but propagated successfully along the epicardial surface until the M region regained excitability. The electrical wave then penetrated to the endocardium and reentered the previously refractory M region to initiate a reentry. (*Adapted from* Akar and Rosenbaum [19]; with permission.)

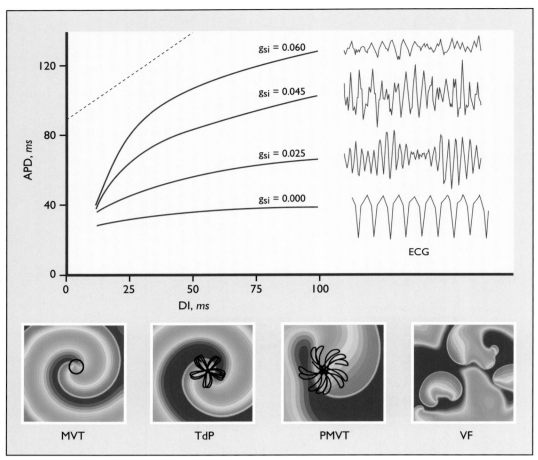

FIGURE 3-9. Causes of wave break: dynamic wave instability. The initiation of a rotor and its degeneration into a fibrillation-like state may occur in the absence of any preexisting tissue heterogeneity [20,21]. In these simulations, every cell in the two-dimensional tissue had identical properties. After wave break was induced by a large premature stimulus, the subsequent behavior was determined by the steepness of the action potential duration (APD) restitution curve (*upper panel*). For the shallowest APD restitution curve (*purple*), the rotor is stationary, producing monomorphic ventricular tachycardia (MVT). The *left lower panel* shows a snapshot of membrane voltage and illustrates the circular trajectory of the rotor's tip in *black*. For a somewhat steeper APD restitution curve (*blue*), the rotor now meandered, and its gradually shifting electrical axis produced an ECG pattern resembling torsades des pointes (TdP). A voltage snapshot and tip trajectory are illustrated in the *second lower panel*. For still steeper APD restitution slope (*green*), the meander became more violent (*lower third panel*), producing an ECG pattern resembling polymorphic ventricular tachycardia (PMVT). With very steep APD restitution, the rotor was so unstable that the process of wave break repeated itself, resulting in ventricular fibrillation (VF).

Thus, dynamic wave instability, in this case caused by steep APD restitution, may result in a fibrillation-like state in the absence of any preexisting tissue heterogeneity. Electrical restitution refers to the dependence of the APD and conduction velocity on the preceding diastolic interval (DI). Generally, shorter DIs produce shorter action potentials, which serves the important physiologic role of preserving the diastolic filling period and coronary flow when heart rate accelerates. The steepness of this relationship between APD and DI turns out to be a critical parameter for wave stability. When the slope of the APD restitution curve is steep (*ie*, exceeds 1), small changes in DI get magnified into larger changes in APD, which get translated into larger changes in wavelength. For a succession of waves, this creates yet a larger change in DI for the next wave, and so forth. This positive feedback, analogous to an amplifier with gain greater than 1, causes wavelength oscillations to grow progressively until the DI becomes too short for the wave to propagate, resulting in wave break. In contrast, an APD restitution slope less than 1 attenuates perturbations in the wave, causing the wavelength oscillations to stabilize rather than grow larger. Although steep APD restitution slope as a cause of APD alternation during pacing [22] and unstable reentry around anatomic obstacles [23] had long been appreciated, its role in destabilizing rotors was not elucidated until Karma [20] showed that steep APD restitution slope could cause spiral wave breakup into a fibrillation-like state, even in completely homogeneous tissue in which every cell had identical properties.

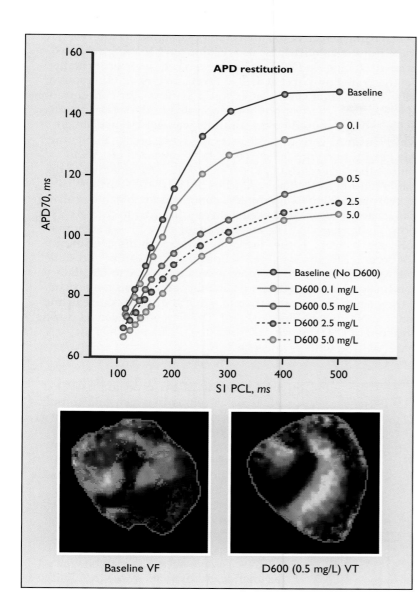

APD restitution

Baseline
0.1
0.5
2.5
5.0

— Baseline (No D600)
— D600 0.1 mg/L
— D600 0.5 mg/L
---○--- D600 2.5 mg/L
---○--- D600 5.0 mg/L

APD70, ms

SI PCL, ms

Baseline VF

D600 (0.5 mg/L) VT

FIGURE 3-10. Experimental validation of the importance of action potential duration (APD) restitution slope as a factor regulating dynamic wave stability in ventricular fibrillation (VF). These computer simulations suggest that drugs that flatten APD restitution slope might be useful as antifibrillatory agents (the restitution hypothesis). This prediction was subsequently validated experimentally in several VF models in normal hearts [24–27]. The figure shows an example in normal rabbit ventricle. The *top panel* shows APD restitution curves under control conditions and during infusion of the calcium channel blocker D600 at various doses indicated. The *bottom panel* shows a voltage snapshot during VF under control conditions, illustrating multiple wave fronts that circulate in complex patterns. With exposure to 0.5 mg/mL D600 to flatten APD restitution slope, the *bottom right panel* shows that VF converted to a stable double rotor producing monomorphic ventricular tachycardia (VT). Whether this strategy will be useful in diseased ventricles remains to be established. (*Adapted from* Wu *et al.* [18]; with permission.)

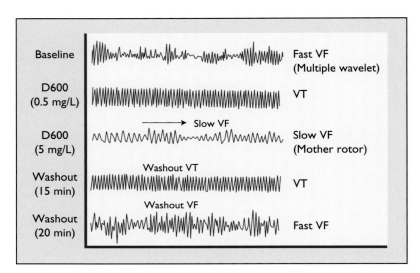

FIGURE 3-11. Conduction velocity (CV) restitution and dynamic wave stability in ventricular fibrillation (VF). CV restitution also plays an important role in promoting wave instability. Just as wave back instability may arise from action potential duration

(APD) being sensitive to small changes in diastolic interval (DI), wave front instability may also result from CV being sensitive to small changes in DI. This has been recently experimentally demonstrated by Wu *et al.* [18], who characterized two types of VF in intact rabbit ventricles exposed to increasing concentrations of D600. Fast VF (*top trace*, corresponding to the *bottom left panel* of Fig. 3-10) is caused by the multiple wavelet mechanism, in which steep APD restitution generates wave break. Flattening APD restitution with 0.5 mg/mL D600 converted fast VF to ventricular tachycardia (VT) (*second trace*, corresponding to the stable rotor in the *bottom right panel* of Fig. 3-10). Further increasing D600 to 5 mg/mL to a concentration blocking calcium (Na) channels decreased excitability sufficiently to convert VT to slow VF (*third trace*). The mechanism of slow VF is the mother rotor mechanism. Under the latter low excitability conditions, CV becomes highly sensitive to both wave curvature and static heterogeneities, which promote wave breaks due to fibrillatory conduction block. Such low excitability conditions may occur during acute or chronic ischemia, or with drug toxicity causing marked Na current blockade [18]. The sequence reversed during washout of D600 (*fourth and fifth traces*). (*Adapted from* Wu *et al.* [18]; with permission.)

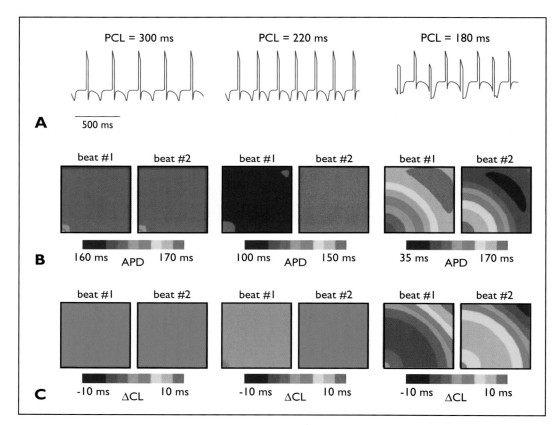

FIGURE 3-12. T-wave alternans: an index of dynamic wave instability. Action potential duration (APD) alternans, in which successive waves alternate between short and long APD, is also a natural consequence of steep APD restitution and has been linked, through its clinical manifestation as EGC T-wave alternans, as a risk factor for ventricular arrhythmias [28]. Concordant and discordant APD alternans are shown in simulated two-dimensional cardiac tissue. **A,** As pacing cycle length (PCL) is decreased, the simulated ECG transitions from periodic (*left*) at 300 ms, to T-wave alternans at 220 ms, to both QRS and T-wave alternans at 180 ms. **B** and **C,** The corresponding spatial distributions of APD and the difference between the PCL and the interbeat interval (ΔCL), respectively, for alternate paced beats. At 300 ms, APD and ΔCL are uniform from beat to beat throughout

the tissue. At 220 ms, concordant APD alternans develops, in which APD throughout the tissue is uniformly short on beat #1 and uniformly long on beat #2. CL also alternates slightly. At 180 ms, discordant APD develops, in which both APD and CL alternate spatially throughout the tissue as well as temporally from beat to beat. During discordant alternans, the same wave has a short APD in one region and a long APD in another region, equivalent to dispersion of refractoriness.

Thus, T-wave alternans may be viewed as an index of dynamic wave instability [29]. APD-driven wave instability and conduction velocity (CV)-driven wave instability act synergistically to promote wave break. Without CV restitution, each wave by definition propagates at identical velocity, so that steep APD restitution can promote temporal alternans (*ie,* concordant alternans) but not spatiotemporal alternans (*ie,* discordant alternans) in homogeneous tissue. With CV restitution, however, changes in wave front velocity cause the same wave to experience a variable diastolic interval, so that wavelength can vary in space. A wave that has a short wavelength in some areas and a long wavelength in others translates to enhanced dispersion of refractoriness, making it more likely that a properly timed extrasystole can induce functional reentry [30–32]. Thus, APD and CV restitution properties interact synergistically to promote spatiotemporal wave instability. (*Adapted from* Qu *et al.* [29]; with permission.)

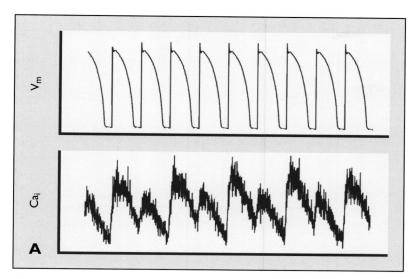

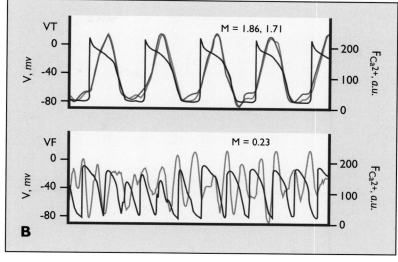

FIGURE 3-13. Intracellular calcium cycling and dynamic wave instability. Although electrical restitution is currently the best understood factor regulating dynamic wave stability, other factors including intracellular Ca cycling, short-term cardiac memory, and diffusive current effects also play important roles. Intracellular Ca levels affect Ca-sensitive ionic currents, such as the L-type Ca current, electrogenic sodium-calcium exchange, and the Ca-activated nonselective cation current. These currents in turn affect action potential duration (APD), which affects wavelength. Ca cycling by the sarcoplasmic reticulum is a dynamically active process in its own right. **A**, Rabbit ventricular myocyte voltage-clamped with a fixed action potential waveform to prevent APD alternans. Despite the fixed voltage waveform, the Ca_i transient amplitude (F_{Ca}) alternates from beat to beat, indicating that intrinsic Ca_i cycling dynamics, rather than steep APD restitution slope, is causing the Ca_i alternans. **B**, Simultaneous recording of membrane voltage (V_m) and intracellular Ca_i fluorescence (F_{Ca}) in isolated porcine ventricle. During ventricular tachycardia (VT; *upper trace*), V_m and Ca_i track each other closely. During ventricular fibrillation (VF; *lower trace*), this close association is lost. Mutual information (MI), a statistical measure of the extent to which V_m and Ca_i are associated, is high during VT and low during VF [33]. These observations raise the possibility that intracellular Ca dynamics may contribute to ongoing wave break during VF [34]. (*Panel A adapted from* Chudin et al. [33]. *Panel B adapted from* Omichi et al. [34].)

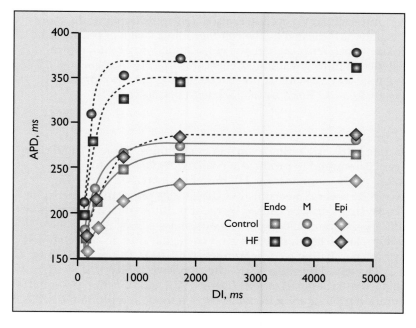

FIGURE 3-14. Effects of heart failure (HF) on dynamic wave instability: action potential duration (APD) restitution steepness. In addition to increasing preexisting tissue heterogeneity, HF also increases dynamic wave instability. The first effect is steepening of APD restitution slope. These APD restitution curves correspond to the same action potential data shown for the canine HF model and illustrate that APD restitution slope at short diastolic intervals (DI) increases in all three myocardial layers in HF (*dotted lines*) compared with normal hearts (*solid lines*). Moreover, the high sympathetic state of HF may exacerbate steep APD restitution, since β-blockade has been shown to decrease APD restitution slope [35].

Dynamic wave instability is also promoted by calcium channel remodeling in ischemic HF through its effects on conduction velocity restitution [36]. Na channel density is reduced, and recovery from inactivation is slowed. In addition to slowing CV, the latter effect broadens CV restitution, facilitating the onset of discordant alternans and the ability of rapid pacing to initiate wave break and reentry. Endo—endocardium; Epi—epicardium.

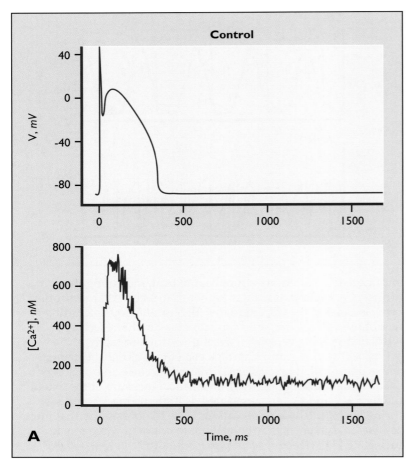

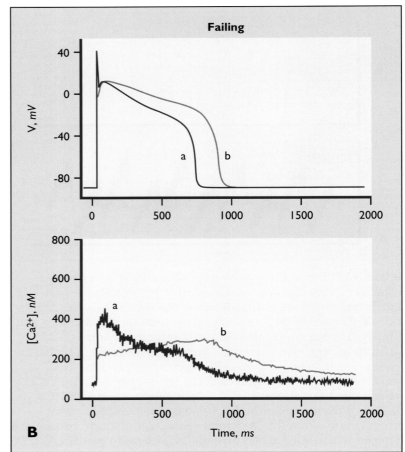

FIGURE 3-15. Effects of heart failure (HF) on dynamic wave instability: intracellular calcium cycling. Changes in intracellular Ca cycling during HF may also play an important role in enhancing dynamic wave instability. As previously illustrated in Figure 3-13*A*, intracellular Ca cycling in cardiac cells constitutes a dynamically active excitable subsystem. Intracellular Ca cycling is coupled to the action potential (and hence wavelength) through Ca-sensitive ionic currents, such as L-type Ca channels, the sodium-calcium exchanger, and Ca-activated nonselective cation and chloride channels. **A** and **B**, Intracellular Ca transient becomes abnormal in HF. Intracellular Ca cycling is also likely to be dynamically more unstable, as indicated by the common clinical sign of pulsus para-doxus, which reflects alternans of the underlying cellular intracellular Ca transient at normal heart rates. The consequences on dynamic wave instability are just beginning to be explored. (*Adapted from* O'Rourke *et al.* [37]; with permission.)

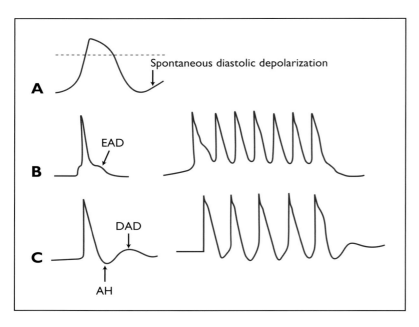

FIGURE 3-16. Triggering events in heart failure (HF). A triggering event is required to produce a localized wave break to form a rotor. At the cellular level, HF promotes increased triggering events by several mechanisms. Classically, premature ventricular extrasystoles may be caused by reentry, automaticity, or triggered activity. Automaticity (spontaneous phase 4 diastolic depolarization) and triggered activity in ventricular muscle are promoted by high circulating catecholamines in HF (**A**). Triggered activity may be caused by either early afterdepolarizations (EADs) (**B**) or delayed afterdepolarizations (DADs) (**C**). In HF, action potential duration prolongation from electrical remodeling promotes EADs, analogous to long QT syndromes, and abnormal Ca_i cycling in heart failure promotes DADs. Recently, it has been reported that hyperphosphorylation of calcium release channels (ryanodine receptors) and associated proteins (*eg*, FK binding protein) alter sarcoplasmic reticulum (SR) Ca release properties [38]. Specifically, SR Ca release is less efficient and the SR becomes leaky during diastole, promoting Ca_i overload and activation of transient inward currents (I_{ti}) underlying triggered activity.

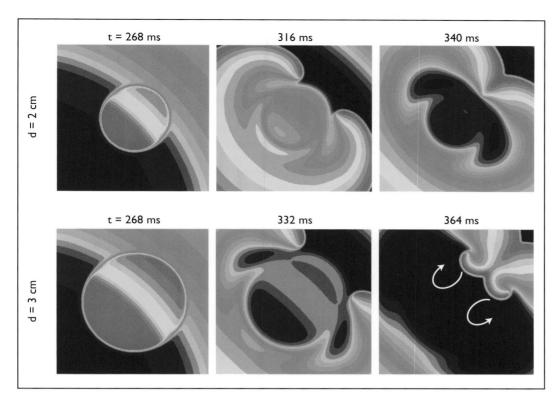

FIGURE 3-17. Triggering events and induction of reentry. Why don't premature ventricular extrasystoles, which are common in normal hearts, cause rotors to form? For a rotor to form, the tip of the broken wave must have enough excitable tissue available to complete a rotation before colliding with inexcitable barrier or refractory tissue. In the u*pper panels*, electrical depolarization of a small area (*red circle*, diameter [d] = 2 cm) in the wake of a previous repolarizing wave (*green in upper right corner*) creates two broken wave tips, but they are not spaced far enough apart to reenter through a common pathway. In the *lower panels*, however, a larger area is depolarized (diameter d = 3 cm) and the separation of the two broken wave tips is sufficient to permit reentry through a common central pathway. *Red* indicates the most depolarized tissue, changing from *yellow* to *green* to the most repolarized in *blue*. *t* refers to the time after the last paced beat.

When a rotor is induced in a normal heart, it almost always leads to fibrillation. The *upper right tracing* shows that a modestly suprathreshold premature extrastimulus initiates a propagated response but not reentry, whereas a large extrastimulus initiates reentry that degenerates into ventricular fibrillation (VF). Fortunately, physiologic triggers such as spontaneous premature extrasystoles are incapable of inducing localized wave break with enough adjacent excitable tissue for a self-sustaining rotor (*ie*, the distance separating the newly formed wave tips is too short to allow reentry). However, when a ventricular extrasystole is induced electrically by a large current pulse (50 to 100 times

threshold) sufficient to depolarize a large area, rotors can be induced that then spontaneously degenerate to VF in all normal human hearts (*lower right panel*). This is known as the VF threshold. Very rapid ventricular pacing may also cause a wave break that induces rotors in normal ventricles by promoting discordant alternans. In the setting of HF, the increased pre-existing tissue heterogeneity and dynamic wave instability due to structural and electrical remodeling increase the probability of rotor formation. In addition, the number of potential triggering events, such as single, coupled, and multiple ventricular extrasystoles, is increased. Even so, the probability remains extremely low. For example, spontaneous ventricular ectopy at a rate of two per minute, equivalent to approximately 1 million ventricular extrasystoles per year, is common in patients with cardiomyopathy. However, the rate of sudden death episodes in such patients is typically measured in months to years, rather than minutes.

Structural remodeling also enhances the probability that automaticity and triggered activity at the cellular level will propagate in tissue. In normal, well-coupled ventricular tissue, a single myocyte faces too large a source-sink mismatch to depolarize enough surrounding cells to initiate a propagated impulse. Indeed, synchronous depolarization of a critical mass of myocytes is required. In HF, gap junction remodeling reduces connectivity and decreases the critical mass of myocytes required to initiate a propagated response.

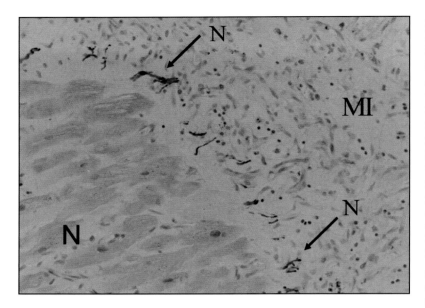

FIGURE 3-18. Sympathetic tone and arrhythmias in heart failure (HF). Despite the high level of ventricular ectopy in HF patients, providing potentially millions of triggering events, the probability that any individual triggering event will induce rotor formation, ventricular fibrillation (VF), and sudden cardiac death (SCD) is very low. This observation suggests that the interaction between potential triggering events and substrate is not stable, but changes dynamically over time. The sympathetic nervous system has important effects on both triggering events and substrate, and is an important factor causing dynamic modulation of the arrhythmogenic substrate. In HF, the autonomic system undergoes remodeling, both structurally and functionally. The figure shows a histologic section of ventricular myocardium at the border zone of a 2-week-old canine infarct. Antibody against S-100 protein identifies Schwann cells, which colocalize with cardiac sympathetic nerves and stain brown. Note the high density of sympathetic nerves in the border region between normal tissue (N) and the myocardial infarction (MI), indicating that nerve sprouting has caused this region to become hyperinnervated. This juxtaposition of hyper-innervated, normally innervated, and denervated myocardium results in a very heterogeneous electrophysiologic response when the sympathetic tone increases, and promotes wave break by increasing preexisting tissue heterogeneity. The local hyper-innervated areas may play an especially important role because during sympathetic stimulation, they may be exposed to supra-physiologic catecholamine levels. Local catecholamine toxicity may promote intracellular calcium overload, enhanced automaticity, and triggered activity such as delayed afterdepolarizations, which then serve as triggers inducing lethal reentrant arrhythmias. The ability of β-blockers to consistently reduce SCD in HF from many etiologies provides a strong clue that sympathetic activity plays a key role in modulating the risk of lethal ventricular arrhythmias in HF. Enhanced sympathetic tone and depressed vagal tone predict increased cardiac risk. Furthermore, animal and human studies have shown that sympathetic denervation is not just a feature of ischemic heart disease, but occurs in nonischemic heart disease as well. In humans, both ischemic and nonischemic cardiomyopathic hearts have depressed sympathetic neurotransmitter uptake on meta-iodobenzylguanidine (MIBG) scans [39,40], and in animal models, pacing-induced cardiomyopathy has been directly shown to reduce sympathetic nerve density in ventricular muscle [41]. (*From* Chen *et al.* [42]; with permission.)

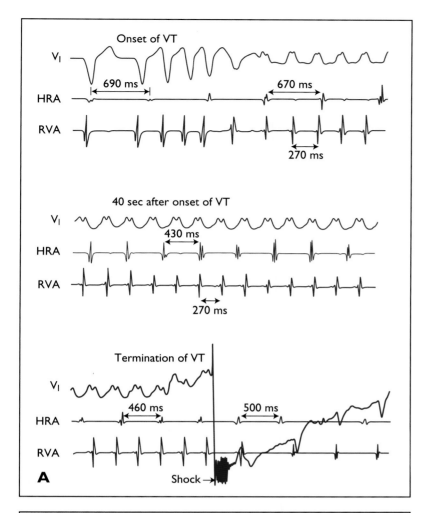

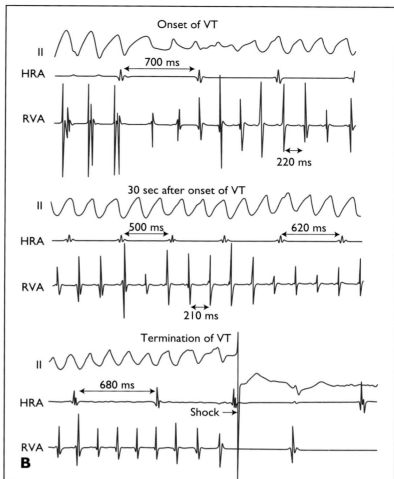

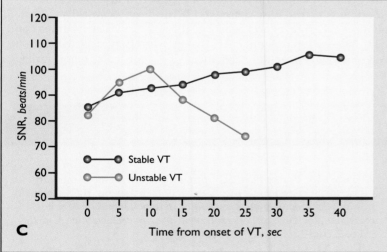

FIGURE 3-19. Functional neural remodeling. In heart failure (HF) patients who develop sustained ventricular tachycardia (VT), the response of the autonomic nervous system plays a key role in hemodynamic outcome. Although left ventricular ejection fraction and VT rate are important, hemodynamic collapse during VT is often associated with inappropriate sympathetic withdrawal. Here are shown recordings from two patients with hemodynamically stable (**A**) and unstable VT (**B**) induced by programmed electrical stimulation. Both patients had ventriculoatrial block, so the sinus rate could be recorded as an index of autonomic tone. In both patients, VT induction initially caused the sinus rate to increase. In the hemodynamically stable patient, sinus rate remained high, reflecting maintained sympathetic stimulation. In the hemodynamically unstable patient, however, the sinus rate then slowed, reflecting sympathetic withdrawal, and blood pressure fell,

requiring defibrillation. Average responses in hemodynamically stable versus unstable patients are summarized (**C**).

The mechanism may involve a competition between arterial and cardiopulmonary baroreceptors, whose stimulation by stretch causes sympathetic withdrawal and vagal stimulation. During VT, the fall in systolic blood pressure inhibits the arterial baroreceptors in the carotid body and aortic arch, signaling increased sympathetic tone and vagal withdrawal. However, cardiac filling pressures increase during VT, stretching cardiopulmonary baroreceptors in the ventricular walls, signaling sympathetic withdrawal and vagal stimulation. In hemodynamically unstable VT, the latter effect appears to predominate, causing sinus rate to slow and blood pressure to fall.

Responses of baroreceptors and metaboreceptors that regulate sympathetic/parasympathetic balance have been extensively characterized in both animal and human models of HF. Their dysfunction, as manifested by blunted baroreceptor sensitivity and heart rate variability, predicts increased SCD risk [43]. Heightened sympathetic activity has well-known proarrhythmic consequences, including increased ventricular ectopy, decreased VF threshold [44], and increased inherent dynamic instability of cardiac wave propagation (as indexed, for example, by microvolt T wave alternans [45] and steepened action potential duration restitution slope [35].

It is intriguing that interventions proven to protect against SCD in HF, including aldosterone inhibition and statin therapy, reverse aspects of cardiac autonomic dysfunction in the diseased heart. Aldosterone antagonists have been shown to preserve baroreceptor sensitivity and sympathetic innervation in both ischemic and non-ischemic heart disease [40,41]. In animal models, statins preserve baroreceptor sensitivity in heart failure [46,47]. The effects of statins may be independent of their lipid-lowering effects, because hyper-cholesterolemia, which induces sympathetic nerve sprouting [48], confers lower risk in severe HF [49,50]. (*Adapted from* Liu *et al.* [51].)

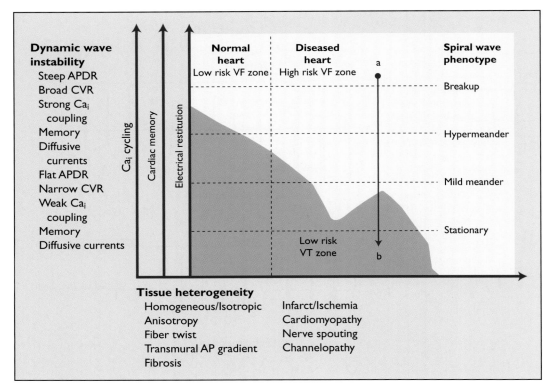

Dynamic wave instability
- Steep APDR
- Broad CVR
- Strong Ca_i coupling
- Memory
- Diffusive currents
- Flat APDR
- Narrow CVR
- Weak Ca_i coupling
- Memory
- Diffusive currents

Ca_i cycling
Cardiac memory
Electrical restitution

Normal heart
Low risk VF zone

Diseased heart
High risk VF zone

Spiral wave phenotype
- Breakup
- Hypermeander
- Mild meander
- Stationary

Low risk VT zone

Tissue heterogeneity

Homogeneous/Isotropic	Infarct/Ischemia
Anisotropy	Cardiomyopathy
Fiber twist	Nerve spouting
Transmural AP gradient	Channelopathy
Fibrosis	

FIGURE 3-20. Conclusions. Heart failure (HF) promotes ventricular arrhythmias and sudden cardiac death (SCD) by increasing the likelihood that a cardiac electrical wave will break to form a rotor, which subsequently breaks up into ventricular fibrillation (VF). This increased tendency to wave break is promoted synergistically by an interplay between dynamic factors and tissue heterogeneity, as summarized here. The incidence of triggering events increases as a result of enhanced automaticity, greater susceptibility to triggered activity mediated by both delayed and early afterdepolarizations, and increased dynamic wave instability promoting discordant alternans. Through a combination of structural and electrical remodeling, HF increases both preexisting and dynamically generated tissue heterogeneity. *Preexisting tissue heterogeneity* refers to the degree of dispersion of electrophysiologic and anatomic features throughout the ventricles. *Dynamically generated tissue heterogeneity* refers to dynamic factors that regulate wave stability, including electrical restitution, intracellular calcium cycling, short-term cardiac memory, and other factors. Together, preexisting tissue heterogeneity and dynamic wave instability are synergistic at promoting wave break. Superimposed on cardiac remodeling, neural remodeling in HF further dynamically enhances the triggers and substrate for ventricular arrhythmias and SCD. AP—action potential; APDR—AP duration restitution; CVR—coronary vascular resistance; VT—ventricular tachycardia.

REFERENCES

1. Gutstein DE, Liu FY, Meyers MB, *et al.*: The organization of adherens junctions and desmosomes at the cardiac intercalated disc is independent of gap junctions. *J Cell Sci* 2003, 116:875–885.

2. Fenton F, Karma A: Vortex dynamics in three-dimensional continuous myocardium with fiber rotation: filament instability and fibrillation. *Chaos* 1998, 8:20–47.

3. Qu Z, Kil J, Xie F, *et al.*: Scroll wave dynamics in a three-dimensional cardiac tissue model: roles of restitution, thickness, and fiber rotation. *Biophys J* 2000, 78:2761–2775.

4. Krinsky VI: Spread of excitation in an inhomogeneous medium. *Biofizika* 1966, 11:776–784.

5. Gul'ko FB, Petrov AA: Mechanisms of the formation of closed pathways of conduction in excitable media. *Biofizika* 1972, 17:261–270.

6. Winfree AT: *When Time Breaks Down.* Princeton, NJ: Princeton University Press; 1987.

7. Allessie MA, Bonke FIM, Schopman FJC: Circus movement in rabbit atrial muscle as a mechanism of tachycardia. *Circ Res* 1973, 33:54–77.

8. Allessie MA, Bonke FIM, Schopman FJC: Circus movement in rabbit atrial muscle as a mechanism of tachycardia. II. The role of nonuniform recovery of excitability in the occurrence of unidirectional block as studied with multiple microelectrodes. *Circ Res* 1976, 39:168-181.

9. Allessie M, Bonke F, Schopman F. Circus movement in rabbit atrial muscle as a mechanism of tachycardia. *Circ Res* 1977, 41:9–18.

10. Davidenko JM, Pertsov AV, Salomonsz JR, *et al.*: Stationary and drifting spiral waves of excitation in isolated cardiac muscle. *Nature* 1992, 355:349–351.

11. Gray RA, Jalife J, Panfilov AV, *et al.*: Mechanisms of cardiac fibrillation. *Science* 1995, 270:1222–1223.

12. Jais P, Haissaguerre M, Shah DC, *et al.*: A focal source of atrial fibrillation treated by discrete radiofrequency ablation. *Circulation* 1997, 95:572–576.

13. Chen PS, Wu TJ, Hwang C, *et al.*: Thoracic veins and the mechanisms of non-paroxysmal atrial fibrillation. *Cardiovasc Res* 2002, 54:295–301.

14. Moe GK, Rheinboldt WC, Abildskov JA: A computer model of atrial fibrillation. *Am Heart J* 1964;67:200–220.

15. Allessie MA, Lammers WJEP, Bonke FIM, Hollen J: Experimental evaluation of Moe's multiple wavelet hypothesis of atrial fibrillation. In *Cardiac Arrhythmias*. Edited by Zipes DP, Jalife J. New York: Grune & Stratton; 1985:265–276.

16. Lee JJ, Kamjoo K, Hough D, *et al.*: Reentrant wave fronts in Wiggers' stage II ventricular fibrillation. Characteristics and mechanisms of termination and spontaneous regeneration. *Circ Res* 1996, 78:660–675.

17. Zaitsev AV, Berenfeld O, Mironov SF, *et al.*: Distribution of excitation frequencies on the epicardial and endocardial surfaces of fibrillating ventricular wall of the sheep heart [see comments]. *Circ Res* 2000, 86:408–417.

18. Wu TJ, Lin SF, Weiss JN, *et al.*: Two types of ventricular fibrillation in isolated rabbit hearts: importance of excitability and action potential duration restitution. *Circulation* 2002, 106:1859–1866.

19. Akar FG, Rosenbaum DS: Transmural electrophysiological hetero-geneities underlying arrhythmogenesis in heart failure. *Circ Res* 2003, 93:638–645.

20. Karma A: Spiral breakup in model equations of action potential propagation in cardiac tissue. *Phys Rev Lett* 1993, 71:1103–1106.

21. Qu Z, Xie F, Garfinkel A, Weiss JN: Origins of spiral wave meander and breakup in a two-dimensional cardiac tissue model. *Ann Biomed Eng* 2000, 28:755–771.

22. Nolasco JB, Dahlen RW: A graphic method for the study of alternation in cardiac action potentials. *J Appl Physiol* 1968, 25:191–196.

23. Frame LH, Simson MB: Oscillations of conduction, action potential duration, and refractoriness. A mechanism for spontaneous termination of reentrant tachycardias. *Circulation* 1988, 78:1277–1287.

24. Riccio ML, Koller ML, Gilmour RF Jr: Electrical restitution and spatiotemporal organization during ventricular fibrillation. *Circ Res* 1999, 84:955–963.

25. Garfinkel A, Kim YH, Voroshilovsky O, *et al.*: Preventing ventricular fibrillation by flattening cardiac restitution [see comments]. *Proc Natl Acad Sci U S A* 2000, 97:6061–6066.

26. Lee MH, Lin SF, Ohara T, *et al.*: Effects of diacetyl monoxime and cytochalasin D on ventricular fibrillation in swine right ventricles. *Am J Physiol Heart Circ Physiol* 2001, 280:H2689–H2696.

27. Omichi C, Zhou S, Lee MH, *et al.*: Effects of amiodarone on wave front dynamics during ventricular fibrillation in isolated swine right ventricle. *Am J Physiol Heart Circ Physiol* 2002, 282:H1063–H1070.

28. Rosenbaum DS: T wave alternans: a mechanism of arrhyth-mogenesis comes of age after 100 years. *J Cardiovasc Electrophysiol* 2001, 12:207–209.

29. Qu ZL, Garfinkel A, Chen PS, Weiss JN: Mechanisms of discordant alternans and induction of reentry in simulated cardiac tissue. *Circulation* 2000, 102:1664–1670.

30. Pastore JM, Girouard SD, Laurita KR, *et al.*: Mechanism linking T-wave alternans to the genesis of cardiac fibrillation. *Circulation* 1999;99:1385–1394.

31. Qu Z, Garfinkel A, Chen PS, Weiss JN: Mechanisms of discordant alternans and induction of reentry in simulated cardiac tissue. *Circulation* 2000, 102:1664–1670.

32. Watanabe MA, Fenton FH, Evans SJ, *et al.*: Mechanisms for discordant alternans. [see comment in]. *J Cardiovasc Electrophysiol* 2001, 12:196–206.

33. Chudin E, Goldhaber J, Garfinkel A, *et al.*: Intracellular Ca(2+) dynamics and the stability of ventricular tachycardia. *Biophys J* 1999, 77:2930–2941.

34. Omichi C, Lamp ST, Lin SF, *et al.*: Intracellular Ca dynamics in ventricular fibrillation. *Am J Physiol Heart Circ Physiol* 2004, 286:H1836–H1844.

35. Taggart P, Sutton P, Chalabi Z, *et al.*: Effect of adrenergic stimulation on action potential duration restitution in humans. *Circulation* 2003, 107:285–289.

36. Qu Z, Karagueuzian HS, Garfinkel A, Weiss JN: Effects of Na+ channel and cell coupling abnormalities on vulnerability to reentry: a simulation study. *Am J Physiol Heart Circ Physiol* 2004, 286:H1310–H1321.

37. O'Rourke B, Kass DA, Tomaselli GF, *et al.*: Mechanisms of altered excitation-contraction coupling in canine tachycardia-induced heart failure, I: experimental studies. *Circ Res* 1999, 84:562–570.

38. Marx SO, Marks AR: Regulation of the ryanodine receptor in heart failure. *Basic Res Cardiol* 2002, 97(Suppl 1):I49–I51.

39. Kasama S, Toyama T, Kumakura H, *et al.*: Effect of spironolactone on cardiac sympathetic nerve activity and left ventricular remodeling in patients with dilated cardiomyopathy. *J Am Coll Cardiol* 2003,41:574–581.

40. Barr CS, Lang CC, Hanson J, *et al.*: Effects of adding spironolactone to an angiotensin-converting enzyme inhibitor in chronic congestive heart failure secondary to coronary artery disease. *Am J Cardiol* 1995, 76:1259–1265.

41. Himura Y, Felten SY, Kashiki M, *et al.*: Cardiac noradrenergic nerve terminal abnormalities in dogs with experimental congestive heart failure. *Circulation* 1993, 88:1299–1309.

42. Chen PS, Chen LS, Cao JM, *et al.*: Sympathetic nerve sprouting, electrical remodeling and the mechanisms of sudden cardiac death. *Cardiovasc Res* 2001, 50:409–416.

43. Huikuri HV, Zaman L, Castellanos A, *et al.*: Changes in spontaneous sinus node rate as an estimate of cardiac autonomic tone during stable and unstable ventricular tachycardia. *J Am Coll Cardiol* 1989, 13:646–652.

44. Woo MA, Stevenson WG, Moser DK, Middlekauff HR: Complex heart rate variability and serum norepinephrine levels in patients with advanced heart failure. *J Am Coll Cardiol* 1994, 23:565–569.

45. Jalife J: Ventricular fibrillation: mechanisms of initiation and maintenance. *Ann Rev Physiol* 2000, 62:25–50.

46. Rashba EJ, Cooklin M, MacMurdy K, *et al.*: Effects of selective autonomic blockade on T-wave alternans in humans. *Circulation* 2002, 105:837–842.

47. Pliquett RU, Cornish KG, Peuler JD, Zucker IH: Simvastatin normalizes autonomic neural control in experimental heart failure. *Circulation* 2003, 107:2493–2498.

48. Pliquett RU, Cornish KG, Zucker IH: Statin therapy restores sympathovagal balance in experimental heart failure. *J Appl Physiol* 2003, 95:700–704.

49. Horwich TB, Hamilton MA, Maclellan WR, Fonarow GC: Low serum total cholesterol is associated with marked increase in mortality in advanced heart failure. *J Card Fail* 2002, 8:216–224.

50. Rauchhaus M, Coats AJ, Anker SD: The endotoxin-lipoprotein hypothesis. *Lancet*. 2000, 356:930–933.

51. Liu YB, Wu CC, Lu LS, *et al.*: Sympathetic nerve sprouting, electrical remodeling, and increased vulnerability to ventricular fibrillation in hypercholesterolemic rabbits. *Circ Res* 2003, 92:1145–1152.

THE ELECTROCARDIOGRAM IN HEART FAILURE

Hein J. Wellens and Subramaniam C. Krishnan

The increasing incidence of heart failure (HF) has resulted in a growing need for inexpensive tools to diagnose the presence of HF, to risk stratify the patients, and to direct their management. The electrocardiogram (ECG), to an extent, fulfills these requirements, being inexpensive, noninvasive, easily repeatable, and without peer in diagnosing cardiac arrhythmias, which are frequently present in the patient with HF and often of prognostic significance. In this chapter we discuss information that can be obtained from the 12-lead ECG and help in the management of the HF patient.

The clinician analyzing the ECG should review the rhythm including sinus rhythm or atrial and ventricular arrhythmias, the P wave and PR interval, the QRS complex, and the ST segment. Our chapter is also organized along these lines. Sinus tachycardia in the patient with HF indicates increased sympathetic stimulation and represents the likelihood of poor prognosis. Atrial arrhythmias occur frequently in HF, increasing in prevalence with the severity of symptomatic status. Atrial fibrillation (AF) is the most common atrial arrhythmia. Although its presence is of little prognostic significance, it may contribute to worsening of the clinical status in mild or moderate HF. Similar to AF, ventricular arrhythmias are common in HF, especially increasing with the severity of HF, but are poor predictors of sudden death.

The P wave provides clues about the presence of conduction abnormalities and enlargement of the atria. An appropriate PR interval during sinus rhythm is essential for optimal filling of the ventricle, with a decrease when the PR interval becomes more than 200 ms. On the other hand, the QRS complex not only indicates the etiology of impaired cardiac function such as the Q wave from a previous myocardial infarction or the QRS changes in ventricular hypertrophy, but also gives prognostic information. Bundle branch block is an important mechanism of QRS widening, and an inverse relationship has been demonstrated between QRS width and life expectancy. Finally, dynamic changes in ST segment represent cardiac insult. Importantly, presence of persistent ST-segment elevation indicates abnormal wall motion or ventricular aneurysm formation, and persistent T-wave negativity indicates chronic myocardial damage.

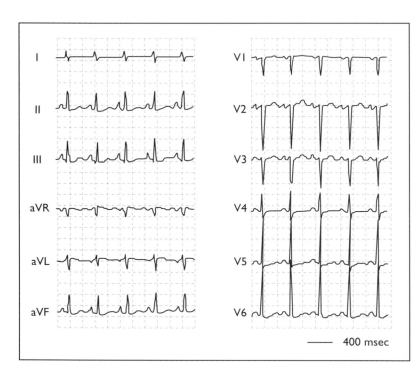

FIGURE 4-1. Electrocardiogram of a 42-year-old man with a non-ischemic dilated cardiomyopathy. The sinus rate is 140 beats per minute; biatrial and biventricular hypertrophy is present. The presence of sinus tachycardia in the patient with heart failure (HF) indicates that increased sympathetic stimulation is trying to assure adequate cardiac output. Sinus tachycardia is a marker of poor prognosis [1]. It is of interest, however, that the ability to slow the sinus rate by a pharmacologic intervention predicts a better long-term outcome. An example is given by the GESICA study [1,2]. When a high sinus rate was present that decreased below 90 beats per minute during amiodarone, the patient had a significantly lower 6-month mortality compared with the patient receiving placebo (21.7% vs 53.8% [$P < 0.002$]). If no decrease in sinus rate occurred after amiodarone, no difference in mortality was observed [2]. In the GESICA study many patients had a nonischemic cause of HF. Improvement has also been described in ischemic HF following a reduction in sinus rate during the administration of a beta-blocking agent [3,4]. These observations were made in patients with left ventricular systolic dysfunction and a markedly reduced left ventricular ejection fraction. Approximately half of the HF patients [5] have left ventricular diastolic dysfunction with preserved or mildly impaired systolic function. Unfortunately, we have little information about sinus rate behavior and the value of its prognostic response to interventions in patients with diastolic left ventricular dysfunction.

ATRIAL ARRHYTHMIAS

Atrial arrhythmias occur frequently in HF, with its prevalence increasing in relation to the New York Heart Association (NYHA) class [6,7]. The most common atrial arrhythmia is AF. The increased propensity of AF in HF can be explained by structural atrial changes, abnormalities of conduction, sinus node dysfunction, and increased refractoriness in the atria, promoting the genesis of AF [8]. Recently it was shown that there are racial variations in the prevalence of AF in HF with a lesser incidence in African-Americans [9]. There are many studies on the significance of AF on prognosis of the HF patient [7,10–14]. The data are not uniform but suggest that the presence of AF is of little significance for prognosis in the patient with severe HF, but worsening of the clinical status has been described in patients with mild or moderate HF. The latter implies that especially in case of asymptomatic or mild HF with AF it makes sense to try to convert AF and to attempt to keep the patient in sinus rhythm.

This is supported by data from the AFFIRM and RACE studies [15,16] where patients with mild HF did better in the rhythm control group compared with patients in whom the ventricular rate was controlled by pharmacologic means during persistent AF. Again, as with sinus tachycardia, we have no information on the prognostic importance of the restoration of sinus rhythm comparing diastolic and systolic HF. Of the antiarrhythmic drugs in HF, amiodarone and dofetilide [17,18] are the two drugs that are most successful in converting AF patients and keeping them in sinus rhythm. Converting the patient to sinus rhythm improved survival [17]. The Atrial Fibrillation and Congestive Heart Failure (AF-CHF) trial, which is in progress, will answer the question as to the best antiarrhythmic drug treatment strategy in patients with HF and AF [19]. Since AF will more easily recur in the HF patient, anticoagulant therapy is essential after the patient has converted to sinus rhythm.

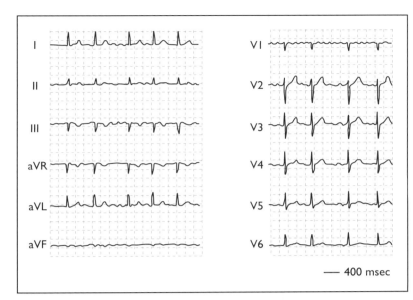

FIGURE 4-2. Atrial arrhythmias in congestive heart failure. In an unknown number of patients, heart failure (HF) may be the consequence of atrial fibrillation (AF), a so-called *tachycardia-mediated cardiomyopathy*. This electrocardiogram is from a 52-year old man presenting with AF and a left ventricular ejection fraction (LVEF) of 40%. The QRS is normal. Three months after electrical conversion of AF to sinus rhythm the LVEF value was 58%.

The incidence of the development of HF following an episode of AF is prospectively being analyzed in the REVERSE study. This possbility has to be considered, especially in the non-ischemic HF patient with AF [20]. Recently, improvement of ventricular function by restoration of sinus rhythm through catheter ablation of AF has been reported [21,22]. Another approach used in patients with AF and HF is catheter ablation of the atrioventricular (AV) junction and ventricular pacing. The best results were obtained in patients with nonischemic AF in whom the ventricular rate could not be controlled by pharmacologic means [23–25]. In patients in whom AV nodal ablation is performed, more information is needed as to the best pacing sites in the ventricles because of potential detrimental effects of desynchronization of right and left ventricular contraction by pacing from the right ventricular apex [26]. An important finding in the management of HF patients with AF is that drugs used in HF that are not primarily antiarrhythmic drugs reduce the occurrence of AF and promote conversion of AF to sinus rhythm. This has been shown for angiotensin-converting enzyme inhibitors and angiotensin receptor blockers [27–30]. Several factors may play a role here, such as the improvement in cardiac function, but also the preventive effect of these drugs on collagen and fibrosis formation. Fibrosis formation in the atrium is a factor promoting AF by creating the electrophysiologic "milieu" for multiple sites of reentry in the atrium.

VENTRICULAR ARRHYTHMIAS

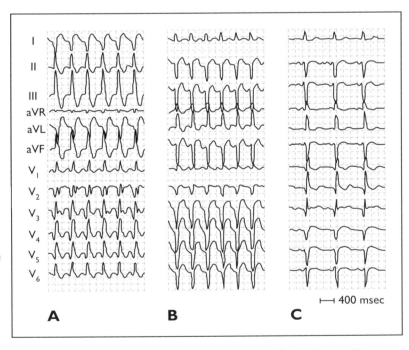

FIGURE 4-3. **A** and **B**, Monomorphic ventricular tachycardias (VT) that occurred in a patient with severe heart failure (HF). **C**, Right bundle branch block and left anterior hemiblock following a large anteroseptal myocardial infarction during sinus rhythm. Ventricular arrhythmias are common in HF and, like in atrial fibrillation (AF), their prevalence increases with the severity of HF. However, even in the presence of severe HF, they are poor predictors of sudden death [31–33].

Important when discussing the prognostic significance of spontaneously occurring ventricular arrhythmias are the answers to two questions 1) are the ventricular arrhythmias symptomatic; and 2) is a sustained VT inducible during an electrophysiologic study? Dizziness and syncope in the HF patient are frequently based on ventricular arrhythmias and carry a poor prognosis [34]. That information is therefore of value in decision making about (nonpharmacologic) protection against sudden cardiac death.

The MADIT I [34] and the MUSST studies [35] showed that induction of a sustained VT in patients with left ventricular systolic dysfunction also identifies patients with an increased risk of dying from an arrhythmia compared with patients with the same degree of ventricular dysfunction but no inducible ventricular arrhythmias. The ability of antiarrhythmic drugs to prevent sudden death in these patients has been disappointing, including when drug selection was guided by serial drug testing [35]. Increased mortality was found in patients receiving class IC drugs and d-sotalol because of proarrhythmic effects from these drugs [36,37]. In a meta-analysis, amiodarone did result in a slightly better outcome than placebo in patients with impaired left ventricular function caused by ischemic or nonischemic heart disease [38]. Equal effects on mortality were seen with the class III drugs dofetilide [18] and azimilide [39]. Recent information from the SCD-HeFT study [40] revealed better outcome as to mortality from an implantable cardioverter-defibrillator than from amiodarone in patients with HF based on systolic dysfunction, irrespective of the severity of ventricular arrhythmias. Importantly, a number of drugs that were not developed as antiarrhythmic drugs decrease arrhythmic death in the HF population. They include β-blockers, angiotensin-converting enzyme inhibitors, angiotensin receptor blockers, lipid lowering agents, aldosterone receptor antagonists, polyunsaturated fatty acids, and aspirin [41].

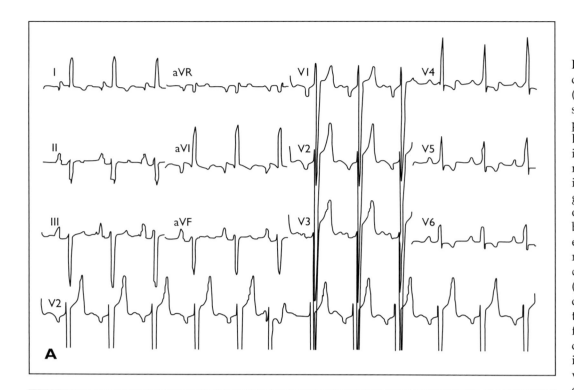

A

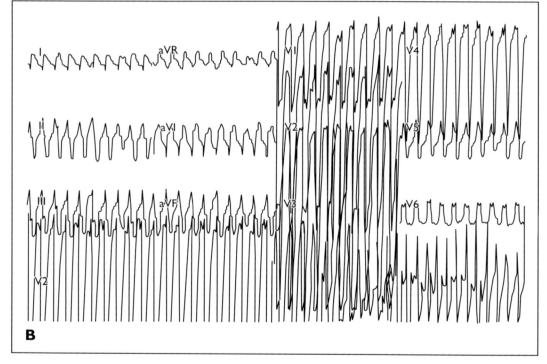

B

FIGURE 4-4. A, Sustained ventricular tachycardia (VT) due to bundle branch reentry (BBR-VT). A discussion on VTs seen in the setting of heart failure would be incomplete without a mention being made of BBR-VT, the most characteristic VT associated with patients with dilated cardiomyopathy and heart failure [42]. An important component of the arrhythmogenic substrate for this VT is the presence of conduction system disease, and the baseline electrocardiogram often shows either a left bundle branch block or a nonspecific intraventricular conduction delay often with a prolonged PR interval (**A**). The HV interval during SR is often characteristically prolonged. The circuit for this arrhythmia has been well defined, and for the typical form of this arrhythmia consists of a macroreentrant circuit involving the conduction system of the ventricle with antegrade conduction occurring over the right bundle branch and retrograde conduction occurring over one of the fascicles of the left bundle branch. Therefore, the QRS morphology seen in the typical form of BBR-VT (**B**) can resemble that seen in supraventricular arrhythmias with aberrant conduction. Another electrocardiographic feature of the arrhythmia is that the QRS during VT and SR can be identical. This arrhythmia is important to recognize since catheter ablation of the right bundle branch is curative. Especially in patients with valvular heart disease, BBR-VT can occur with a right bundle branch block (RBBB) morphology and the circuit may be a counterpart of the typical form where the direction of impulse propagation may be reversed along the right and left bundle branches [43]. BBR-VT with a RBBB morphology may also be due to a variant of this arrhythmia termed *interfascicular tachycardia*, where the left bundle branch fascicles are components of the circuit and the right bundle branch is activated passively [44,45].

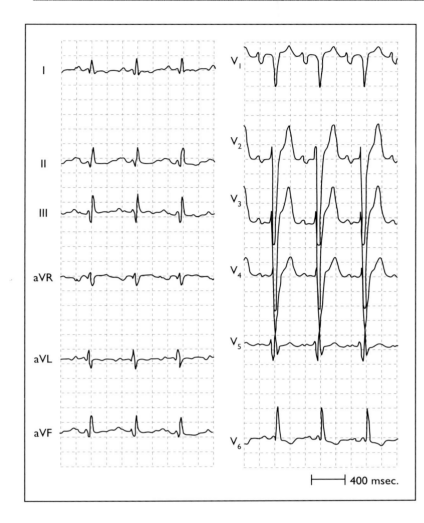

⊢———⊣ 400 msec.

FIGURE 4-5. The P wave in congestive heart failure. Width and axis of the sinus P wave give information about the presence of conduction abnormalities in and/or enlargement of the atria. There are three electrocardiogram findings indicative of left atrial disease: 1) increased width (more than 100 ms) of the P wave that can be caused by delayed intra-atrial conduction and/or left atrial enlargement; 2) terminal P wave negativity in lead V1, the product of the surface of the negative part (width x depth) being more than 1 mm; and 3) terminal P-wave positivity in lead aVL. These P-wave changes can be found in diastolic and systolic left ventricular dysfunction.

Isolated right atrial enlargement results in right axis deviation of the P wave in the frontal plane leading to increased P-wave height in the inferior leads II, III, and aVF. There is no increased width of the P wave unless there is marked dilatation of the right atrium.

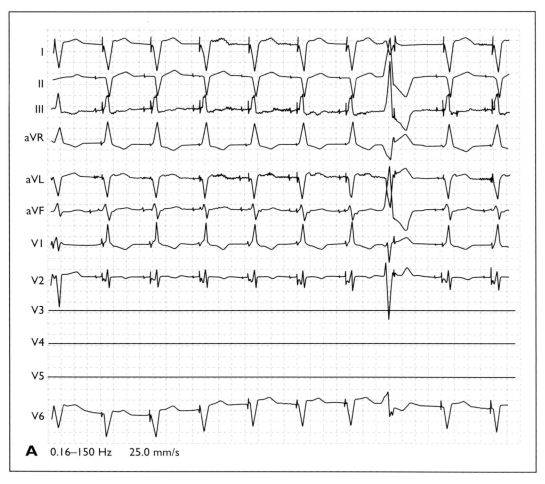

A 0.16–150 Hz   25.0 mm/s

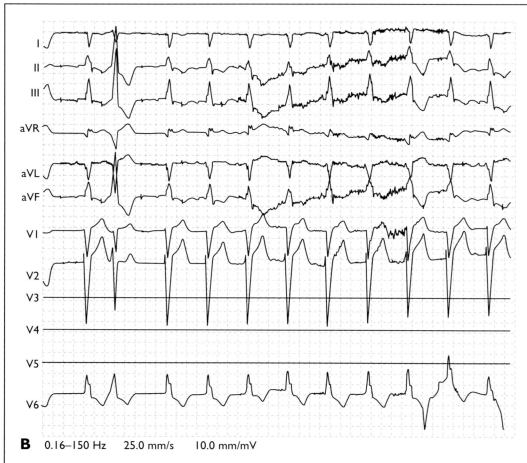

B 0.16–150 Hz   25.0 mm/s   10.0 mm/mV

FIGURE 4-6. A–D, The effects of prolonged interatrial conduction on hemodynamics in heart failure patients. **A,** An electrocardiogram (ECG) from a 70-year-old man with atherosclerotic heart disease, severe systolic dysfunction, and heart failure who had a dual chamber implantable cardioverter-defibrillator (ICD) implanted. He was entirely pacemaker dependent and it was apparent that his heart failure had been worsening. An upgrade to a dual chamber defibrillator with biventricular pacing was performed. In this postprocedure ECG, with a paced atrioventricular (AV) delay of 100 ms following the atrial pacing spike, a P wave (evidence of atrial capture) is not seen. **B,** Upon changing the programming in the ICD to the atrial inhibited pacing (AAI) mode, following the atrial pacing spike a P wave is seen 240 ms following the pacing stimulus. This finding is consistent with very slow intra- and interatrial conduction and delayed activation of the left atrium. Since most biventricular pacemakers tend to have short AV delays programmed (to decrease presystolic mitral regurgitation), there is a concern that a delayed activation of the left atrium can result in its contraction against a closed mitral valve with a possible worsening of the heart failure.

Continued on next page

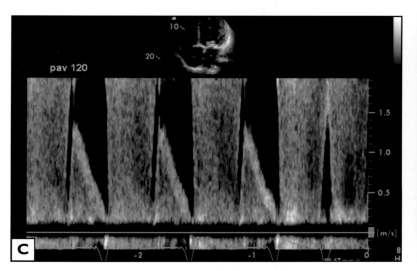

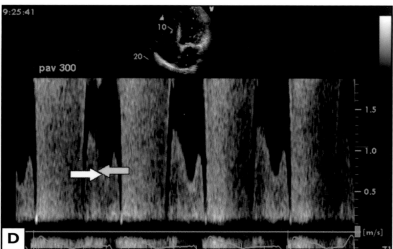

FIGURE 4-6. *(Continued)* **C**, Doppler tracings of blood flow across the mitral valve. Programming an AV delay of 120 ms results in suboptimal flow across the structure. **D**, Extending the paced AV delay to 300 ms, possibly allowing the left atrium to contract against a mitral valve that is open, shows more optimal transmitral filling pattern. This was also associated with a significant resolution of heart failure symptoms in this patient. Patients with prolonged interatrial conduction who receive dual chamber or biventricular pacemakers should have consideration given to placing the atrial lead close to the Bachman's bundle to advance left atrial activation.

ATRIOVENTRICULAR CONDUCTION ABNORMALITIES

An appropriate PR interval during sinus rhythm is essential for optimal filling of the ventricle. Prolongation of the PR interval above 200 ms decreases ventricular function because of a reduction in filling time and presystolic mitral incompetence. This is more marked on the left side of the heart when left bundle branch block is present. Normalization of the PR interval may result in better ventricular function in patients with HF. This was shown in several studies when the effect of synchronous atrioventricular (AV) pacing was evaluated using an optimized AV delay in patients with a prolonged PR [46–49]. These studies preceded those in which not only an optimized AV delay was selected, but also ventricular activation resynchronized by pacing in the appropriate ventricle in case of bundle branch block [50–53].

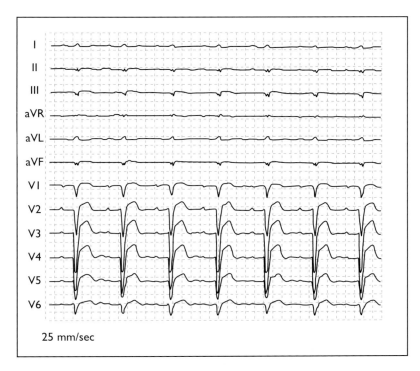

25 mm/sec

FIGURE 4-7. An electrocardiogram from a 62-year-old man with severe systolic heart failure shows sinus rhythm with a prolonged PR interval and complete left bundle branch block. Note the low voltage of the QRS in the limb leads and the rS complex in lead V6, both indicating marked biventricular enlargement.

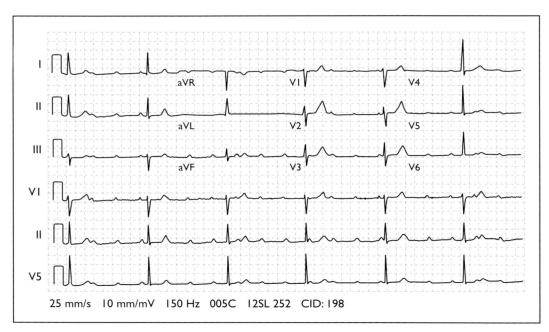

25 mm/s 10 mm/mV 150 Hz 005C 12SL 252 CID: 198

FIGURE 4-8. Congestive heart failure due to complete heart block. Marked bradycardia in patients with underlying heart disease and even in the absence of heart disease is a well recognized cause of depression of cardiac output and cause of or worsening of heart failure. Stroke volume in these conditions may be maximal and cannot rise further to maintain cardiac output. A loss of atrioventricular (AV) synchrony due to the loss of the atrial booster pump mechanism can impair ventricular filling, lower cardiac output and increase atrial pressures [54]. This is especially true in patients with impairments of ventricular filling due to cardiac hypertrophy. This figure shows an example of heart failure due to acquired AV block. This tracing was recorded from an 82-year-old man with hypertensive heart disease and normal ventricular systolic function who developed heart failure symptoms including exercise intolerance, exertional dyspnea, orthopnea, and pedal edema. All his symptoms resolved following implantation of a dual chamber pacemaker. Patients who exhibit signs and symptoms of sinus node disease and chronotropic incompetence should have consideration given to implantation of a rate-responsive pacemaker that can restore physiologic heart rates during physical activity.

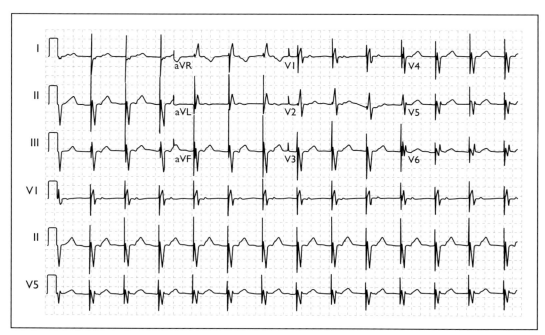

FIGURE 4-9. Pacemaker syndrome. From the early days of pacing when single chamber pacing was the only mode available, it was noted that several patients developed a hemodynamic decline with single chamber ventricular pacing. It was established that the hemodynamic impairment was due to ventriculoatrial conduction and/or contraction against a closed atrioventricular (AV) valve. The resulting symptoms constitute the pacemaker syndrome [55]. It can be manifested by a variety of symptoms including weakness, exercise intolerance and dyspnea, presyncope, and syncope. In addition to VVI pacing, any pacing mode with loss of AV synchrony can produce the syndrome. This figure shows an example of ventriculoatrial (VA) conduction in a patient with pacemaker syndrome. This patient had a dual chamber pacemaker with biventricular pacing implanted for refractory heart failure. Due to malfunction of the atrial lead, sensing and pacing functions in the atrium were lost. Pure ventricular pacing results in VA conduction with retrograde P waves seen in the inferior leads. The symptoms resolved with a revision of the atrial lead and restoration of AV synchrony.

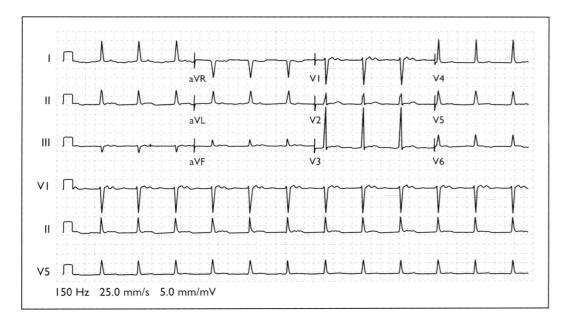

150 Hz 25.0 mm/s 5.0 mm/mV

FIGURE 4-10. Pseudopacemaker syndrome. A pacemaker syndrome–like picture can also be seen in patients with a markedly prolonged PR interval with atrial systole effectively occurring during or immediately after ventricular systole [56]. A dual chamber pacemaker with a standard atrioventricular delay is a very effective treatment for this condition.

THE QRS COMPLEX

In the HF patient, the QRS complex not only indicates the etiology of impaired cardiac function such as the Q wave from a previous myocardial infarction or the QRS changes in ventricular hypertrophy, but also gives prognostic information. When Q waves and notching of the QRS complex are present, they point to extensive myocardial scarring and indicate an increased likelihood for the occurrence of serious ventricular arrhythmias. Already in 1989 Wilensky *et al.* [57] reported on the relation between QRS width and prognosis indicating an inverse relation between QRS width and life expectancy. This has more recently been confirmed in several publications [58–61]. QRS widening can be based on several mechanisms, such as intra- and interventricular conduction delay, ventricular hypertrophy, ventricular dilatation, and scar. Bundle branch block is an important mechanism of QRS widening. Twenty-five years ago, epidemiologic studies indicated that in the nonhospital population, the presence of left bundle branch block (LBBB) but not right bundle branch block predicted a shorter life span [62,63], the reason being that LBBB results in important asynchrony of ventricular contraction [64]. Recently, endocardial mapping studies in patients with LBBB showed that the ventricular activation sequence may vary from patient to patient. LBBB, as depicted in Figure 4-11, may not only result in different patterns of ventricular contraction, but also in different degrees of mitral incompetence [65,66].

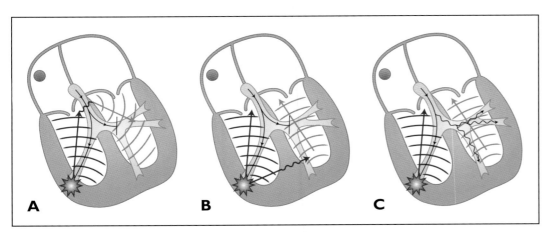

FIGURE 4-11. Examples of right and left ventricular activation in left bundle branch block (LBBB). **A,** Septal breakthrough of the activation front coming from the right ventricle occurs in the superior part of the interventricular septum. This results in desynchronized contraction of both ventricles with the right ventricle contracting in an apico-basal direction and the left ventricle in a baso-apical direction. **B,** Septal breakthrough takes place in the inferior portion of the interventricular septum. Right and left ventricular contraction are desynchronized but both occur an in apico-basal direction. **C,** There is no true LBBB but markedly delayed conduction in the left bundle branch. Right and left ventricular contraction are desynchronized but both occur in an apico-basal direction.

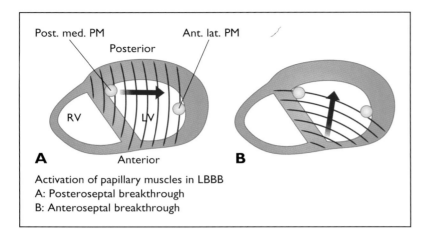

A

B

Activation of papillary muscles in LBBB
A: Posteroseptal breakthrough
B: Anteroseptal breakthrough

FIGURE 4-12. A cross section of the right and left ventricle (RV and LV) in the horizontal plane shows how during left bundle branch block the site of septal breakthrough may affect desynchronized contraction of the two papillary muscles (PM) resulting in mitral incompetence. **A,** Desynchronization of the papillary muscles is most marked in posteroseptal breakthrough. **B,** More synchronized activation of the papillary muscles occurs in case of anteroseptal breakthrough.

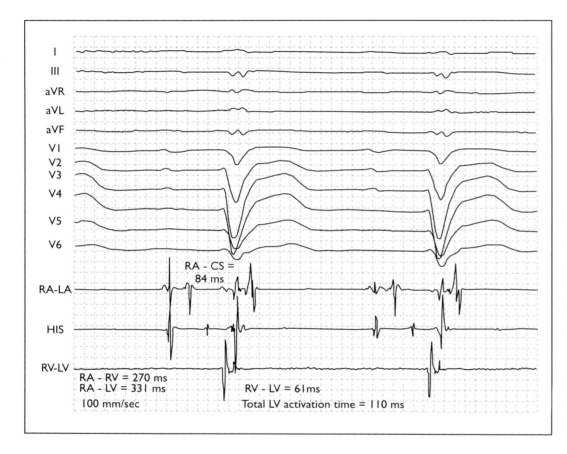

FIGURE 4-13. Intracardiac recordings. For optimal resynchronization of ventricular contraction in patients with left bundle branch block, information about the time intervals between contraction of the different components of the different ventricles is essential. This information can be obtained by intracardiac recordings and intracardiac activation mapping [66,67]. This figure, which is from the same patient as in Figure 4-7, shows how this is done by a bipolar recording from the right and left side of the heart. The purpose of such a study is to determine not only the most appropriate site for stimulation and time interval between left and right ventricular stimulation, but also the best time interval between atrial and ventricular contraction.

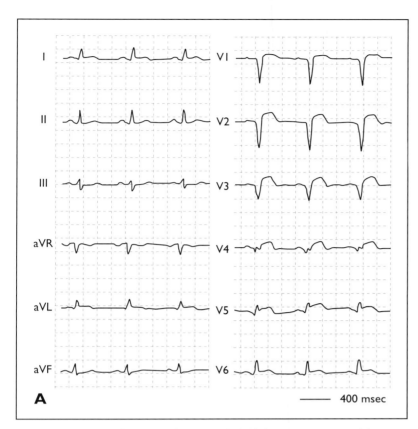

A

———— 400 msec

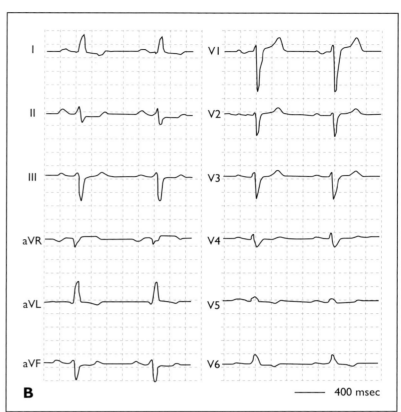

B

———— 400 msec

FIGURE 4-14. **A**, Electrocardiogram (ECG) from a 73-year-old man with an extensive anterior wall myocardial infarction. As shown in **B**, those ECG changes completely disappear when left bundle branch block (LBBB) develops. LBBB will also "mask" changes in the QRS complex that are present when observed when the intraventricular conduction system is intact.

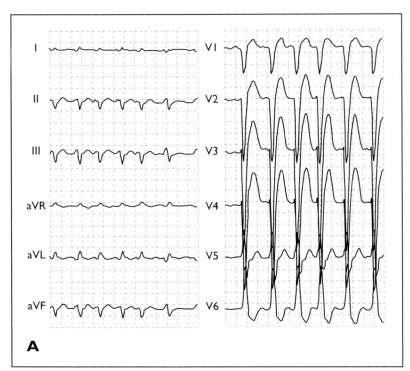

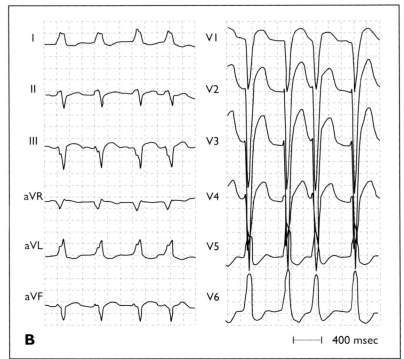

A

B

├──────┤ 400 msec

FIGURE 4-15. Electrocardiogram (ECG) from a 67-year-old woman with severe systolic heart failure. In patients with heart failure and left bundle branch block (LBBB), apart from QRS width, there are two other important ECG findings. The ECG on admission shows atrial fibrillation with a ventricular rate of approximately 130/minute (**A**). LBBB is present with a QRS width of 180 ms, indicating additional causes for QRS widening other than LBBB alone, such as ventricular dilatation, hypertrophy, or scarring, alone or in combination. There is a marked discrepancy in voltage between the extremity (low voltage) and precordial high voltage leads. The decreased voltage in the bipolar limb leads is the result of an increased intracardiac blood pool, which is present between the two leads [68–70]. In contrast, the precordial unipolar leads record the voltage of the tissue under the electrode. Presence of biventricular enlargement is supported by the frontal QRS axis of -90 degrees, indicating the late activation of the base and outflow tract of the right and left ventricle after ventricular activation starting at the exit of the right bundle branch (*see* Fig. 4-11). **B**, Two days later, after a fluid loss of 10 L, two important changes are noted: 1) marked diminution of the voltage difference between extremity and precordial leads, and 2) a shift of the frontal QRS axis to -30 degrees. These changes indicate a marked decrease in intracardiac volume, especially of the right ventricle.

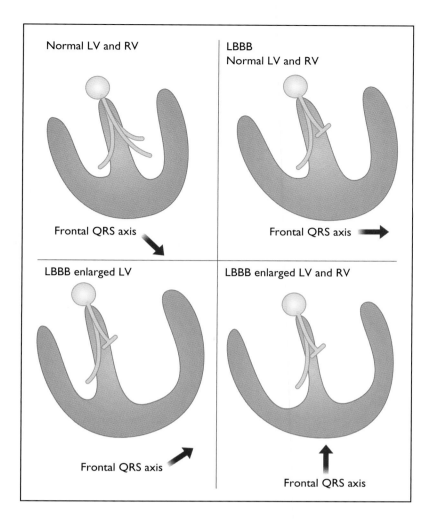

FIGURE 4-16. Frontal plane axis and severity of heart disease in left bundle branch block (LBBB). When a superior QRS axis is present in the frontal plane during LBBB, there is not only left ventricular but also right ventricular dilatation. As shown in this figure, in LBBB the frontal plane QRS axis changes from intermediate to a more horizontal direction when the heart is otherwise normal. However, when left ventricular dilatation and LBBB are present, the frontal plane QRS axis moves further to the left (*lower left panel*). In case of biventricular enlargement and LBBB, ventricular activation goes from apex to base resulting in a superior direction of the frontal plane QRS axis. Patients with LBBB showing this frontal plane axis do not seem to respond well to cardiac resynchronization pacing, the presence of right ventricular failure being a marker for poor prognosis.

EFFECT OF RIGHT VENTRICULAR PACING ON VENTRICULAR DYSSYNCHRONY

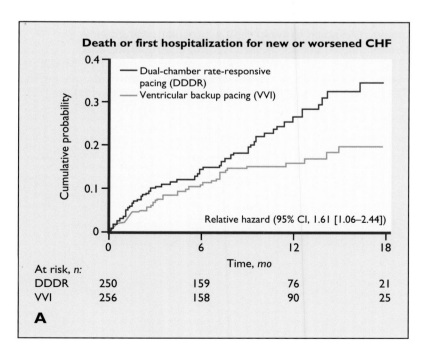

FIGURE 4-17. A–C, Results of the DAVID trial. Right ventricular pacing has been reported to be deleterious in patients who do not have a primary indication for bradycardia pacing. This question was addressed by the DAVID trial investigators [71]. They studied 506 patients with ventricular systolic dysfunction who had an indication for implantable cardioverter-defibrillator (ICD) therapy but no primary indications for bradycardia pacing. The patients received a combined ICD and a dual chamber pacemaker and were randomized to receive either

Continued on next page

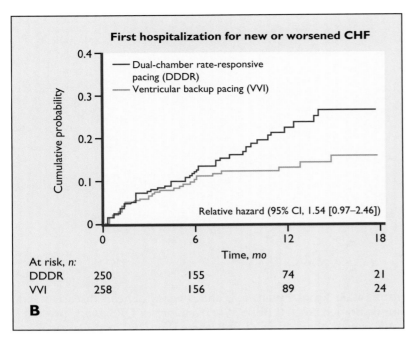

First hospitalization for new or worsened CHF

— Dual-chamber rate-responsive pacing (DDDR)
— Ventricular backup pacing (VVI)

Relative hazard (95% CI, 1.54 [0.97–2.46])

At risk, *n*:

DDDR	250	155	74	21
VVI	258	156	89	24

B

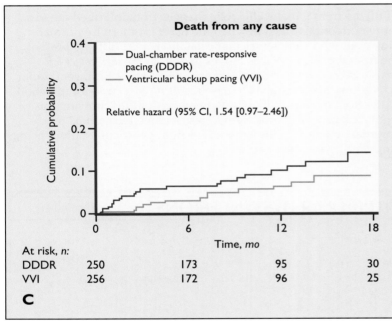

Death from any cause

— Dual-chamber rate-responsive pacing (DDDR)
— Ventricular backup pacing (VVI)

Relative hazard (95% CI, 1.54 [0.97–2.46])

At risk, *n*:

DDDR	250	173	95	30
VVI	256	172	96	25

C

FIGURE 4-17. *(Continued)* 1) ventricular-only backup pacing (VVI-40) with a lower rate of 40 beats per minute, or 2) dual chamber rate responsive pacing with a lower rate of 70 beats per minute (DDDR-70). In the VVI-40 group, pacing accounted for approximately 1% of all beats. In the DDDR-70 group, nearly 60% of all the beats were paced. At the 18-month follow-up, DDDR-70 patients had about a 60% higher relative probability of death or hospitalization for new or worsened heart failure as compared with VVI-40 patients (*P* < 0.03). Component endpoints were just short of statistical significance but trended significantly. Likely due to the eliciting of mechanical dyssynchrony, the DAVID study conclusively demonstrated the deleterious effects of right ventricular only pacing in patients with ventricular dysfunction. This led to widespread changes in how the pacemaker settings are programmed in patients with systolic dysfunction (designed to avoid right ventricular pacing unless a demonstrative need for antibradycardia pacing is present).

The findings of the DAVID study were corroborated by a MADIT-II substudy that also showed that chronic right ventricular pacing in ICD patients increases the risk of new or worsened heart failure [72].

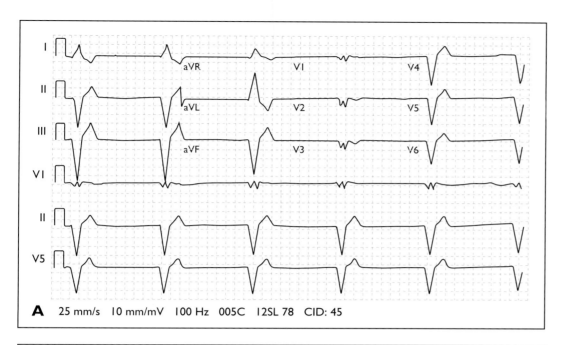

A 25 mm/s 10 mm/mV 100 Hz 005C 12SL 78 CID: 45

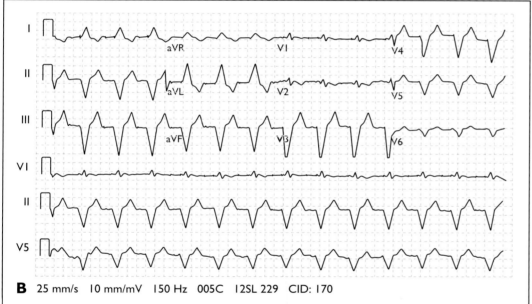

B 25 mm/s 10 mm/mV 150 Hz 005C 12SL 229 CID: 170

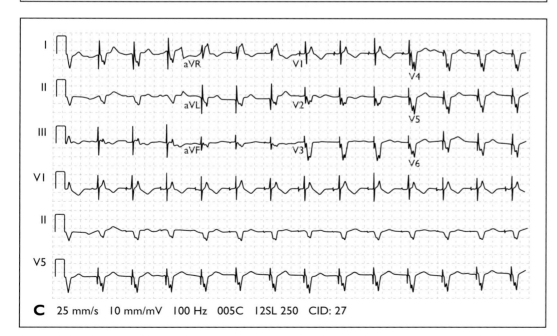

C 25 mm/s 10 mm/mV 100 Hz 005C 12SL 250 CID: 27

FIGURE 4-18. **A–C**, Electrocardiograms from a 67-year-old woman with atherosclerotic coronary heart disease and severe ventricular systolic dysfunction and heart failure who is also pacemaker dependent (**A**). This figure illustrates that in patients with ventricular systolic dysfunction who also have a primary indication for antibradycardia pacing, right ventricular only pacing is not sufficient and these patients require biventricular pacing. **B**, Atrioventricular sequential pacing resulted in only minimal to mild relief of heart failure symptoms. **C**, Upgrading her pacemaker system to include biventricular pacing resulted in complete resolution of heart failure symptoms.

It is well known that the ST-T segment is the part of the ECG showing dynamic changes in case of acute cardiac damage, the typical example being the behavior of the ST-T segment during cardiac ischemia. In HF patients there are two stable ST-T segment abnormalities indicating a poor prognosis. First is the presence of persistent ST-segment elevation, indicating abnormal wall motion or ventricular aneurysm formation in the area under the ECG lead. Second is persistent T-wave negativity, indicating chronic cardiac damage in the area represented by the respective ECG leads.

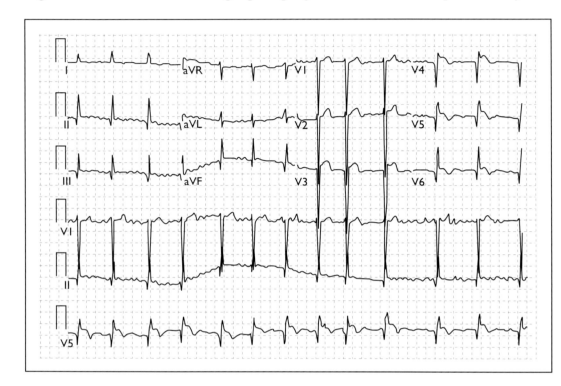

FIGURE 4-19. Electrocardiogram of a 70-year-old woman with atherosclerotic coronary heart disease due to a prior inferior infarction, and persistent atrial fibrillation with class IV heart failure. The persistent ST-segment elevation seen in leads V3–V6 indicates an apical aneurysm, confirmed in this patient by multiple imaging studies. Aneurysm resection in this patient may result in improvement of systolic function.

THE ELECTROCARDIOGRAM IN HEART FAILURE DUE TO DIASTOLIC DYSFUNCTION AND RESTRICTIVE CARDIOMYOPATHY

Although cardiac hypertrophy may be an effective mechanism to sustain emptying of the overloaded ventricle, it may interfere with the heart's diastolic properties and impair ventricular filling. Abnormalities of the heart's diastolic characteristics constitute a very important cause of HF, and a discussion on HF would be incomplete without an analysis of mechanisms and disease conditions underlying diastolic dysfunction. This section will focus on the ECG recognition of two entities, *ie*, cardiac amyloidosis and hypertrophic cardiomyopathy.

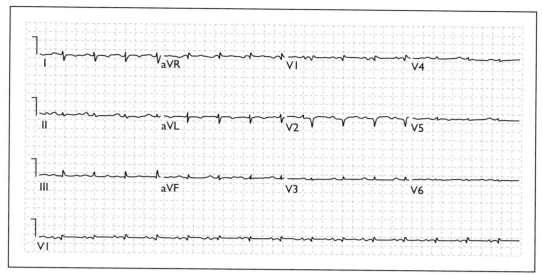

FIGURE 4-20. A typical amyloid electrocardiogram (ECG) with diffuse low voltage. Cardiac amyloidosis refers to a group of diseases involving extracelluar deposition of pathologic insoluble fibrillar proteins in organs and tissues. Cardiac tissue specimens display a characteristic red to apple green appearance with Congo red stain and polarized light. Patients with cardiac amyloidosis can present in a number of ways including pericardial effusions, orthostatic hypotension, valvular disorder, or systolic dysfunction. The characteristic presentation involves diastolic dysfunction and heart failure with a restrictive cardiomyopathy picture [73]. A distinctive characteristic of amyloid heart disease is an inverse relationship between the QRS voltage in the ECG and the left ventricular (LV) mass [74]. A combination of low voltage in the ECG and increased septal and posterior LV wall thickness are highly specific for amyloid heart disease. Other characteristic ECG findings of cardiac amyloid include atrioventricular conduction abnormalities, atrial arrhythmias, and a pseudo infarct pattern.

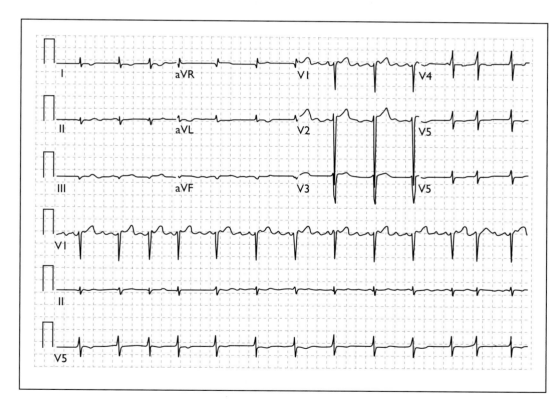

FIGURE 4-21. A typical electrocardiogram in a 57-year-old woman with biopsy-proven cardiac amyloid and no epicardial occlusive coronary artery disease with a characteristic atrial fibrillation and a pseudo infarct pattern. In a recent study, Rahman *et al.* [75] found a pseudo infarct pattern in 60% of patients and a low voltage pattern in 56% of patients with biopsy-proven cardiac amyloidosis.

HYPERTROPHIC CARDIOMYOPATHY

The term *hypertrophic cardiomyopathy* refers to a primary myocardial abnormality characterized by inappropriate myocardial hypertrophy often predominating on the interventricular septum with supranormal function [76]. The most characteristic pathophysiologic abnormality in hypertrophic cardiomyopathy is diastolic dysfunction [77]. The abnormally stiff ventricle results in impaired ventricular filling and an elevated left ventricular end-diastolic pressure, with resulting dyspnea and congestive heart failure.

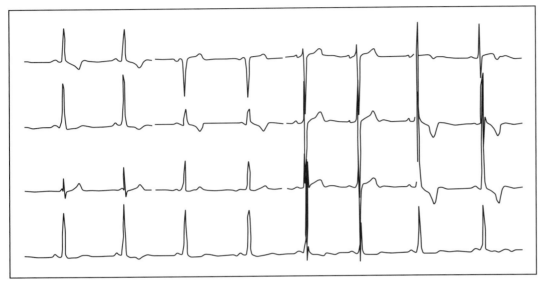

FIGURE 4-22. A typical electrocardiogram (ECG) of a 17-year-old boy with hypertrophic cardiomyopathy. A spectrum of ECG abnormalities may be seen in hypertrophic cardiomyopathy including 1) evidence of large voltages in the limb and precordial leads with secondary repolarization changes, 2) evidence of chamber enlargement in the atria especially the left atrium, 3) marked left axis deviation, and 4) deep and narrow Q waves in the leftward-oriented leads [78,79]. It should be noted that 15% of patients, especially those who have only localized hypertrophy, may have normal ECGs. Giant negative T waves in the midprecordial leads may be found in patients of Japanese descent and are characteristic of hypertrophic cardiomyopathy involving the apex [80]. Prominent Q waves on the inferior and lateral leads can be seen in 20% to 50% of patients. They appear to be due to depolarization of the myopathic cells of the septum. (*Courtesy of* Dr. Robert Myerburg, University of Miami, Miami, FL.)

OTHER SPECIFIC HEART MUSCLE DISEASES

There are many conditions under this category that can present as heart failure. However, we will mention one condition, *ie*, Chagas disease, a protozoal myocarditis caused by *Trypanosoma cruzi* prevalent in Central and South America where it continues to be a major public health problem. The major cardiac manifestation is an extensive myocarditis, and advanced cases present as chronic progressive HF that is often predominantly right sided. Patients with chronic Chagas disease as a rule demonstrate ECG changes, with right bundle branch block and a left anterior hemiblock being the most common changes [81].

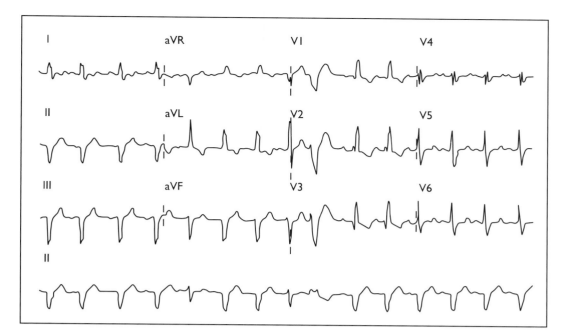

Figure 4-23. Electrocardiogram (ECG) of a 56-year-old woman from Brazil with Chagas disease with typical ECG features of Chagasic cardiomyopathy showing evidence of trifascicular disease. She has severe impairment of left ventricular systolic function (ejection fraction 20%) with class II congestive heart failure and a history of syncope and sustained monomorphic ventricular tachycardia. Ventricular tachyarrhythmias are a prominent feature of the disease. (*Courtesy of* Dr. Rodrigo Mendonca, Institute du Curacao, University of Sao Paulo Medical School, Sao Paulo, Brazil.)

References

1. Zuanetti G, Mantini L, Hernandez-Bernal F, *et al.*: Relevance of heart rate as a prognostic factor in patients with acute myocardial infarction: insights from the GISSI-2 study. *Eur Heart J* 1998, 19(Suppl F):F19–26.

2. Doval HC, Nul DR, Grancelli HO, *et al.*: Randomised trial of low-dose amiodarone in severe congestive heart failure. Grupo de Estudio de la Sobrevida en la Insuficiencia Cardiaca en Argentina (GESICA). *Lancet* 1994, 344:493–498.

3. Lechat P, Packer M, Chalon S, *et al.*: Clinical effects of beta-adrenergic blockade in chronic heart failure: a meta-analysis of double-blind, placebo-controlled, randomized trials. *Circulation* 1998, 98:1184–1191.

4. The MERIT-HF Investigators: Effect of metoprolol CR/XL in chronic heart failure: Metoprolol CR/XL Randomised Intervention Trial in Congestive Heart Failure (MERIT-HF). *Lancet* 1999, 353:2001–2007.

5. Hogg K, Swedberg K, McMurray J: Heart failure with preserved left ventricular systolic function; epidemiology, clinical characteristics, and prognosis. *J Am Coll Cardiol* 2004, 43:317–327.

6. Crijns HJ, Tjeerdsma G, de Kam PJ, *et al.*: Prognostic value of the presence and development of atrial fibrillation in patients with advanced chronic heart failure. *Eur Heart J* 2000, 21:1238–1245.

7. Mahoney P, Kimmel S, DeNofrio D, *et al.*: Prognostic significance of atrial fibrillation in patients at a tertiary medical center referred for heart transplantation because of severe heart failure. *Am J Cardiol* 1999, 83:1544–1547.

8. Sanders P, Morton JB, Davidson NC, *et al.*: Electrical remodeling of the atria in congestive heart failure: electrophysiological and electroanatomic mapping in humans. *Circulation* 2003, 108:1461–1468.

9. Ruo B, Capra AM, Jensvold NG, Go AS: Racial variation in the prevalence of atrial fibrillation among patients with heart failure: the Epidemiology, Practice, Outcomes, and Costs of Heart Failure (EPOCH) study. *J Am Coll Cardiol* 2004, 43:429–435.

10. Carson PE, Johnson GR, Dunkman WB, *et al.*: The influence of atrial fibrillation on prognosis in mild to moderate heart failure. The V-HeFT Studies. The V-HeFT VA Cooperative Studies Group. *Circulation* 1993, 87(Suppl 6):VI102–VI110.

11. Cha YM, Redfield MM, Shen WK, Gersh BJ: Atrial fibrillation and ventricular dysfunction: a vicious electromechanical cycle. *Circulation* 2004, 109:2839–2843.

12. Dries DL, Exner DV, Gersh BJ, *et al.*: Atrial fibrillation is associated with an increased risk for mortality and heart failure progression in patients with asymptomatic and symptomatic left ventricular systolic dysfunction: a retrospective analysis of the SOLVD trials. Studies of Left Ventricular Dysfunction. *J Am Coll Cardiol* 1998, 32:695–703.

13. Mathew J, Hunsberger S, Fleg J, *et al.*: Incidence, predictive factors, and prognostic significance of supraventricular tachyarrhythmias in congestive heart failure. *Chest* 2000, 118:914–922.

14. Wang TJ, Larson MG, Levy D, *et al.*: Temporal relations of atrial fibrillation and congestive heart failure and their joint influence on mortality: the Framingham Heart Study. *Circulation* 2003, 107:2920–2925.

15. van Gelder IC, Hagens VE, Bosker HA, *et al.*: A comparison of rate control and rhythm control in patients with recurrent persistent atrial fibrillation. *N Engl J Med* 2002, 347:1834–1840.

16. Wyse DG, Waldo AL, DiMarco JP, *et al.*: A comparison of rate control and rhythm control in patients with atrial fibrillation. *N Engl J Med* 2002, 347:1825–1833.

17. Deedwania PC, Singh BN, Ellenbogen K, *et al.*: Spontaneous conversion and maintenance of sinus rhythm by amiodarone in patients with heart failure and atrial fibrillation: observations from the veterans affairs congestive heart failure survival trial of antiarrhythmic therapy (CHF-STAT). The Department of Veterans Affairs CHF-STAT Investigators. *Circulation* 1998, 98:2574–2579.

18. Torp-Pedersen C, Moller M, Bloch-Thomsen PE, *et al.*: Dofetilide in patients with congestive heart failure and left ventricular dysfunction. Danish Investigations of Arrhythmia and Mortality on Dofetilide Study Group. *N Engl J Med* 1999, 341:857–865.

19. The AF-CHF Trial Investigators: Rationale and design of a study assessing treatment strategies of atrial fibrillation in patients with heart failure: the Atrial Fibrillation and Congestive Heart Failure (AF-CHF) trial. *Am Heart J* 2002, 144:597–607.

20. Grogan M, Smith HC, Gersh BJ, Wood DL: Left ventricular dysfunction due to atrial fibrillation in patients initially believed to have idiopathic dilated cardiomyopathy. *Am J Cardiol* 1992, 69:1570–1573.

21. Chen MS, Marrouche NF, Khaykin Y, *et al.*: Pulmonary vein isolation for the treatment of atrial fibrillation in patients with impaired systolic function. *J Am Coll Cardiol* 2004, 43:1004–1009.

22. Hsu LF, Jais P, Sanders P, *et al.*: Catheter ablation for atrial fibrillation in congestive heart failure. *N Engl J Med* 2004, 351:2373–2383.

23. Brignole M, Menozzi C, Gianfranchi L, *et al.*: Assessment of atrioventricular junction ablation and VVIR pacemaker versus pharmacological treatment in patients with heart failure and chronic atrial fibrillation: a randomized, controlled study. *Circulation* 1998, 98:953–960.

24. Jensen SM, Bergfeldt L, Rosenqvist M: Long-term follow-up of patients treated by radiofrequency ablation of the atrioventricular junction. *Pacing Clin Electrophysiol* 1995, 18(9 Pt 1):1609–1614.

25. Rodriguez LM, Smeets JL, Xie B, *et al.*: Improvement in left ventricular function by ablation of atrioventricular nodal conduction in selected patients with lone atrial fibrillation. *Am J Cardiol* 1993, 72:1137–1141.

26. Leclercq C, Victor F, Alonso C, *et al.*: Comparative effects of permanent biventricular pacing for refractory heart failure in patients with stable sinus rhythm or chronic atrial fibrillation. *Am J Cardiol* 2000, 85:1154–1156.

27. Bosch J, Yusuf S, Pogue J, *et al.*: Use of ramipril in preventing stroke: double blind randomised trial. *BMJ* 2002, 324:699–702.

28. Madrid AH, Bueno MG, Rebollo JM, *et al.*: Use of irbesartan to maintain sinus rhythm in patients with long-lasting persistent atrial fibrillation: a prospective and randomized study. *Circulation* 2002, 106:331–336.

29. Pedersen OD, Bagger H, Kober L, Torp-Pedersen C: Trandolapril reduces the incidence of atrial fibrillation after acute myocardial infarction in patients with left ventricular dysfunction. *Circulation* 1999, 100:376–380.

30. Vermes E, Tardif JC, Bourassa MG, *et al.*: Enalapril decreases the incidence of atrial fibrillation in patients with left ventricular dysfunction: insight from the Studies Of Left Ventricular Dysfunction (SOLVD) trials. *Circulation* 2003, 107:2926–2931.

31. Meinertz T, Hoffman T, Kasper W, *et al.*: Significance of ventricular arrhythmias in idiopathic dilated cardiomyopathy. *Am J Cardiol* 1988, 63:138–140.

32. Packer M: Lack of relation between ventricular arrhythmias and sudden death in patients with chronic heart failure. *Circulation* 1992, 85(Suppl I):I50–I56.

33. Teerlink JR, Jalaluddin M, Anderson S, Kukin ML, *et al.*: Ambulatory ventricular arrhythmias in patients with heart failure do not specifically predict an increased risk of sudden death. PROMISE (Prospective Randomized Milrinone Survival Evaluation) Investigators. *Circulation* 2000, 101:40–46.

34. Moss AJ, Hall WJ, Cannom DS, *et al.*: Improved survival with an implanted defibrillator in patients with coronary disease at high risk for ventricular arrhythmia. Multicenter Automatic Defibrillator Implantation Trial Investigators. *N Engl J Med* 1996, 335:1933–1940.

35. Buxton AE, Lee KL, Fisher JD, *et al.*: A randomized study of the prevention of sudden death in patients with coronary artery disease. Multicenter Unsustained Tachycardia Trial Investigators. *N Engl J Med* 1999, 341:1882–1890.

36. The Cardiac Arrhythmia Suppression Trial Investigators: Preliminary report: effect of encainide and flecainide on mortality in a randomized trial of arrhythmia suppression after myocardial infarction. The Cardiac Arrhythmia Suppression Trial (CAST) Investigators. *N Engl J Med* 1989, 321:406–412.

37. Hennekens CH, Albert CM, Godfried SL, *et al.*: Adjunctive drug therapy of acute myocardial infarction—evidence from clinical trials. *N Engl J Med* 1996, 335:1660–1667.

38. Effect of prophylactic amiodarone on mortality after acute myocardial infarction and in congestive heart failure: meta-analysis of individual data from 6500 patients in randomised trials. Amiodarone Trials Meta-Analysis Investigators. *Lancet* 1997, 350:1417–1424.

39. Camm AJ, Pratt CM, Schwartz PJ, *et al.*: Mortality in patients after a recent myocardial infarction: a randomized, placebo-controlled trial of azimilide using heart rate variability for risk stratification. *Circulation* 2004, 109:990–996.

40. The SCD HeFT study. *The American College of Cardiology Meeting.* New Orleans, LA. March 7–10 2004.

41. Linseman JV, Bristow MR: Drug therapy and heart failure prevention. *Circulation* 2003, 107:1234–1236.

42. Blanck Z Sra J, Dhala A, *et al.*: Bundle branch reentry: mechanisms, diagnosis and treatment. In *Cardiac Electrophysiology: From the Cell to the Bedside*. Edited by Zipes DP. Philadelphia: WB Saunders; 2000:656–661.

43. Narasimhan C , Jazayeri M, Sra J, *et al.*: Ventricular tachycardia in valvular heart disease. Facilitation of sustained bundle branch reentry by valve surgery. *Circulation* 1997, 96:4307–4313.

44. Jazayeri M Sra J, Dhala A, *et al.*: Interfascicular reentrant ventricular tachycardia: Utility of bundle branch potentials in diagnosis and catheter ablation [abstract]. *Circulation* 1992, 4:2065.

45. Lopera G, Stevenson WG, *et al.*: Identification and ablation of three types of ventricular tachycardia involving the His-Purkinje system in patients with heart disease. *J Cardiovasc Electrophysiol* 2004, 15:52–58.

46. Auricchio A, Stellbrink C, Block M, *et al.*: Effect of pacing chamber and atrioventricular delay on acute systolic function of paced patients with congestive heart failure. The Pacing Therapies for Congestive Heart Failure Study Group. The Guidant Congestive Heart Failure Research Group. *Circulation* 1999, 99:2993–3001.

47. Gold MR, Feliciano Z, Gottlieb SS, Fisher ML: Dual-chamber pacing with a short atrioventricular delay in congestive heart failure: a randomized study. *J Am Coll Cardiol* 1995; 26:967–973.

48. Kass DA, Chen CH, Curry C, *et al.*: Improved left ventricular mechanics from acute VDD pacing in patients with dilated cardiomyopathy and ventricular conduction delay. *Circulation* 1999, 99:1567–1573.

49. Linde C, Gadler F, Edner M, *et al.*: Results of atrioventricular synchronous pacing with optimized delay in patients with severe congestive heart failure. *Am J Cardiol* 1995, 75:919–923.

50. Auricchio A, Stellbrink C, Butter C, *et al.*: Clinical efficacy of cardiac resynchronization therapy using left ventricular pacing in heart failure patients stratified by severity of ventricular conduction delay. *J Am Coll Cardiol* 2003, 42:2109–2116.

51. Bradley DJ, Bradley EA, Baughman KL, *et al.*: Cardiac resynchronization and death from progressive heart failure: a meta-analysis of randomized controlled trials. *JAMA* 2003, 289:730–740.

52. Bristow MR, Saxon L, Boehmer J, *et al.*: Cardiac resynchronization therapy (CRT) reduces hospitalizations, and CRT + an implantible defibrillator (CRT-D) reduces mortality in chronic heart failure: preliminary results of the COMPANION trial. Available at http://www.uchsc.edu/cvi/clb.pdf.

53. Lupi G, Brignole M, Oddone D, *et al.*: Effects of left ventricular pacing on cardiac performance and on quality of life in patients with drug refractory heart failure. *Am J Cardiol* 2000, 86:1267–1270.

54. Braunwald E, Frahm C: Studies on Starling's law of the heart. IV. Observations on the hemodynamic functions of the left atrium in man. *Circulation* 1962, 24:633.

55. Ausubel K, Furman S: The pacemaker syndrome. *Ann Intern Med* 1985, 103:420–429.

56. Kim YH, O'nunain S, Trouton T, *et al.*: Pseudopacemaker syndrome following inadvertent fast pathway ablation for atrioventricular nodal re-entrant tachycardia. *J Cardiovasc Electrophysiol* 1993, 4:178–182.

57. Wilensky R, Yudelman P, Cohen AL, *et al*.: Serial electrocardiographic changes in idopathic dilated cardiomyopathy confirmed at necropsy. *Am J Cardiol* 1989, 62:276–283.

58. Baldasseroni S, Opasich C, Gorini M, *et al*.: Left bundle-branch block is associated with increased 1-year sudden and total mortality rate in 5517 outpatients with congestive heart failure: a report from the Italian network on congestive heart failure. *Am Heart J* 2002, 143:398–405.

59. Iuliano S, Fisher SG, Karasik PE, *et al*.: QRS duration and mortality in patients with congestive heart failure. *Am Heart J* 2002, 143:1085–1091.

60. Shamim W, Francis DP, Yousufuddin M, *et al*.: Intraventricular conduction delay: a prognostic marker in chronic heart failure. *Int J Cardiol* 1999, 70:171–178.

61. Shenkman HJ, Pampati V, Khandelwal AK, *et al*.: Congestive heart failure and QRS duration: establishing prognosis study. *Chest* 2002, 122:528–534.

62. Kulbertus HE, de Leval-Rutten F, Albert A, *et al*.: Electrocardiographic changes occurring with age. In *What's New in Electrocardiography?* Edited by Wellens H, Kulbertus HE. The Haque: Martinus Nijhoff; 1981:300–314.

63. Schneider JF, Thomas HE Jr, Sorlie P, *et al*.: Comparative features of newly acquired left and right bundle branch block in the general population: the Framingham study. *Am J Cardiol* 1981, 47:931–940.

64. Grines CL, Bashore TM, Boudoulas H, *et al*.: Functional abnormalities in isolated left bundle branch block. The effect of interventricular asynchrony. *Circulation* 1989, 79:845–853.

65. Rodriguez LM, Timmermans C, Nabar A, *et al*.: Variable patterns of septal activation in patients with left bundle branch block and heart failure. *J Cardiovasc Electrophysiol* 2003, 14:135–141.

66. Wellens HJ: Cardiac arrhythmias: the quest for a cure: a historical perspective. *J Am Coll Cardiol* 2004, 44:1155–1163.

67. Auricchio A, Fantoni C, Regoli F, *et al*.: Characterization of left ventricular activation in patients with heart failure and left bundle-branch block. *Circulation* 2004, 109:1133–1139.

68. Brody DA: A theoretical analysis of intracavitary blood mass influence on the heart-lead relationship. *Circ Res* 1956, 4:731–738.

69. Goldberger AL, Dresselhaus T, Bhargava V: Dilated cardiomyopathy: utility of the transverse: frontal plane QRS voltage ratio. *J Electrocardiol* 1985, 18:35–40.

70. Wellens HJ, Gorgels AP: The electrocardiogram 102 years after Einthoven. *Circulation* 2004, 109:562–564.

71. The DAVID trial investigators: Dual chamber pacing or ventricular back up pacing in patients with an implantable defibrillator: the Dual chamber and VVI implantable defibrillator (DAVID) trial. *JAMA* 2002, 288:3115–3123.

72. Predictive value of ventricular pacing in the MADIT-II study. In *NASPE Scientific Sessions*. Washington, DC; 2003.

73. Falk RH, Comenzo RL, Skinner M: The systemic amyloidoses. *N Engl J Med* 1997, 377:898–907.

74. Carroll JD Gaasch W, MacAdam KP: Amyloid cardiomyopathy: characterization by a distinctive voltage/mass relation. *Am J Cardiol* 1982, 49:9–13.

75. Rahman JE Helou EF, Gelzer-Bell R, *et al*.: Noninvasive diagnosis of biopsy-proven cardiac amyloidosis. *J Am Coll Cardiol* 2004, 43:410–415.

76. Maron BJ, Bonow R, Canon R, *et al*.: Hypertrophic cardiomyopathy: Interrelations of clinical manifestations, pathophysiology and therapy. *N Engl J Med* 1987, 316:780.

77. Braunwald E: Hypertrophic cardiomyopathy- continued progress. *N Engl J Med* 1989, 320:800.

78. Bahl OP, Massie E: Electrocardiographic and vectorcardiographic patterns in cardiomyopathy. *Cardiovasc Clin* 1972, 4:95.

79. Spodick DH: Hypertrophic obstructive cardiomyopathy of the left ventricle (idiopathic hypertrophic subaortic stenosis). *Cardiovasc Clin* 1972, 4:133–165.

80. Alfonso F, Annopoulos PN, Stewart J, *et al*.: Clinical significance of giant negative T waves seen in hypertrophic cardiomyopathy. *J Am Coll Cardiol* 1990, 15:965.

81. Casado J, Davila DF, Donis J, *et al*.: Electrocardiographic abnormalities and left ventricular systolic function in Chagas' heart disease. *Int J Cardiol* 1990; 27:55.

IMPACT OF MEDICAL THERAPIES ON THE MANAGEMENT OF ARRHYTHMIC RISK OF HEART FAILURE

Gregg C. Fonarow

Arrhythmias often complicate heart failure and substantially contribute to mortality and morbidity [1]. The incidence of sudden death increases with the severity of heart failure from 2% to 6% per year for patients with mild to moderate heart failure (class I or II) to as much as 5% to 12% per year for patients with moderate to severe heart failure (class III or IV) [1–3]. As the severity of heart failure increases, the proportion of deaths caused by pump failure increases, and the proportion of mortality caused by sudden death decreases, 50% to 80% for mild to moderate heart failure and 5% to 30% for severe heart failure [1,2]. Despite potential differences in arrhythmic mechanisms between ischemic and nonischemic heart failure, the risk of sudden death is generally similar [1,3].

The electrophysiologic abnormalities of ventricular dilation and hypertrophy in chronic heart failure are associated with a decrease in repolarizing currents and prolongation of the action potential duration and QT interval [1,4]. Activation of the sympathetic nervous system and renin-angiotensin-aldosterone systems contribute to significant myocardial structural and functional changes in heart failure. Electrical coupling between myocytes is reduced as a consequence of interstitial fibrosis and decreased gap junction surface area, slowing conduction and potentially promoting reentry [4]. These changes likely play a role in heart failure arrhythmic risk, facilitating polymorphic ventricular tachycardias and ventricular fibrillation. Neurohumoral activation and diuretic-induced electrolyte perturbations further promote arrhythmias [1]. Clinically unrecognized acute coronary syndromes are a frequent precipitating cause of sudden death in heart failure, being present in 42% of autopsies in patients with heart failure who die suddenly [5]. In addition, not all sudden deaths in heart failure are caused by primary ventricular arrhythmias. Severe bradyarrhythmias may occur as a result of conduction system disease. Furthermore, bradycardias and pulseless electrical activity may be caused by hyperkalemia, myocardial ischemia, pulmonary emboli, or stroke [1].

Antiarrhythmic drug options for patients with heart failure are limited. Ventricular dysfunction is one of the primary risk factors for development of ventricular proarrhythmia in patients taking antiarrhythmic drugs [6]. In randomized clinical trials of antiarrhythmic drugs in patients with heart failure, these agents have been associated with a significant increased risk of sudden death and overall mortality, or at best a neutral effect [7–11]. Patients with heart failure who were receiving class I drugs for atrial fibrillation had an increase by a factor of three in the risk of both death and death from arrhythmia [7]. Class I sodium channel–blocking drugs (mexiletine, tocainide, procainamide, quinidine, disopyramide, flecainide, and propafenone) should be avoided because of negative inotropic effects, the potential for proarrhythmia, and an increased risk of mortality [1]. These agents should be reserved for control of frequent arrhythmias in heart failure patients with implanted cardioverter-defibrillators when other drug options have failed. Amiodarone blocks cardiac sodium, potassium, and calcium currents, and has sympatholytic effects. Randomized trials of amiodarone in heart failure have demonstrated no increase but also no decrease in mortality [9]. The suggestion from non–placebo-controlled trials and observational data that amiodarone is beneficial when administered concomitantly with β-blocker therapy has not been confirmed in recent placebo-controlled trials. The type III antiarrhythmic drug dofetilide has a neutral effect on mortality in heart failure; the D-isomer of sotalol increased mortality; and sotalol, which also has nonselective β-adrenergic blocking activity, has not been well studied in this patient population [10,11].

In striking contrast to antiarrhythmic medications, neurohumoral antagonists have been consistently demonstrated to reduce mortality in patients with heart failure due to left ventricular systolic dysfunction. In more than 50 placebo-controlled trials involving more than 25,000 patients with left ventricular systolic dysfunction (ejection fraction < 0.35 to 0.45), ACE inhibitors, aldosterone antagonists, and β-blockers have been shown to alleviate symptoms, improve clinical status, reduce the risk of death, and decrease hospitalizations [12]. The clinical trials have included a variety of patients, including women, the elderly, diabetics, and those with a wide range of underlying heart failure etiologies and severities of left ventricular systolic dysfunction [13]. ACE inhibitors have reduced the risk of sudden death in some, but not all, clinical trials [14]. Significant reductions in the incidence of new-onset atrial fibrillation have been observed [15]. The angiotensin receptor antagonist candesartan has been demonstrated to reduce the risk of sudden death when added to other standard heart failure treatments, including ACE inhibitors and β-blockers, and also to reduce the incidence of new-onset atrial fibrillation [16,17]. Aldosterone antagonists have resulted in substantial reductions in sudden death in patients with mild as

well as severe heart failure [18,19]. β-Blockers have been demonstrated to be the single most effective heart failure medication for reducing the risk of sudden death [2,20–22]. There have been consistent reductions in sudden death observed in the clinical trials of β-blockers in heart failure in the range of 41% to 55%.

ACE inhibitors and/or angiotensin receptor antagonists, aldosterone antagonists, and β-blockers have thus emerged as evidence-based, life-prolonging treatments for heart failure in a spectrum of patients, including those at high risk for developing left ventricular systolic dysfunction and those with asymptomatic and symptomatic left ventricular systolic dysfunction [23]. Antiarrhythmic medications do not decrease, and in many circumstances may increase, the risk of sudden death and all-cause mortality. Use of implantable cardioverter-defibrillators to reduce arrhythmia risk has been shown to be superior to antiarrhythmic medications or standard therapy alone. Placement of an implantable cardioverter-defibrillator in conjunction with optimal use of neurohumoral antagonists thus represents the best protection from death caused by ventricular arrhythmias. Based on this evidence, guidelines put forth by the American College of Cardiology/American Heart Association and the Heart Failure Society of America recommend the use of ACE inhibitors and/or angiotensin receptor antagonists, aldosterone antagonists, and β-blockers for the treatment of chronic stable heart failure as part of the standard of care [23,24]. Despite the compelling scientific evidence that ACE inhibitors and/or angiotensin receptor antagonists, aldosterone antagonists, and β-blockers reduce hospitalizations and mortality in patients with heart failure, these life-prolonging therapies continue to be underutilized. Every effort should be made to improve the use of these therapies in eligible patients, without contraindications or intolerance.

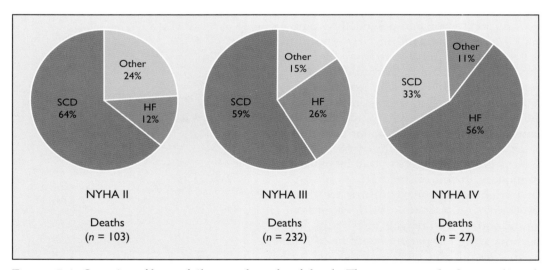

FIGURE 5-1. Severity of heart failure and mode of death. The Metoprolol CR/XL Randomized Intervention Trial in Congestive Heart Failure (MERIT-HF) study evaluated the effects of metoprolol succinate extended release on mortality in patients with decreased ejection fraction and symptoms of heart failure [2]. A post hoc analysis of the MERIT-HF study looked at the total mortality and mode of death relative to the New York Heart Association (NYHA) functional classification. Overall, sudden death occurred in nearly 60% of patients who died. The proportion of sudden cardiac deaths (SCD), however, decreased with increasing severity of NYHA functional class. As seen in this

and other studies, the proportion of mortality caused by sudden death decreases from 50% to 80% for mild to moderate heart failure and 5% to 35% for severe heart failure. The proportion of patients who died from worsening heart failure increased with increasing functional class. Patients with heart failure thus remain at substantially increased risk for ventricular dysrhythmias and sudden cardiac death. Clearly, there are unmet needs in the management of patients with heart failure. HF— mortality secondary to worsening heart failure. (*Adapted from* MERIT-HF Study Group [2].)

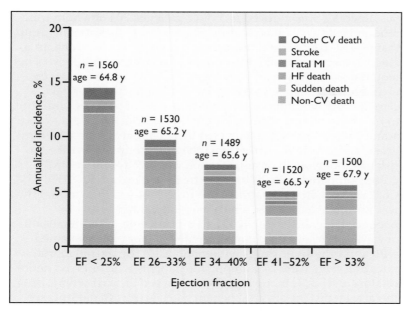

FIGURE 5-2. Relationship between ventricular function and cause-specific mortality. In heart failure (HF), as the left ventricular ejection fraction (LVEF) is decreased, the rate of sudden death and pump dysfunction death as well as overall mortality increases. In this study, data from the Candesartan in Heart Failure: Assessment of Reduction in Mortality and morbidity (CHARM) Program trial was analyzed by baseline LVEF and rates of death were compared [16,25]. The CHARM trials were parallel, randomized, double-blind clinical trials comparing candesartan with placebo in three distinct populations: patients with LVEF of 40% or less who were not receiving ACE inhibitors because of previous intolerance or who were currently receiving ACE inhibitors, and patients with LVEF higher than 40%. Overall, 7601

patients were randomly assigned to candesartan (titrated to 32 mg once daily) or matching placebo and followed up for at least 2 years. The primary outcome of the overall program was all-cause mortality and for all the component trials was cardiovascular (CV) death or hospital admission for worsening heart failure. As illustrated here, death due to myocardial infarction (MI), stroke, and noncardiac causes were similar across the spectrum of ejection fraction. The absolute rates of sudden death and heart failure pump dysfunction death increased with decreasing LVEF, as did total mortality. In addition, the proportions of death due to heart failure and sudden death increased markedly in the population with ejection fractions lower than 40%. (*Adapted from* Solomon *et al.* [16].)

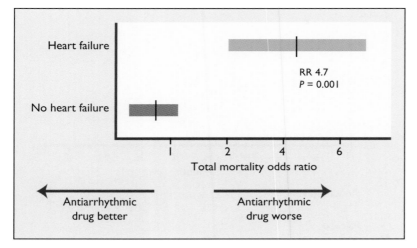

FIGURE 5-3. Increased risk of mortality with antiarrhythmic drugs in patients with heart failure and atrial fibrillation. The relation between cardiac mortality and antiarrhythmic drug administration was analyzed in 1330 patients enrolled in the Stroke Prevention in Atrial Fibrillation Study, a randomized clinical trial comparing warfarin, aspirin, and placebo for the prevention of ischemic stroke or systemic embolism in patients with nonvalvular atrial fibrillation [7]. Patients who received antiarrhythmic drug therapy for atrial fibrillation in this study were compared with patients not receiving antiarrhythmic agents. The antiarrhythmic medications assessed in this study were predominately class I: quinidine (*n* = 127), pro-cainamide (*n* = 57), disopyramide (*n* = 15), flecainide (*n* = 34), encainide (*n* = 20), and amiodarone (*n* = 7). In patients receiving antiarrhythmic drug therapy, cardiac mortality was increased 2.5-fold (95% CI, 1.3–4.9; *P* = 0.006) and arrhythmic death was

increased 2.6-fold (95% CI, 1.2–5.6; *P* = 0.02). Among patients with a history of congestive heart failure, those given antiarrhythmic medications had a relative risk of cardiac death of 4.7 (*P* < 0.001; 95% CI, 1.9–11.6) compared with that of patients not so treated. Patients without a history of congestive heart failure had no increased risk of cardiac mortality during antiarrhythmic drug therapy. After adjustment for other variables predictive of cardiac death, in patients with a history of heart failure who received antiarrhythmic drug therapy, the relative risk of cardiac death was 3.3 (*P* = 0.05; 95% CI, 0.99–11.1) and that of arrhythmic death was 5.8 (*P* = 0.009; 95% CI, 1.5–21.7) compared with the risk in patients not taking antiarrhythmic medications. Although antiarrhythmic drug therapy was not randomly assigned in this trial, the data suggest that in patients with heart failure, antiarrhythmic drug therapy is associated with a substantial increased risk of mortality. (*Adapted from* Flaker *et al.* [7].)

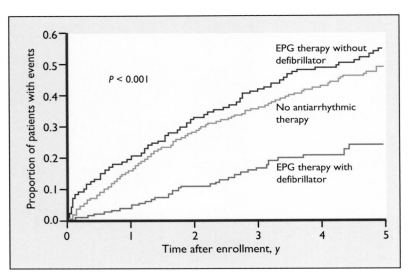

FIGURE 5-4. Mortality with antiarrhythmic drugs versus electrophysiologic-guided (EPG) therapy. Patients with depressed left ventricular systolic function and nonsustained ventricular tachycardia (VT) who were inducible for VT on electrophysiologic testing have substantially increased mortality if treated with antiarrhythmic drugs as compared with an implantable cardioverter-defibrillator (ICD). The Multicenter Unsustained Tachycardia Trial (MUSTT) evaluated 2202 patients with left ventricular dysfunction (ejection fraction < 0.40) who had a history of nonsustained VT [8].

Sustained VT was induced in 35% of patients, 704 of whom were randomized to no antiarrhythmic therapy or to a treatment group that received antiarrhythmic drugs or an ICD if at least one drug failed at electrophysiologic testing. Although heart failure was not required for inclusion and advanced heart failure patients were excluded, the mean left ventricular ejection fraction was 0.30, class II or III symptoms were present in 63% of patients, and 72% to 75% were treated with ACE inhibitors. β-Blockers were administered to 51% of patients in the no-antiarrhythmic therapy group and 29% in the arrhythmia therapy group. At 5 years, the risk of sudden death or resuscitation was 32% for the control group compared with 25% for the treatment group (RR, 0.73; 95% CI, 0.53–0.99). In the treatment group, the reduction in mortality was attributable to ICDs, which were implanted in 46% of patients. Patients with an ICD had a 5-year rate of sudden death or cardiac arrest of 9% compared with 37% for patients treated with antiarrhythmic drugs without an ICD. The overall mortality rates at 5 years were 24% among the patients who received defibrillators and 55% among those who received antiarrhythmic drug therapy alone. The survival benefit associated with defibrillator treatment relative to antiarrhythmic drug therapy remained significant (P < 0.001) after Cox regression analysis, in which adjustments were made for all available prognostic clinical factors. Patients with electrophysiologic-guided drug therapy were four times more likely to have arrhythmic events and 2.5 times more likely to die than patients who received defibrillators. (*Adapted from* Buxton *et al.* [8].)

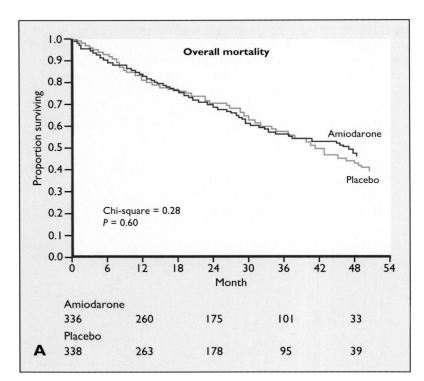

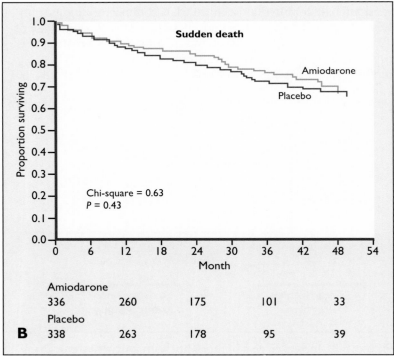

FIGURE 5-5. Kaplan-Meier estimates of the impact of amiodarone compared with placebo in patients with heart failure and systolic dysfunction on overall mortality (**A**) and sudden death (**B**) from cardiac causes. The results of several small studies had suggested that amiodarone may be beneficial in the treatment of patients after acute myocardial infarction, and it was hypothesized that arrhythmia suppression in patients with heart failure would be beneficial. The Veterans Affairs Congestive Heart Failure Antiarrhythmic Trial (CHF-STAT) was conducted to determine whether amiodarone can reduce overall mortality in patients with congestive heart failure and asymptomatic ventricular arrhythmias [9]. In this study, 674 patients with symptoms of congestive heart failure, 10 or

more premature ventricular contractions per hour, and a left ventricular ejection fraction of 40% or less were randomly assigned to receive amiodarone or placebo. Over a median follow-up of 45 months, there was no significant difference in overall mortality between the two treatment groups. The 2-year actuarial survival rate was 69.4% for the patients in the amiodarone group and 70.8% for those in the placebo group (P = 0.60). At 2 years, the rate of sudden death was 15% in the amiodarone group and 19% in the placebo group (P = 0.43). Although amiodarone was effective in suppressing ventricular arrhythmias and improving ventricular function in patients with heart failure, it did not reduce the incidence of sudden death or prolong survival. (*Adapted from* Singh *et al.* [9].)

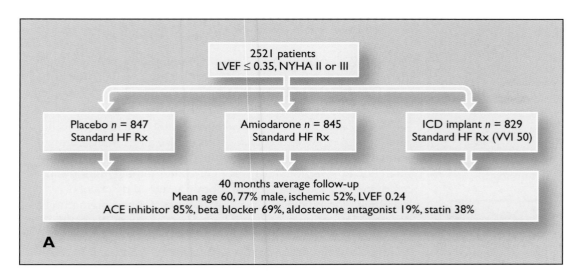

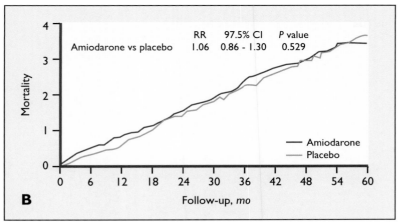

FIGURE 5-6. Impact of amiodarone versus placebo on survival when added to standard medical therapy for patients with heart failure (HF) due to systolic dysfunction. **A,** The Sudden Cardiac Death in Heart Failure Trial (SCD-HeFT) enrolled patients with New York Heart Association (NYHA) class II or III heart failure, either ischemic or nonischemic cardiomyopathy, and a left ventricular ejection fraction (LVEF) of 35% or less [26]. There were 2521 patients enrolled in 148 centers in North America and New Zealand. Patients were randomized to best medical therapy, best medical therapy plus amiodarone, or best medical therapy plus the insertion of an implantable cardioverter-defibrillator (ICD). The median age of the 2521 patients was 60 years, 23% were female, the average duration of heart failure was 24 months, and the mean LVEF was 25%. Seventy percent of patients were in NYHA class II; the remainder were in class III. Fifty-two percent of patients had ischemic heart disease, and the mean QRS duration was 112 ms. The baseline use of ACE inhibitors was 85%, 96% if angiotensin receptor blockers were included. β-Blockers were prescribed in 69% of patients at baseline, and this improved to 78% at last follow-up identification. The primary outcome of the trial demonstrated that ICD implantation reduced all-cause mortality 23% when compared with placebo, whereas amiodarone did not improve mortality. The 3-year rates of all-cause mortality for the ICD, amiodarone, and placebo were 17.1%, 24.0%, and 22.3%, respectively; 5-year all-cause mortality was 28.9%, 34.1%, and 35.8%, respectively. **B,** The relative risk of mortality with amiodarone relative to placebo over the 5 years of the study was 1.06 (97.5% CI, 0.86–1.30). Subgroup analysis did not show any favorable interaction between patients treated with β-blockers and randomization to amiodarone. This trial demonstrates that in heart failure and LVEF less than or equal to 35%, and NYHA class II or III heart failure symptoms, amiodarone offers absolutely no survival advantage. (*Adapted from* Bardy *et al.* [26].)

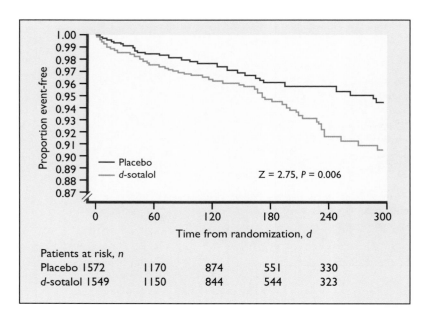

Patients at risk, *n*

Placebo 1572	1170	874	551	330
d-sotalol 1549	1150	844	544	323

FIGURE 5-7. Increased risk of mortality with the type III anti-arrhythmic drug d-sotalol in patients post myocardial infarction with left ventricular dysfunction and/or heart failure. d-Sotalol is a pure potassium-channel blocker (I_{Kr}) with no clinically significant β-blocking activity. The Survival With Oral d-Sotalol (SWORD) trial investigated whether d-sotalol could reduce all-cause mortality in patients with left ventricular dysfunction after recent myocardial infarction or symptomatic heart failure after remote myocardial infarction [10]. Patients were randomly assigned d-sotalol or matching placebo twice daily. The trial was stopped prematurely. Among 1549 patients assigned d-sotalol, there were 78 deaths (5.0%) compared with 48 deaths (3.1%) among the 1572 patients assigned placebo (hazard ratio 1.65; 95% CI, 1.15–2.36; $P = 0.006$). Presumed arrhythmic deaths were substantially increased and the mechanism for the increased risk of overall mortality was seen in this trial. (*Adapted from* Waldo *et al.* [10].)

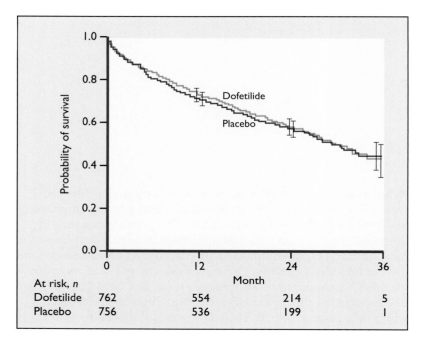

At risk, *n*

Dofetilide	762	554	214	5
Placebo	756	536	199	1

FIGURE 5-8. Impact of dofetilide on mortality in patients with heart failure and reduced systolic function. Dofetilide is a class III anti-arrhythmic drug that blocks a repolarizing potassium current (I_{Kr}), increasing action potential duration in both atrium and ventricle. Dofetilide is approved for therapy of atrial fibrillation. The Danish Investigations of Arrhythmia and Mortality on Dofetilide (DIAMOND-CHF) study randomized 1518 patients with left ventricular dysfunction who had been hospitalized with class III or IV heart failure to therapy with dofetilide or placebo [11]. Survival was similar in dofetilide-treated and placebo groups. During a median follow-up of 18 months, 311 patients in the dofetilide group (41%) and 317 patients in the placebo group (42%) died (hazard ratio, 0.95; 95% CI, 0.81 to 1.11). Dofetilide-treated patients were less likely to be rehospitalized for exacerbation of heart failure (30% vs 38%). Once sinus rhythm was restored, dofetilide was significantly more effective than placebo in maintaining sinus rhythm (hazard ratio for the recurrence of atrial fibrillation, 0.35; 95% CI, 0.22–0.57; $P < 0.001$) during follow-up. The major toxicity of dofetilide is the polymorphic ventricular tachycardia torsades de pointes, which developed in 3.3% of patients as compared with none of the placebo patients. Excretion of dofetilide is partly renal, and the drug dosage must be adjusted according to calculated creatinine clearance. Dofetilide is contraindicated in patients with markedly impaired renal function. Dofetilide must be initiated in-hospital with ECG monitoring for 72 hours. (*Adapted from* Torp-Pedersen *et al.* [11].)

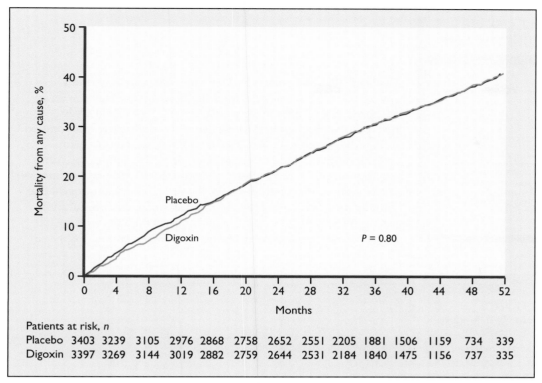

Patients at risk, n

Placebo	3403	3239	3105	2976	2868	2758	2652	2551	2205	1881	1506	1159	734	339
Digoxin	3397	3269	3144	3019	2882	2759	2644	2531	2184	1840	1475	1156	737	335

Figure 5-9. The impact of digoxin on survival in patients with chronic heart failure and normal sinus rhythm. The role of cardiac glycosides in treating patients with chronic heart failure and normal sinus rhythm continues to be controversial. The Digitalis Investigator Group studied the effect of digoxin on mortality and hospitalization in a randomized, double-blind clinical trial. In this study, 6800 patients with left ventricular ejection fractions of 0.45 or less were randomly assigned to digoxin or placebo in addition to diuretics and ACE inhibitors [27]. Digitalis had no impact on all-cause mortality. The mortality rate was 34.8% with digoxin and 35.1% with placebo (risk ratio, 0.99; 95% CI, 0.91–1.07; $P = 0.80$). In the digoxin group, there was a trend toward a decrease in the risk of death attributed to worsening heart failure (risk ratio, 0.88; 95% CI, 0.77–1.01; $P = 0.06$).

There was, however, a statistically significant increase in other cardiovascular death with digitalis (risk ratio, 1.14; 95% CI, 1.01–1.30). There were 6% fewer hospitalizations overall in that group than in the placebo group, and fewer patients were hospitalized for worsening heart failure; however, more patients were hospitalized for myocardial infarction. There was no significant difference between the groups in the number of patients hospitalized for ventricular arrhythmia or cardiac arrest (142 vs 145). Digoxin did not reduce overall mortality, but it reduced the rate of hospitalization both overall and for worsening heart failure. These findings clarified the relatively limited impact digoxin has on clinical outcomes in patients with heart failure and normal sinus rhythm. (*Adapted from* The Digitalis Investigation Group [27].)

A. DISTRIBUTION OF EVENTS ACCORDING TO DIURETIC USE AT BASELINE

	DIURETIC (N = 2901)		NO DIURETIC (N = 3896)		
	N (%)	INCIDENCE*	N (%)	INCIDENCE	P
Death from any cause	1013 (34.9)	12.8	586 (15.0)	5.3	0.001
Cardiovascular death	903 (31.1)	11.4	510 (13.1)	4.6	0.001
Arrhythmic death	241 (8.3)	3.1	183 (4.7)	1.7	0.001

*Incidence is expressed as the number of events per 100 patient-years of follow-up.

Figure 5-10. The association of the use of diuretics in patients with left ventricular dysfunction and the risk of arrhythmic death. Randomized trials to assess the impact of loop diuretics on morbidity and mortality in heart failure have not been conducted, but these medications are in common use and are frequently necessary to address the congested state. Treatment with diuretics has been reported to increase the risk of arrhythmic death in patients with hypertension. The effect of diuretic therapy on arrhythmic death in patients with left ventricular dysfunction has not been well studied, but diuretic-induced neurohumoral activation and electrolyte disturbances are potential mechanisms by which arrhythmic risk

could be increased. The Studies of Left Ventricular Dysfunction (SOLVD) trial was a retrospective analysis performed to assess the relation between diuretic use at baseline and the subsequent risk of arrhythmic death; 6797 patients with an ejection fraction less than or equal to 35% were enrolled in the study [28]. **A,** In this analysis, participants receiving a diuretic at baseline were more likely to have an arrhythmic death than those not receiving a diuretic (3.1% vs 1.7% arrhythmic deaths per 100 person-years, $P = 0.001$). On univariate analysis, diuretic use was associated with an increased risk of arrhythmic death (relative risk 1.85, $P = 0.0001$).

Continued on next page

B. MULTIVARIATE ANALYSIS: RELATIVE RISK OF ARRHYTHMIC DEATH ACCORDING TO DIURETIC USE*

	RR (95% CI)	P
No diuretic	1.00	—
Any diuretic	1.37 (1.08–1.73)	0.009
Non–potassium sparing	1.33 (1.05–1.69)	0.02
Potassium sparing	0.90 (0.61–1.31)	0.6

*The multivariate Cox model also included study drug allocation (enalapril or placebo); age; sex; ejection fraction; New York Heart Association class; history of angina, myocardial infarction, revascularization, hypertension, diabetes, or tobacco use; and baseline use of digoxin, β-blockers, anti-arrhythmic agents, aspirin, or anticoagulants.

FIGURE 5-10. *(Continued)* **B**, After controlling for important covariates, diuretic use remained significantly associated with an increased risk of arrhythmic death (RR 1.37, P = 0.009). Only non–potassium-sparing diuretic use was independently associated with arrhythmic death (RR 1.33, P = 0.02). Use of a potassium-sparing diuretic, alone or in combination with a non–potassium-sparing diuretic, was not independently associated with an increased risk of arrhythmic death (RR 0.90, P = 0.6). These data suggest that diuretic-induced electrolyte disturbances and/or neurohumoral activation may result in fatal arrhythmias in patients with systolic left ventricular dysfunction. (*Adapted from* Cooper *et al.* [28].)

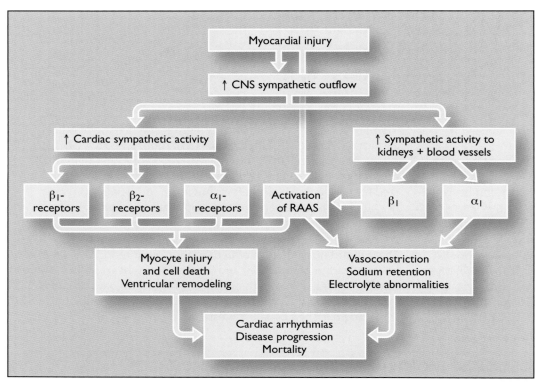

FIGURE 5-11. The role of neurohumoral activation in the pathophysiology of heart failure. The pathophysiology of heart failure involves hemodynamic abnormalities, neurohumoral abnormalities, and myocardial cellular alterations [12]. Left ventricular dysfunction results from myocardial injury. Neurohumoral activation, which includes activation of the sympathetic nervous system and the renin-angiotensin-aldosterone system (RAAS), occurs in response to acute hemodynamic alterations and myocardial injury. This neurohumoral activation is counterproductive in patients with heart failure. Changes occur in cardiac function and the peripheral circulation that contribute to the symptoms and drive the progression of heart failure. Neurohumoral activation results in progressive dilation and dysfunction of the left ventricle (pathologic ventricular remodeling). There are also fundamental abnormalities at the cellular level, including myocyte contractile dysfunction, changes in ion channels and gap junctions, programmed cell death (apoptosis), fetal gene expression, hypertrophy, and myocardial fibrosis. These structural and functional changes contribute not only to progressive ventricular dysfunction but also to ventricular arrhythmias and sudden death.

As a result, neurohumoral antagonists (ACE inhibitors, angiotensin II receptor antagonists, aldosterone antagonists, and β-blockers) could be expected to decrease the risk not only of heart failure pump dysfunction death but also of sudden death in patients with heart failure. CNS—central nervous system. (*Adapted from* Fonarow [12].)

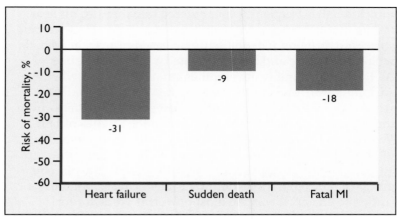

FIGURE 5-12. Risk of cause-specific mortality with ACE inhibitors in heart failure. A pooled analysis of 32 randomized trials of ACE inhibitors in heart failure was conducted by the Collaborative Group on ACE Inhibitors Trials [14]. Eight different ACE inhibitors were compared with placebo in a total of 7105 patients with symptomatic congestive heart failure (CHF). ACE inhibitors reduced total mortality by 23% ($P < 0.01$), lowered the incidence of death or hospitalization for heart failure by 35% ($P < 0.001$), and lowered the risk of CHF hospitalizations. Reductions for total mortality and the combined end point were similar for various subgroups examined (age, sex, etiology, and New York Heart Association class). The greatest effect was seen during the first 3 months, but additional benefit was observed during further treatment. The reduction in mortality was primarily a result of fewer deaths from progressive heart failure (odds ratio [OR], 0.69; 95% CI, 0.58-0.83). There was a trend for reduced risk of sudden death with ACE inhibitors; point estimates for effects on sudden or presumed arrhythmic deaths (OR, 0.91; 95% CI, 0.73–1.12), but this did not reach statistical significance. The risk of fatal myocardial infarction (MI) also showed a trend toward lower risk (OR, 0.82; 95% CI, 0.60–1.11). (*Adapted from* Garg and Yusuf [14].)

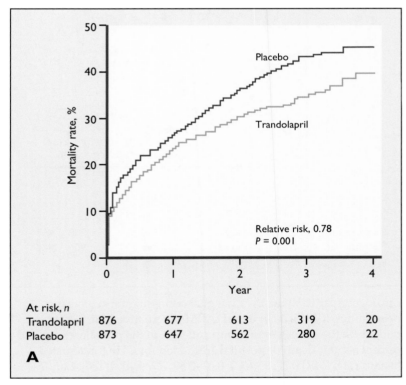

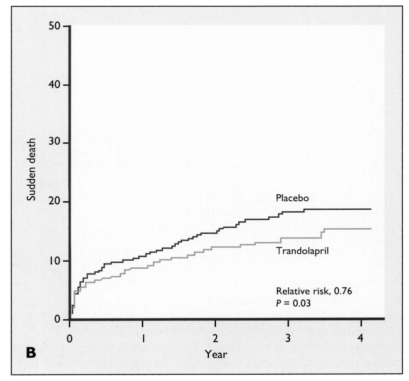

FIGURE 5-13. The impact of ACE inhibitors on all-cause mortality and sudden death in patients with left ventricular systolic dysfunction after acute myocardial infarction. The Trandolapril Cardiac Evaluation (TRACE) study was designed to determine whether patients who have left ventricular dysfunction soon after myocardial infarction benefit from long-term oral ACE inhibition [29]. A total of 1749 patients who had echocardiographic evidence of left ventricular systolic dysfunction (ejection fraction, < 35%) were randomly assigned to receive oral trandolapril or placebo. **A,** During the study period, 34.7% in the trandolapril group died as compared with 42.3% in the placebo group ($P = 0.001$). **B,** Trandolapril also reduced the risk of sudden death (RR, 0.76; 95% CI, 0.59–0.98; $P = 0.03$). Long-term treatment with trandolapril in patients with reduced left ventricular function soon after myocardial infarction significantly reduced the risk of overall mortality and sudden death. (*Adapted from* Kober *et al.* [29].)

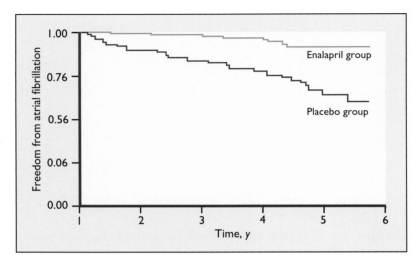

<FIGURE 5-14. Impact of ACE inhibitor therapy on the incidence of atrial fibrillation (AF) in patients with left ventricular dys->

FIGURE 5-14. Impact of ACE inhibitor therapy on the incidence of atrial fibrillation (AF) in patients with left ventricular dys-

function. AF is frequently encountered in patients with heart failure. Recent experimental studies have shown electrical and structural atrial remodeling with increased fibrosis in animals with heart failure and have suggested a preventive effect of ACE inhibitors on the development of AF. To assess whether ACE inhibitors prevent the development of AF in patients with heart failure, a retrospective analysis of the patients from the Montreal Heart Institute included in the Studies of Left Ventricular Dysfunction (SOLVD) trial was performed [15]. Of the 391 patients assessed, 55 had AF during the follow-up: 10 (5.4%) in the enalapril group and 45 (24%) in the placebo group ($P < 0.0001$). By Cox multivariate analysis, randomization to enalapril was the most powerful predictor for risk reduction of AF (hazard ratio, 0.22; 95% CI, 0.11–0.44; $P < 0.0001$). This study indicates that treatment with the ACE inhibitor enalapril markedly reduces the risk of development of AF in patients with left ventricular dysfunction. (*Adapted from* Vermes *et al.* [15].)

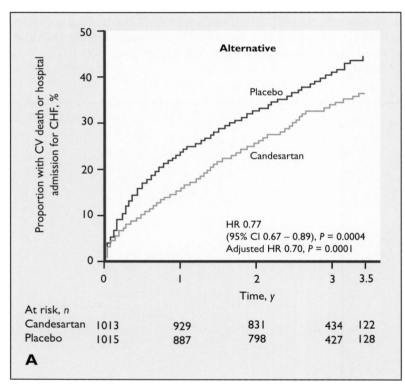

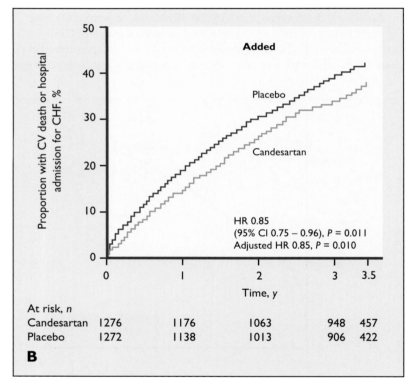

FIGURE 5-15. Impact of angiotensin receptor antagonists on clinical outcomes in heart failure due to systolic dysfunction. The Candesartan in Heart Failure: Assessment of Reduction in Mortality and morbidity (CHARM) Program trials were parallel, randomized, double-blind clinical trials comparing candesartan with placebo in three distinct populations: patients with a left ventricular ejection fraction (LVEF) of 40% or less who were not receiving ACE inhibitors because of previous intolerance (CHARM-Alternative) or who were currently receiving ACE inhibitors (CHARM-Added), and patients with LVEF higher than 40% (CHARM-preserved) [25]. Overall, 7601 patients were randomly assigned candesartan (titrated to 32 mg once daily) or matching placebo and followed up for at least 2 years. The primary outcome for all the component trials was

cardiovascular (CV) death or hospital admission for worsening heart failure (CHF). A, In the CHARM-Alternative trial, 33% of patients in the candesartan group and 40% in the placebo group had cardiovascular death or hospital admission for CHF (unadjusted hazard ratio [HR] 0.77; 95% CI, 0.67–0.89; $P = 0.0004$) [30]. Candesartan was generally well tolerated and reduced cardiovascular mortality and morbidity in patients with symptomatic chronic heart failure and intolerance to ACE inhibitors. B, In the CHARM-Added trial, 38% patients in the candesartan group and 42% in the placebo group experienced the primary outcome (unadjusted hazard ratio 0.85; 95% CI, 0.75–0.96; $P = 0.011$) [31]. The benefits of candesartan were similar in all predefined subgroups, including patients receiving baseline ACE inhibitor plus β-blocker treatment.

Continued on next page

C. NUMBER, PROPORTION, AND ANNUALIZED INCIDENCE OF SUDDEN DEATH IN THE THREE CHARM TRIALS AND THE OVERALL CHARM PROGRAM

CAUSE OF DEATH	CHARM-ALTERNATIVE		CHARM-ADDED		CHARM-PRESERVED		CHARM-OVERALL		HAZARD RATIO AND 95% CI
	CANDESARTAN (N = 1013)	PLACEBO (N = 1015)	CANDESARTAN (N = 1276)	PLACEBO (N = 1272)	CANDESARTAN (N = 1514)	PLACEBO (N = 1508)	CANDESARTAN (N = 3803)	PLACEBO (N = 3796)	
Sudden death	80 (7.9)	111 (10.9)	150 (11.8)	168 (13.2)	69 (4.6)	65 (4.3)	299 (7.9)	344 (9.1)	0.85 (0.73–0.99)
Incidence rate	3.0	4.3	3.9	4.5	1.6	1.5	2.7	3.2	P = 0.036

FIGURE 5-15. *(Continued)* **C,** Candesartan reduced both sudden death (HR 0.85 [0.73–0.99], P = 0.036) and death from worsening heart failure (HR 0.78 [0.65–0.94], P = 0.008). The addition of candesartan to an ACE inhibitor and other treatment leads to a further clinically important reduction in relevant cardiovascular events, including sudden death, in patients with CHF and reduced LVEF. (**A** and **B**, *Adapted from* Granger *et al.* [30] and McMurray *et al.* [31]; **C,** *Adapted from* Solomon *et al.* [32].)

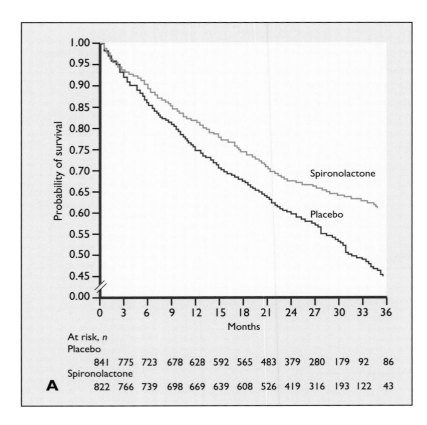

A

FIGURE 5-16. Impact of aldosterone antagonists on mortality and sudden death in patients with severe heart failure due to systolic dysfunction. Aldosterone has an important role in the pathophysiology of heart failure and may also contribute to the arrhythmia and sudden death risk. Aldosterone promotes the retention of sodium, the loss of magnesium and potassium, sympathetic activation, parasympathetic inhibition, myocardial and vascular fibrosis, baroreceptor dysfunction, and vascular damage, and impairs arterial compliance. **A** and **B**, The Randomized Aldactone Evaluation Study (RALES) enrolled 1663 patients who had severe heart failure and a left ventricular ejection fraction of no more than 35% and who were being treated with an ACE inhibitor, a loop diuretic, and, in most cases, digoxin [18]. Patients were randomly assigned to receive 25 mg of spironolactone daily or placebo. The primary end point was death from all causes. The trial was discontinued early, after a mean follow-up period of 24 months for benefit.

Continued on next page

B. RELATIVE RISKS OF DEATH

CAUSE OF DEATH	PLACEBO GROUP (N = 841), N	SPIRONOLACTONE GROUP (N = 822), N	RR (95% CI)	P
Cardiac causes	314	226	0.69 (0.58–0.82)	< 0.001
Progression of heart failure*	189	127	0.64 (0.51–0.80)	< 0.001
Sudden death†	110	82	0.71 (0.54–0.95)	0.02
Myocardial infarction	15	17		
Other cardiac causes	13	12		
Stroke	11	8		
Noncardiovascular causes	41	29		
Unknown	7	9		
Total	386	284	0.70 (0.60–0.82)	< 0.001

* This category includes death due to worsening heart failure (defined as increasing symptoms or signs requiring an increase in treatment).

† This category includes witnessed death from cardiac causes heralded by abrupt loss of consciousness within 1 hour after the onset of symptoms in a patient in whom death was unexpected.

FIGURE 5-16. *(Continued)* The mortality rate was 46% with placebo and 35% with spironolactone (RR of death 0.70; 95% CI, 0.60–0.82; P < 0.001). The reduction in the risk of death was attributed to a lower risk of both death from progressive heart failure and sudden death from cardiac causes. Sudden death was reduced by 29% with aldosterone blockade (RR of sudden death 0.71; 95% CI, 0.54–0.95; P = 0.02). The frequency of hospitalization for worsening heart failure was 35% lower with spironolactone. In addition, patients who received spironolactone had a significant improvement in the symptoms of heart failure, as assessed on the basis of the New York Heart Association functional class (P < 0.001). With the close monitoring provided by virtue of trial participation, the incidence of serious hyperkalemia was low. This trial convincingly demonstrated that blockade of aldosterone receptors by spironolactone, in addition to standard therapy, substantially reduces the risk of sudden death as well as overall mortality among patients with severe heart failure, although only 11% of these patients were on a β-blocker. (*Adapted from* Pitt *et al.* [18].)

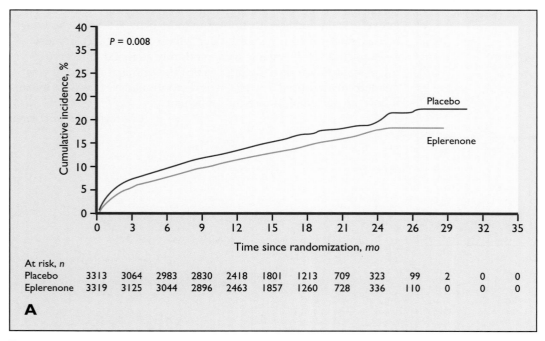

FIGURE 5-17. Impact of selective aldosterone receptor blockade on mortality and sudden death in patients with ventricular dysfunction and mild heart failure post myocardial infarction. Although aldosterone blockade substantially reduced mortality and morbidity among patients with severe heart failure, many questioned if similar benefits would be seen in mild heart failure. The Eplerenone Post–Acute Myocardial Infarction Heart Failure Efficacy and Survival Study (EPHESUS) was designed to test the hypothesis that treatment with eplerenone, an aldosterone blocker that selectively blocks the mineralocorticoid receptor and not glucocorticoid, progesterone, or androgen receptors, reduces overall mortality and cardiovascular mortality or hospitalization for cardiovascular events among patients with acute myocardial infarction complicated by left ventricular dysfunction and heart failure who are receiving optimal medical therapy [19]. A total of 6642 patients were randomly assigned to eplerenone 25 mg per day initially, titrated to a maximum of 50 mg per day, or placebo, in addition to optimal medical therapy. **A,** During a mean follow-up of 16 months, there were 478 deaths in the eplerenone group and 554 deaths in the placebo group (RR, 0.85; 95% CI, 0.75–0.96; P = 0.008). The rate of the other primary end point, death from cardiovascular causes or hospitalization for cardiovascular events, was reduced by eplerenone (RR, 0.87; 95% CI, 0.79–0.95; P = 0.002).

Continued on next page

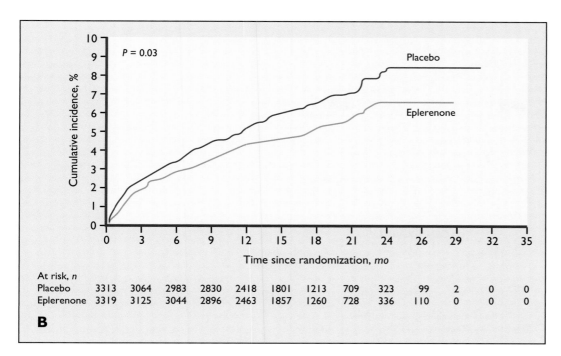

At risk, n

Placebo	3313	3064	2983	2830	2418	1801	1213	709	323	99	2	0	0
Eplerenone	3319	3125	3044	2896	2463	1857	1260	728	336	110	0	0	0

B

FIGURE 5-17. *(Continued)* **B**, There was also a significant reduction in the rate of sudden death from cardiac causes (RR, 0.79; 95% CI, 0.64–0.97; *P* = 0.03). The rate of serious hyperkalemia was 5.5% in the eplerenone group and 3.9% in the placebo group (*P* = 0.002), whereas the rate of hypokalemia was 8.4% in the eplerenone group and 13.1% in the placebo group (*P* < 0.001). This trial demonstrated that the addition of eplerenone to optimal medical therapy reduces morbidity and mortality among patients with acute myocardial infarction complicated by left ventricular dysfunction and heart failure. (*Adapted from* Pitt *et al.* [19].)

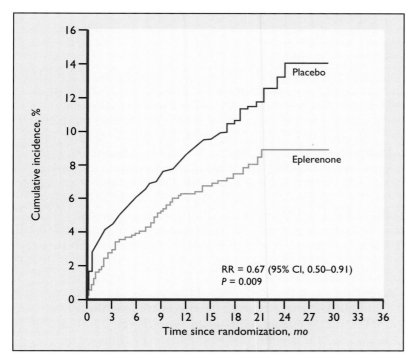

FIGURE 5-18. The impact of eplerenone on sudden death in post–myocardial infarction patients with left ventricular ejection fractions of 30% or less. In a post hoc analysis of the Eplerenone Post–Acute Myocardial Infarction Heart Failure Efficacy and Survival Study (EPHESUS), the impact of aldosterone antagonists on the risk of sudden death in the subgroup of patients with left ventricular ejection fractions of 30% or less was analyzed [19]. In this subgroup of patients, the risk of sudden death was reduced by 33% (RR 0.67; 95% CI, 0.50–0.91; *P* = 0.009). There are multiple mechanisms by which eplerenone may provide sudden death protection in patients with acute myocardial infarction complicated by left ventricular dysfunction and heart failure, but they are not completely clear. Effects of aldosterone blockers on plasma volume and electrolyte excretion may have contributed to the sudden death risk reduction provided by eplerenone as increased ventricular filling pressure and hypokalemia are associated with increased risk of sudden death. Eplerenone also reduces coronary vascular inflammation and oxidative stress, improves endothelial dysfunction, attenuates platelet aggregation, decreases activation of matrix metalloproteinases, and improves ventricular remodeling. In addition, aldosterone blockade decreases sympathetic drive through direct actions in the brain, improves norepinephrine uptake in patients with heart failure, and improves heart rate variability. Irrespective of the exact mechanisms, aldosterone antagonists added to ACE inhibitors and β-blockers substantially reduce the risk of sudden death and overall mortality. (*Adapted from* Pitt *et al.* [19].)

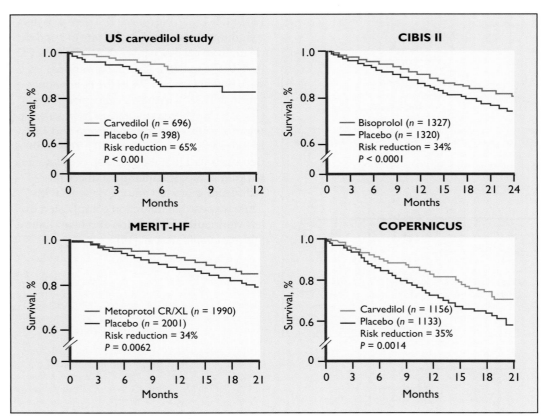

Figure 5-19. Impact of β-blockers on survival in chronic heart failure as demonstrated in the landmark clinical trials. β-Blockers have traditionally been viewed as contraindicated in patients with heart failure. Their inclusion into recent guidelines represents a significant change in the pharmacologic management of heart failure. The CIBIS II, MERIT-HF, and COPERNICUS trials all met predefined stopping rules because of significant mortality benefit in the β-blocker treatment group. Clinical trials have convincingly demonstrated that β-blockers are the single most effective medication for heart failure [2,20–22]. The Metoprolol CR/XL Randomized Intervention Trial in Congestive Heart Failure (MERIT-HF) was a double-blind, placebo-controlled trial on the efficacy of metoprolol CR/XL (controlled release/extended release) involving 3991 patients with symptomatic heart failure (New York Heart Association [NYHA] class II to IV and an ejection fraction ≤ 0.40) stabilized with standard treatment [2]. The results indicated significant risk reductions with metoprolol compared with placebo (P < 0.001) for several outcome measures: all-cause mortality (34%), the combined end point of total mortality or all-cause hospitalization (19%), total mortality or hospitalization due to worsening heart failure (31%), and total mortality or hospitalization or emergency department visit due to worsening heart failure (32%). The Cardiac Insufficiency Bisoprolol Study II (CIBIS-II) compared the effects of bisoprolol (1.25 to 10 mg), a highly selective β₁-antagonist, with placebo in 2647 symptomatic patients (NYHA class III or IV and a left ventricular ejection fraction ≤ 0.35) also taking ACE inhibitors and diuretics [21]. Over a mean of 1.3 years, bisoprolol had a significant 29% reduction in all-cause mortality versus placebo (P < 0.0001). Bisoprolol therapy also resulted in significantly fewer cardiac deaths (P < 0.0049), all-cause hospital admissions (P < 0.0006), and hospital admissions for worsening heart failure (a 32% reduction compared with placebo, P < 0.0001). The efficacy of carvedilol in reducing morbidity and mortality in patients with chronic heart failure has been established in several placebo-controlled trials. A 65% decrease in death was found (P < 0.001) when carvedilol was compared with placebo in chronic heart failure [20]. There was also a large reduction in the risk of death due to sudden death (3.8% for placebo, 1.7% for carvedilol). The Carvedilol Prospective Randomized Cumulative Survival (COPERNICUS) trial evaluated the effects of carvedilol on mortality in 2289 patients with severe heart failure [22]. This trial indicated that the benefits of β-blockade can be obtained by patients with severe chronic heart failure. Carvedilol produced reductions in risk of death; death or hospitalizations; and death, hospitalization, or permanent withdrawal during the first 8 weeks of the trial, and as early as the first 14 to 21 days of treatment. (*Adapted from* MERIT-HF Study Group [2], Packer *et al.* [20,22], and CIBIS-II Investigators and Committees [21].)

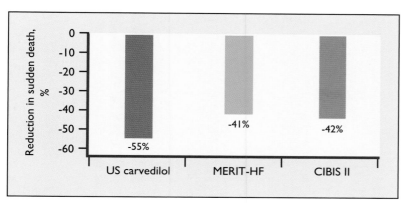

FIGURE 5-20. Impact of β-blockers on sudden death in chronic heart failure as demonstrated in the landmark clinical trials. β-Blockers have been demonstrated to reduce sudden death in patients after myocardial infarction. In the clinical trials of patients with chronic heart failure, the reductions in sudden death with β-blockers have been impressive. In the US Carvedilol Heart Failure Trials Program, there was a 55% reduction in sudden death risk (3.8% [15/398] for placebo vs 1.7% [12/696] for carvedilol) [20]. In the Metoprolol CR/XL Randomized Intervention Trial in Congestive Heart Failure (MERIT-HF), the sudden death risk reduction was 41% [2]. In the Cardiac Insufficiency Bisoprolol Study II (CIBIS-II), bisoprolol therapy reduced sudden death risk by 42% [21]. These trials demonstrate the remarkable ability of β-blockers to reduce the risk of sudden death in patients with heart failure. These benefits were seen irrespective of heart failure etiology and across clinically relevant subgroups of patients. (*Adapted from* MERIT-HF Study Group [2], Packer *et al.* [20,22], and CIBIS-II Investigators and Committees [21].)

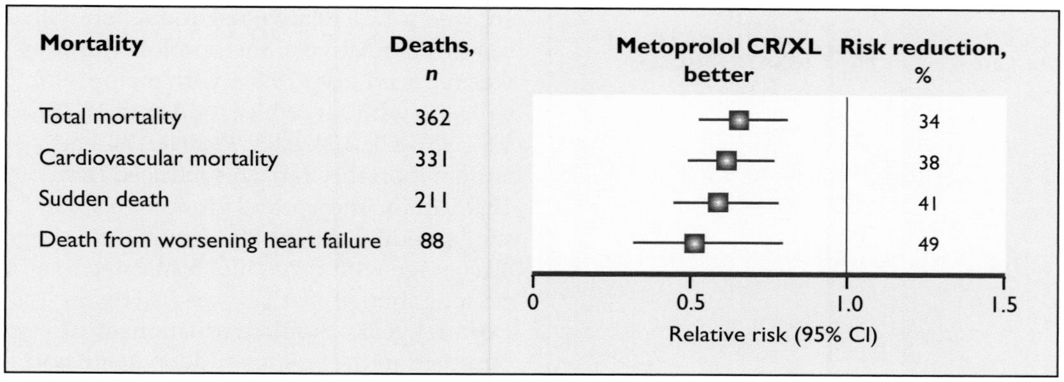

Mortality	Deaths, n	Metoprolol CR/XL better	Risk reduction, %
Total mortality	362		34
Cardiovascular mortality	331		38
Sudden death	211		41
Death from worsening heart failure	88		49

Relative risk (95% CI)

FIGURE 5-21. Impact of metoprolol on total and cause-specific mortality in patients with chronic heart failure. The Metoprolol CR/XL Randomized Intervention Trial in Congestive Heart Failure (MERIT-HF) investigated whether β_1-selective blockade with metoprolol controlled release/extended release (CR/XL) once daily, in addition to standard therapy, would lower mortality in patients with decreased ejection fraction and symptoms of heart failure [2]. This trial enrolled 3991 patients with chronic heart failure in New York Heart Association (NYHA) functional classes II to IV and with ejection fraction of 0.40 or less, stabilized with optimum standard therapy. The target dose was 200 mg once daily, and doses were up-titrated over 8 weeks. All-cause mortality was lower in the metoprolol CR/XL group: 7.2% per patient-year of follow-up as compared with 11.0 % in the placebo group (RR 0.66; 95% CI, 0.53–0.81; $P = 0.00009$). There were significantly fewer sudden deaths in the metoprolol CR/XL group than in the placebo group (79 vs 132; 4.0% vs 6.6%; RR 0.59; 95% CI, 0.45–0.78; $P = 0.0002$). Deaths from worsening heart failure were also lower. This trial demonstrated that metoprolol CR/XL once daily in addition to optimum standard therapy improves survival. (*Adapted from* MERIT-HF Study Group [2].)

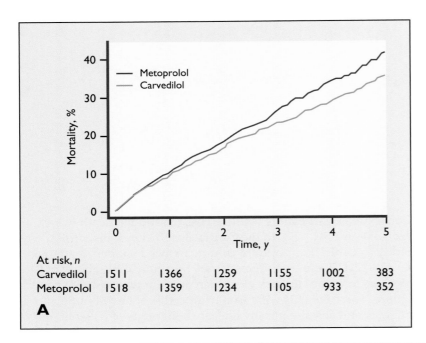

At risk, *n*

Carvedilol	1511	1366	1259	1155	1002	383
Metoprolol	1518	1359	1234	1105	933	352

A

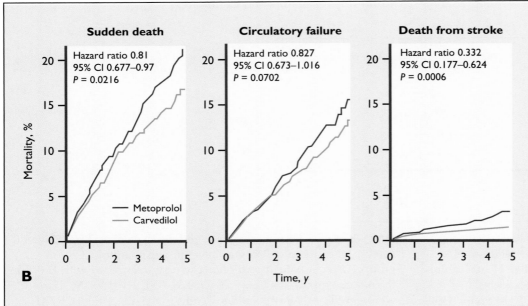

B

11% on spironolactone. A co-primary end point of the trial, all-cause mortality, showed a 17% relative risk reduction with carvedilol relative to metoprolol. Mortality was reduced from 39.5% with metoprolol to 33.9% with carvedilol (odds ratio [OR], 0.87; 95% CI, 0.74–0.93; $P < 0.0017$). The annual mortality rate was reduced from 10.0% in the metoprolol group to 8.3% in the carvedilol group. The survival advantage with carvedilol translated to a prolongation of median survival by an extra 1.4 years. Similar reductions were observed in the risk for sudden death and progressive heart failure deaths with carvedilol. There was greater vascular protection with carvedilol relative to metoprolol, including a 67% reduction in stroke death (95% CI, 0.18–0.62; $P = 0.006$) and a 29% reduction in fatal and nonfatal myocardial infarction (95% CI, 0.52–0.97; $P = 0.03$). There was no significant heterogeneity in response between clinically relevant subgroups of patients, including men and women, those with and without coronary artery disease, and diabetics and nondiabetics. These data suggest that more comprehensive adrenergic receptor blockade with carvedilol provides incremental reductions in heart failure–related mortality compared with this short-acting formulation and dose of a cardioselective β-blocker. (*Adapted from Poole-Wilson et al. [33].*)

FIGURE 5-22. Impact of carvedilol as compared with metoprolol tartrate on overall (**A**) and cause-specific (**B**) mortality in patients with chronic heart failure. β-Blockers have significantly different pharmacologic profiles, which may lead to different clinical outcomes. Metoprolol and bisoprolol have a high specificity for the β_1-adrenergic receptor. Carvedilol blocks β_1-, β_2-, and α_1-adrenergic receptors. Several small clinical studies have suggested that carvedilol is more effective than metoprolol in reversing ventricular remodeling, increasing left ventricular systolic function, and decreasing cardiac sympathetic drive. Whether these differences would translate into differences in survival in patients with chronic heart failure was not previously known. The Carvedilol or Metoprolol European Trial (COMET) was designed to compare directly the effects of carvedilol and a short-acting formulation of metoprolol on mortality and morbidity in patients with mild to severe chronic heart failure [33]. The study enrolled 3029 patients with class II to IV heart failure. Patients were randomized to carvedilol (target dose 25 mg twice daily) or metoprolol tartrate (target dose 50 mg twice daily). Mean left ventricular ejection fraction was 0.26 at baseline; 99% of the patients were already taking diuretics and 98% ACE inhibitors or angiotensin receptor antagonists, with 59% also on digoxin and

FOOTNOTE*

It is not known whether this formulation of metoprolol (tartrate) at any dose or this low dose of metoprolol in any formulation has any effect on survival or hospitalization in patients with heart failure. Thus, this trial extends the time over which carvedilol manifests benefits on survival in heart failure, but it is

not necessarily evidence that carvedilol improves outcome over the long-acting formulation of metoprolol (succinate). *Adapted from the full prescribing information of Coreg (carvedilol) [package insert]. Research Triangle Park, NC: GlaxoSmithKline; May 2005.

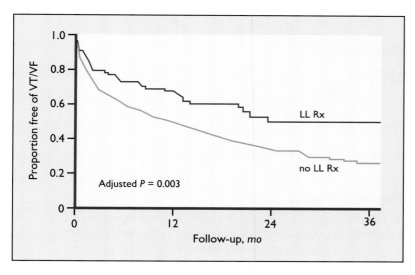

FIGURE 5-23. Kaplan-Meier survival curves for the outcome of freedom from ventricular tachyarrhythmia recurrence in patients with an implantable cardioverter-defibrillator (ICD) as a function of whether lipid-lowering drug therapy (LL Rx) was not used or was used. Randomized trials of lipid-lowering drugs suggest reduction of sudden death in patients with atherosclerotic vascular disease. Because sudden death is usually secondary to ventricular tachycardia/ventricular fibrillation (VT/VF), these findings raise the possibility that lipid-lowering therapy may have direct or indirect antiarrhythmic effects. This study sought to evaluate the antiarrhythmic effects of lipid-lowering drug therapy as assessed by ventricular tachyarrhythmia recurrences recorded by an ICD in patients with atherosclerotic heart disease. The probability of VT/VF recurrence in patients treated with an ICD in the Antiarrhythmics Versus Implantable Defibrillators (AVID) trial who did not receive lipid-lowering drug therapy ($n = 279$) was compared with that in patients who received early and consistent lipid-lowering therapy ($n = 83$) [34]. Baseline mean left ventricular ejection fraction was 32%. Using multivariate analyses, lipid-lowering therapy was associated with a reduction in the relative hazard for VT/VF recurrence of 0.40 (95% CI, 0.15–0.58; adjusted $P = 0.003$) in the ICD subgroup. In patients with atherosclerotic heart disease who have received an ICD, lipid-lowering therapy is associated with reduction in the probability of VT/VF recurrence. These observed effects may be the result of a reduction in ischemia and acute coronary syndrome–induced arrhythmias; however, a more direct antiarrhythmic effect is also possible. (*Adapted from* Mitchell *et al.* [34].)

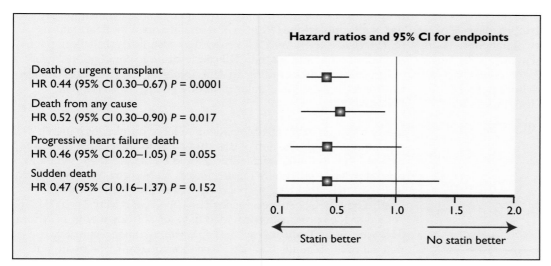

FIGURE 5-24. The risk of death and cause-specific mortality in advanced heart failure patients receiving statins compared with those who are not. Although statins are known to reduce mortality in coronary artery disease, the impact of statin therapy in patients with heart failure had not been well studied. Both the potential risks and benefits of statins in heart failure have been described. Statins have therapeutic properties that are of potential benefit to patients with heart failure of ischemic and nonischemic etiologies, irrespective of lipid levels. Statins may improve endothelial function, inhibit inflammatory cytokines, potentiate nitric oxide synthesis, restore impaired autonomic function, and reverse pathologic myocardial remodeling. This observational study aimed to investigate the impact of statin therapy in patients with advanced heart failure [35]. A cohort of 551 patients with systolic heart failure (left ventricular ejection fraction ≤ 40%) were referred to a single university center for clinical management and/or transplant evaluation. Forty-five percent of the cohort had coronary artery disease, and 45% were receiving statin therapy, including 73% and 22% of coronary artery disease and non–coronary artery disease patients, respectively. Statin use was associated with improved survival in both nonischemic and ischemic heart failure patients (91% vs 72%, $P < 0.001$, and 81% vs 63%, $P < 0.001$, at 1-year follow-up, respectively). After risk adjustment for age, gender, coronary artery disease, cholesterol, diabetes, medications, hemoglobin, creatinine, and New York Heart Association functional class, statin therapy remained an independent predictor of improved survival (hazard ratio [HR] 0.41; 95% CI, 0.18–0.94). There were similar risk reductions in progressive heart failure death and sudden death. This study suggests that statin therapy is associated with markedly improved survival in patients with ischemic and nonischemic heart failure, irrespective of cholesterol levels. Although these finding must be confirmed in randomized clinical trials, statins may represent a novel new therapy to reduce mortality and sudden death risk in patients with heart failure. (*Adapted for* Horwich *et al.* [35].)

CUMULATIVE BENEFITS OF HEART FAILURE THERAPIES

THERAPY*	RELATIVE RISK REDUCTION, %	2-YEAR MORTALITY, %
None		35
ACE inhibitor	23	27
Aldosterone antagonist	30	19
β-Blocker	35	12

*Cumulative risk reduction if all three therapies are used: 63%. Absolute risk reduction: 22%; number needed to treat = 5.

FIGURE 5-25. Cumulative benefits of the evidence-based, guideline-recommended, life-prolonging therapies for heart failure due to systolic dysfunction. There has been a dramatic evolution in heart failure medical therapy. ACE inhibitors, aldosterone antagonists, and β-blockers have emerged as evidence-based, life-prolonging treatments for heart failure in a spectrum of patients, including those at high risk for developing left ventricular systolic dysfunction and those with asymptomatic and symptomatic left ventricular systolic dysfunction. In more than 50 placebo-controlled trials involving more than 25,000 patients with left ventricular systolic dysfunction (ejection fraction < 0.35 to 0.45), ACE inhibitors, aldosterone antagonists, and β-blockers have been shown to alleviate symptoms, improve clinical status, and reduce the risk of death, the combined risk of death and rehospitalization, and, in most studies, the risk of sudden death. The studies have included a variety of patients, including women, the elderly, diabetics, and those with a wide range of underlying heart failure etiologies and severities of left ventricular systolic dysfunction. Based on this evidence, guidelines put forth by the American College of Cardiology/American Heart Association

and the Heart Failure Society of America recommend the use of these agents for the treatment of chronic stable heart failure as part of the standard of care. The benefits of aldosterone antagonists and β-blockers seem to have an additive effect in patients already on ACE inhibitors. Based on the demonstrated risk reduction and additive effects, the cumulative benefit of combining the evidence-based therapies for heart failure are estimated in the figure. Subsequent to the publication of these guidelines, additional information has become available on evidence-based combination therapies. First, is the realization that caution needs to be exercised in adding an aldosterone antagonist, based on the recent publication of the Canadian experience, where there were significant increases in hospitalizations and mortality attributable to hyperkalemia with the use of spironolactone [36]. Second, in patients with heart failure (NYHA Class II–IV) and left ventricular systolic dysfunction, there is evidence that adding the ARB candesartan to conventional heart failure treatments including an ACE inhibitor and β-blocker can also further reduce cardiovascular mortality [17,31]. (*Adapted from* Fonarow [37].)

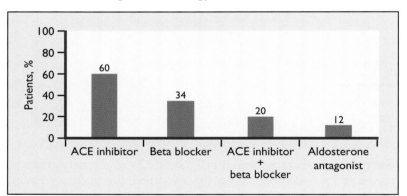

FIGURE 5-26. Use of evidence-based, guideline-recommended therapies in outpatients with chronic heart failure. Despite the demonstration in randomized clinical trials of the benefits of ACE inhibitors, aldosterone antagonists, and β-blockers in reducing mortality and national/international guidelines recommending the

use of these agents in eligible patients, a large number of patients remain untreated. The aim of this study was to assess how primary care physicians think heart failure should be managed and whether this knowledge is actually implemented. The survey was undertaken in 15 countries that had membership in the European Society of Cardiology (ESC) between September 1, 1999, and May 31, 2000 [37]. A total of 1363 physicians provided data for 11,062 patients, of whom 54% were older than 70 years and 45% were women. Eighty-two percent of the patients had had an echocardiogram. The treatment rates in eligible patients with systolic dysfunction heart failure are shown. Results from this survey suggest that treatment seems to be less than optimum and there are substantial variations in practice among countries. A similar treatment gap for heart failure has been demonstrated in the United States. The inconsistencies between physicians' knowledge and the treatment they deliver suggest that improved organization of care for heart failure is urgently required. (*Adapted from* Cleland *et al.* [38].)

REFERENCES

1. Stevenson WG, Stevenson LW, Middlekauff HR, *et al.*: Sudden death prevention in patients with advanced ventricular dysfunction. *Circulation* 1993, 88:2953–2961.

2. MERIT-HF Study Group: Effect of Metoprolol CR/XL in chronic heart failure: Metoprolol CR/XL Randomized Intervention Trial in Congestive Heart Failure. *Lancet* 1999, 353:2001–2007.

3. Narang R, Cleland JGF, Erhardt L, *et al.*: Mode of death in chronic heart failure. *Eur Heart J* 1996, 17:1390–1403.

4. Tomaselli GF, Rose J: Molecular aspects of arrhythmias associated with cardiomyopathies. *Curr Opin Cardiol* 2000, 15:202–208.

5. Uretsky BF, Thygesen K, Armstrong PW, *et al.*: Acute coronary findings at autopsy in heart failure patients with sudden death: results from the assessment of treatment with lisinopril and survival (ATLAS) trial. *Circulation* 2000, 102:611–616.

6. Podrid PJ, Lampert S, Grayboys TB, *et al.*: Aggravation of arrhythmia by antiarrhythmic drugs: incidence and predictors. *Am J Cardiol* 1987, 59:38E–44E.

7. Flaker GC, Blackshear JL, McBride R, *et al.*: Antiarrhythmic drug therapy and cardiac mortality in atrial fibrillation. The Stroke Prevention in Atrial Fibrillation Investigators. *J Am Coll Cardiol* 1992, 20:527–532.

8. Buxton AE, Lee KL, Fisher JD, *et al.*: A randomized study of the prevention of sudden death in patients with coronary artery disease. *N Engl J Med* 1999, 341:1882–1890.

9. Singh SN, Fletcher RD, Fisher SG, *et al.*: Amiodarone in patients with congestive heart failure and asymptomatic ventricular arrhythmia. Survival Trial of Antiarrhythmic Therapy in Congestive Heart Failure. *N Engl J Med* 1995, 333:77–82.

10. Waldo AL, Camm AJ, deRuyter H, *et al.*, for the SWORD Investigators: Effect of d-sotalol on mortality in patients with left ventricular dysfunction after recent and remote myocardial infarction. *Lancet* 1996, 348:7–12.

11. Torp-Pedersen C, Moller M, Bloch-Thomsen PE, *et al.*: Dofetilide in patients with congestive heart failure and left ventricular dysfunction. *N Engl J Med* 1999, 341:857–865.

12. Fonarow GC: Pathogenesis and treatment of cardiomyopathy. *Adv Intern Med* 2001, 47:1–45.

13. Shekelle PG, Rich MW, Morton SC, *et al.*: Efficacy of angiotensin-converting enzyme inhibitors and beta-blockers in the management of left ventricular systolic dysfunction according to race, gender, and diabetic status: a meta-analysis of major clinical trials. *J Am Coll Cardiol* 2003, 41:1529–1538.

14. Garg R, Yusuf S: Overview of randomized trials of angiotensin-converting enzyme inhibitors on mortality and morbidity in patients with heart failure. Collaborative Group on ACE Inhibitor Trials. *JAMA* 1995, 273:1450–1456.

15. Vermes E, Tardif JC, Bourassa MG, *et al.*: Enalapril decreases the incidence of atrial fibrillation in patients with left ventricular dysfunction: insight from the Studies Of Left Ventricular Dysfunction (SOLVD) trials. *Circulation* 2003, 107:2926–2931.

16. Solomon S, Olofsson B, Finn P, *et al.*: Cause of death across full spectrum of ventricular function in patients with heart failure: the CHARM study [abstract]. *J Am Coll Cardiol* 2004, 45:180A.

17. Young JB, Dunlap ME, Pfeffer MA, *et al.*: Morbidity and mortality reduction with candesartan in patients with chronic heart failure and left ventricular systolic dysfunction: results of CHARM low-left ventricular ejection fraction trials. *Circulation* 2004, 110:2618–2626.

18. Pitt B, Zannad F, Remme WJ, *et al.*: The effect of spironolactone on morbidity and mortality in patients with severe heart failure. *N Engl J Med* 1999, 341:709–717.

19. Pitt B, Remme W, Zannad F, *et al.*; Eplerenone Post-Acute Myocardial Infarction Heart Failure Efficacy and Survival Study Investigators: Eplerenone, a selective aldosterone blocker, in patients with left ventricular dysfunction after myocardial infarction. *N Engl J Med* 2003, 348:1309–1321.

20. Packer M, Bristow MR, Cohn JN, *et al.*: The effect of carvedilol on morbidity and mortality in patients with chronic heart failure. U.S. Carvedilol Heart Failure Study Group. *N Engl J Med* 1996, 334:1349–1355.

21. CIBIS-II Investigators and Committees: The Cardiac Insufficiency Bisoprolol Study II (CIBIS-II): a randomised trial. *Lancet* 1999, 353:9–13.

22. Packer M, Coats AJ, Fowler MB, *et al.*: Effect of carvedilol on survival in severe chronic heart failure. *N Engl J Med* 2001, 344:1651–1658.

23. Hunt SA, Baker DW, Chin MH, *et al.*: ACC/AHA guidelines for the evaluation and management of chronic heart failure in the adult: executive summary. A report of the American College of Cardiology-/American Heart Association Task Force on Practice Guidelines (Committee to revise the 1995 Guidelines for the Evaluation and Management of Heart Failure). *J Am Coll Cardiol* 2001, 38:2101–2113.

24. Heart Failure Society of America: Heart Failure Society of America (HFSA) practice guidelines. HFSA guidelines for management of patients with heart failure caused by left ventricular systolic dysfunction—pharmacological approaches. *J Card Fail* 1999, 5:357–382.

25. Pfeffer MA, Swedberg K, Granger CB, *et al.*; CHARM Investigators and Committees: Effects of candesartan on mortality and morbidity in patients with chronic heart failure: the CHARM-Overall programme. *Lancet* 2003, 362:759–766.

26. Bardy GH, Lee KL Mark DB, *et al.*: Amiodarone or an implantable cardioverter-defibrillator for congestive heart failure. *N Engl J Med* 2005, 352:225–237.

27. The Digitalis Investigation Group: The effect of digoxin on mortality and morbidity in patients with heart failure. *N Engl J Med* 1997, 336:525–533.

28. Cooper HA, Dries DL, Davis CE, *et al.*: Diuretics and risk of arrhythmic death in patients with left ventricular dysfunction. *Circulation* 1999, 100:1311–1315.

29. Kober L, Torp-Pedersen C, Carlsen JE, *et al.*: A clinical trial of the angiotensin-converting-enzyme inhibitor trandolapril in patients with left ventricular dysfunction after myocardial infarction. Trandolapril Cardiac Evaluation (TRACE) Study Group. *N Engl J Med* 1995, 333:1670–1676.

30. Granger CB, McMurray JJ, Yusuf S, *et al.*; CHARM Investigators and Committees: Effects of candesartan in patients with chronic heart failure and reduced left-ventricular systolic function intolerant to angiotensin-converting-enzyme inhibitors: the CHARM-Alternative trial. *Lancet* 2003, 362:772–776.

31. McMurray JJ, Ostergren J, Swedberg K, *et al.*; CHARM Investigators and Committees: Effects of candesartan in patients with chronic heart failure and reduced left-ventricular systolic function taking angiotensin-converting-enzyme inhibitors: the CHARM-Added trial. *Lancet* 2003, 362:767–771.

32. Solomon SD, Wang D, Finn P, *et al.*: Effect of candesartan on cause-specific mortality in heart failure patients: the Candesartan in Heart failure Assessment of Reduction in Mortality and morbidity (CHARM) program. *Circulation* 2004, 110:2180–2183.

33. Poole-Wilson PA, Swedberg K, Cleland JG, *et al.*: Comparison of carvedilol and metoprolol on clinical outcomes in patients with chronic heart failure in the Carvedilol Or Metoprolol European Trial (COMET): randomised controlled trial. *Lancet* 2003, 362:7–13.

34. Mitchell LB, Powell JL, Gillis AM, *et al.*; AVID Investigators: Are lipid-lowering drugs also antiarrhythmic drugs? An analysis of the Antiarrhythmics Versus Implantable Defibrillators (AVID) trial. *J Am Coll Cardiol* 2003, 42:81–87.

35. Horwich TB, MacLellan WR, Fonarow GC: Statin therapy is associated with improved survival in ischemic and non-ischemic heart failure. *J Am Coll Cardiol* 2004, 43:642–648.

36. Juurlink DN, Mamdani MM, Lee DS, *et al.*: Rates of hyperkalemia after publication of the Randomized Aldactone Evaluation Study. *N Engl J Med* 2004, 351:543–551.

37. Fonarow GC: Heart failure: recent advances in prevention and treatment. *Rev Cardiovasc Med* 2000, 1:25–33.

38. Cleland JG, Cohen-Solal A, Aguilar JC, *et al.*; IMPROVEMENT of Heart Failure Programme Committees and Investigators: Management of heart failure in primary care (the IMPROVEMENT of Heart Failure Programme): an international survey. *Lancet* 2002, 360:1631–1639.

MECHANICAL DYSSYNCHRONY IN HEART FAILURE AND RESYNCHRONIZATION THERAPY

David A. Kass

The function of the intact heart involves a complex integration of properties spanning from the molecular motors themselves, the signaling systems that regulate them, and the structural surround that encompasses them within and external to the myocyte, to organ-level geometry, vascular tree, and fiber organization. As with any assembly of functional units, the successful generation of cardiac force and output requires coordination among the motor units, and for excitable tissues, this means synchronized electrical activation. This is accomplished by both a specialized conduction system for rapid communication between geographically distant regions of the chamber, facilitated cell-to-cell conduction through specialized regions known as gap junctions, and fiber organization that further enhances this signaling.

The consequences of having regions of myocardium fail to contract with coordinated timing are a decline in the performance of the heart as a chamber, a fall in its mechanical efficiency, and heterogeneous abnormalities that evolve as the likely result of the disparate loading that accompanies the resulting contractile dyssynchrony. First studied decades ago, initial physiologic assessment of this phenomenon was based on single-site pacing studies in which myocardial conduction replaced normal His-Purkinje activation, generating premature and late-activated regions of the heart. Virtually all of these studies were performed in normal hearts—typically of sufficient size for simultaneous regional and global mechanical functional assessment. The effect of generating pacemaker-induced dyssynchrony in normal hearts was significant yet modest, leading to the impression that this would have only a minor net impact.

Some 20 to 30 years later, investigators once again began to examine the impact of cardiac dyssynchrony in failing hearts. Here there are several features that could exacerbate the functional defects associated with electro/mechanical discoordination. The failing heart is much larger—so the time required to activate a distant region via intramyocardial conduction would be longer, even if cell-to-cell conduction properties were normal. In fact, such conduction was abnormal, with reduced gap junction function and delayed conduction velocity providing even greater disparity in the time that one region would be stimulated relative to another. Furthermore, the failing heart was a virtual stew of abnormal signaling, involving calcium, enzymes that regulate cardiac function, remodeling, and metabolism—all of which might render the organ more susceptible to the adverse consequences of discoordinate contraction. By the mid 1990s, initial studies had revealed intriguing benefits of resynchronizing contraction, using a simple pacing method that concomitantly activated two point electrodes, one on the right heart and one on the left. What followed was the rapid evolution and ultimately clinical testing of a new nonpharmacologic therapy for cardiac failure, which in appropriately selected individuals, may provide substantial benefit and improve mortality.

This chapter reviews the underlying pathophysiology of dyssynchrony and mechanisms by which cardiac resynchronization therapy is understood to improve the failing heart. In a separate chapter, the results of recent clinical trials are reviewed.

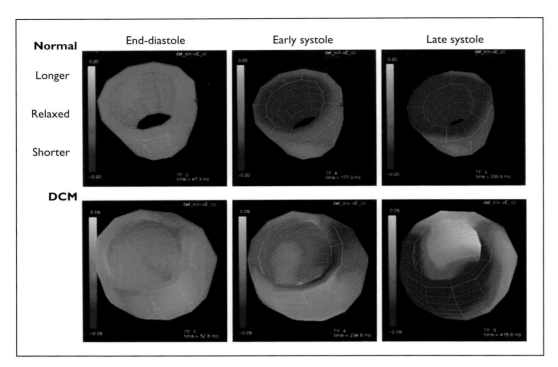

FIGURE 6-1. Cardiac dyssynchrony viewed by magnetic resonance imaging (MRI) in humans. MRI scans were obtained using a method known as tissue tagging, to quantify circumferential strain (analogous to shortening, but dimensionless) in multiple segments and slices throughout the heart. The reconstructed images are shown at end diastole, early systole, and late systole. Segments are color coded to be red in the diastolic starting strain, blue when shortening is occurring, and yellow if the segments are being stretched. For the control normal heart (*top*), all segments display fairly similar shortening at a point in time. In contrast, the *lower panels* display a heart from a patient with dilated cardiomyopathy (DCM) and a left bundle–type conduction delay. Here, the septum shortens in early systole, but the lateral wall only starts to shorten by the tail end of systole, when the septum is now being reciprocally stretched. It takes nearly the full systolic period for mechanical activation to appear in the late-stimulated lateral wall—virtually dividing the heart into two functional regions.

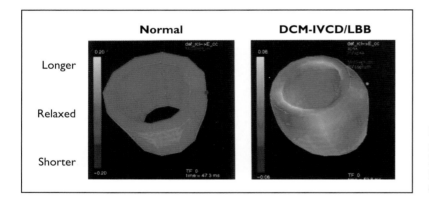

FIGURE 6-2. Dyssynchrony in the human heart; magnetic resonance image–tagging strain analysis. This is a cine version of Figure 6-1. DCM—dilated cardiomyopathy; IVCD—interventricular conduction delay; LBB—left bundle branch. (*Adapted from* Curry *et al.* [1].)

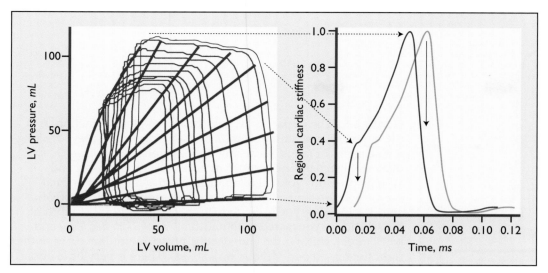

FIGURE 6-3. Dyssynchrony—the basic mechanism of regional disparity of mechanical activation. The contraction of the heart behaves much like the stiffness of a time-varying spring—or elastance. As shown on the *left*, when viewed as a series of pressure-volume loops, cardiac contraction involves a property of chamber (muscle) stiffening and destiffening with each cycle. This time-varying elastance is shown by the slopes of the individual isochrones superimposed on the loops, and to the *right* by the time plot of elastance (chamber stiffness) versus time. Normally, all regions of the heart would develop stiffness synchronously.

However, in the discoordinate heart, the late-activated territory is delayed mechanically—so its time-varying elastance time course is phase shifted to the right. Differences in stiffening between regions will result in reciprocal shortening and stretch at various times in the cardiac cycle. As shown by the *arrows*, these differences become particularly prominent very early in systole, and again near end-systole into early relaxation. This is important to remember because this has an impact on methods now under development to record this dyssynchrony by various imaging modalities. LV—left ventricular.

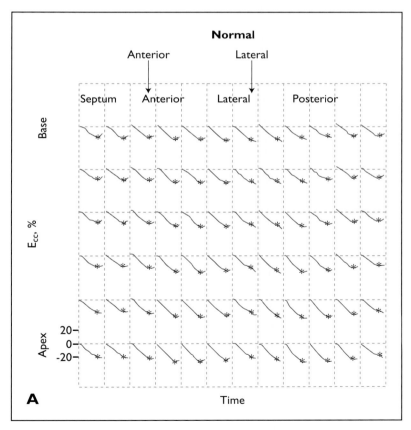

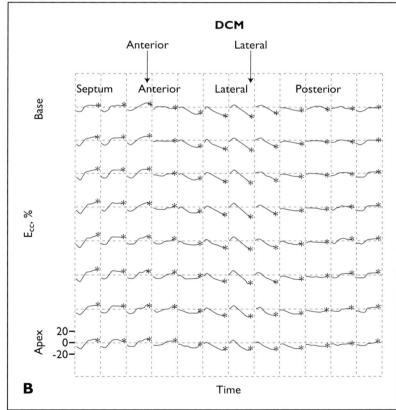

FIGURE 6-4. Magnetic resonance image–derived strain maps showing normal regional strains (**A**) and strain patterns in a dyssynchronous failing heart (**B**). Data are from human subjects. The normal strain pattern is homogenous throughout multiple layers (*top to bottom*) and regions (*right to left* from septum to posterolateral wall). In contrast, there is marked heterogeneity of motion in the failing dyssynchronous heart. These patterns show early septal shortening followed by septal stretch, and early lateral wall stretch followed by delayed shortening. DCM—dilated cardiomyopathy. (*Adapted from* Nelson *et al*. [2].)

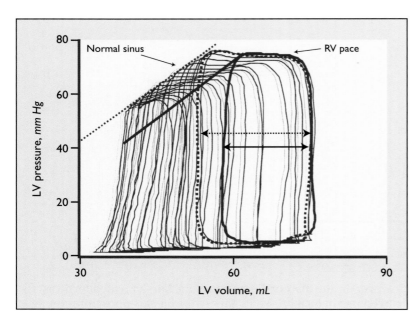

FIGURE 6-5. The impact of dyssynchrony on global function. A resting pressure-volume loop (*thick dotted lines*) is displayed, along with a series of loops at varying preload volumes (*thin dotted lines*) that establish baseline systolic and diastolic function (*eg*, end-systolic pressure-volume relationship, *dotted line*) for a normal canine heart in sinus rhythm. With acute right ventricular (RV) apex pacing, dyssynchrony reduces net stroke volume (width of the *solid loop*—compared with width of the *thick dotted loop*) and work (area), shifting the end-systolic pressure-volume point to the right (increased end-systolic wall stress). There is very little impact on diastolic properties—shown by the lower boundary (diastolic compliance) and unaltered maximal volume (end-diastolic volume, *arrow*). LV—left ventricular.

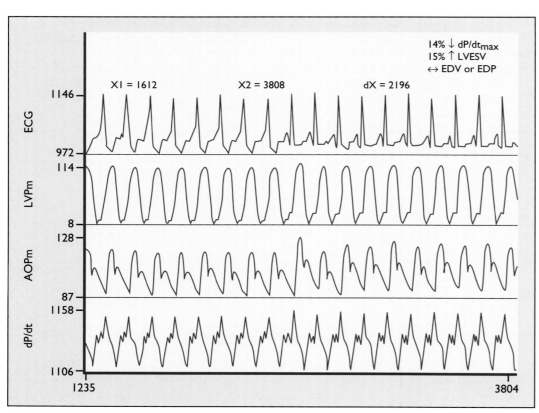

FIGURE 6-6. Evidence for reduced systolic function by acutely generated dyssynchrony in humans. Prior publications have reported declines in ejection fraction, with a rise in end-systolic volume and reduced maximal rate of pressure rise (dP/dt_{max}) with acute right ventricular (RV) pacing. An example of this effect is shown in the hemodynamic tracings in this figure. The patient's heart is being paced from the RV apex at the start of the tracings (*left*), then pacing is terminated, restoring normal sinus rhythm (*arrow*) for the latter half. There is an acute rise in dP/dt_{max}, and an increase in the arterial pulse pressure (*second line from bottom*) that accompanies the restoration of synchrony. On average, our studies observed a 14% decline in dP/dt_{max} with acute dyssynchrony in the normal heart, and a 15% increase in left ventricular end-systolic volume (LVESV). As with the example in Figure 6-5, there was no change in either end-diastolic volume (EDV) or pressure (EDP) [3,4].

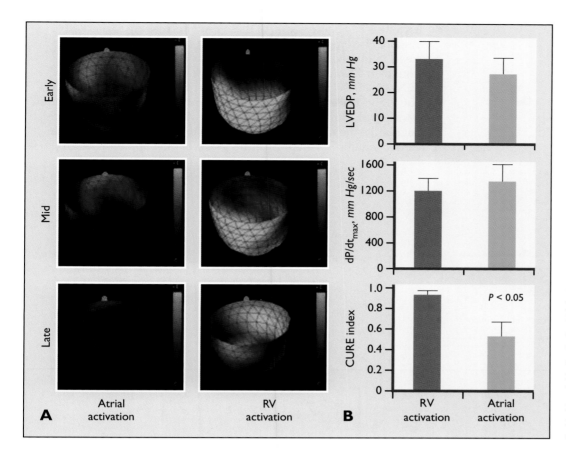

FIGURE 6-7. Animal model of cardiac dyssynchrony with heart failure. **A,** Dyssynchrony similar to that observed in human subjects (Fig. 6-1) in a canine model in which the right ventricular (RV) free wall or atria were rapidly paced for 3 to 4 weeks to induce heart failure with or without dyssynchrony. **B,** This resulted in a similar elevation of left ventricular end-diastolic pressure (LVEDP) and a decline in maximal rate of pressure rise (dP/dt_{max}) (normal for a dog is >2500 mm Hg/sec) but marked differences in discoordination, as determined by a circumferential uniformity ratio (CURE) index between pacing modes. This model was then used to determine regional molecular changes in the wall that might occur as a result of differential timing of contraction versus heart failure itself.

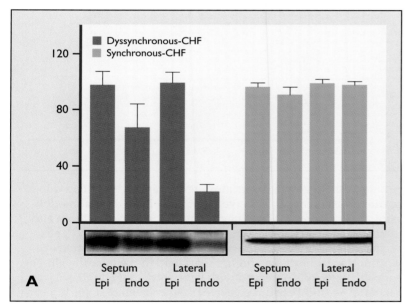

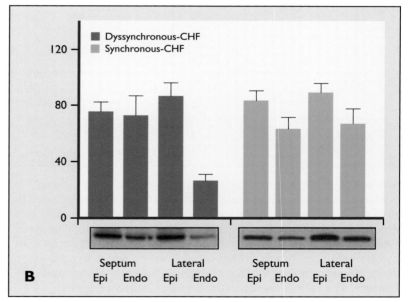

FIGURE 6-8. Molecular polarization induced by dyssynchrony in an animal model of heart failure with or without discoordination. The data show examples and summary Western blots for a calcium handling protein (phospholamban) (**A**), gap junction protein (connexin 43) (**B**), and mitogen-activated kinase (extracellular response kinase, ERK) (**C**).

Continued on next page

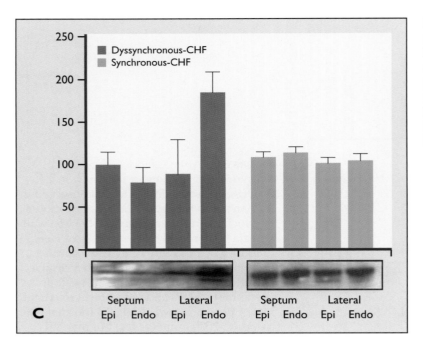

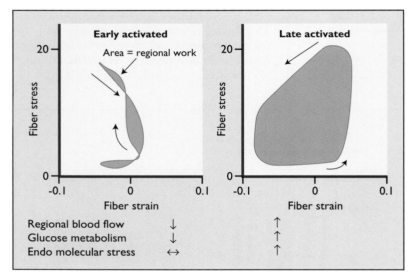

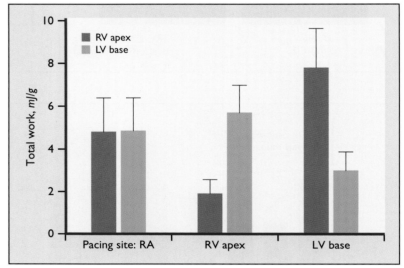

Figure 6-8. *(Continued)* All these proteins displayed marked regional heterogeneity of expression in the discoordinate congestive heart failure (CHF) hearts—with reduced phospholamban and connexin 43 and increased ERK in the lateral endocardium (ENDO). This is the late-stimulated territory that would be under the highest stress. In contrast, such disparities were not observed in hearts with similar cardiac failure but without dyssynchrony, which highlights the role of dyssynchrony in this behavior and regional heterogeneity. Epi—epicardium. (*Adapted from* Spragg *et al.* [5].)

Figure 6-9. Influence of dyssynchrony on regional wall stress, workload, and associated metabolism and coronary perfusion. The plots show stress-strain loops as based on regional strain- and stress-calculated data for the early-activated versus late-activated regions. The *arrows* show the reciprocal early change in stress with late-activated prestretch, which is followed by late-activated shortening (higher stress) that re-extends the early stimulated territory. The area of the stress-strain loops reflects regional workload and is markedly different in both regions. Reduced work in the early-activated zone corresponds to less local blood flow and reduced glucose metabolism, whereas both are increased in the higher stress, late-activated wall. It is in the latter (particularly in the endocardium) that major changes in molecular signaling appear to occur.

Figure 6-10. Regional disparities in myocardial workload due to cardiac dyssynchrony. Data were obtained in an animal model using magnetic resonance imaging methods to assess strain and estimated regional workload. With right ventricular (RV) apex pacing, there is a decline in workload in the early-activated septum that is offset by a higher workload in the lateral wall. The opposite pattern is observed with left ventricular (LV) basal pacing. RA—right atrium. (*Adapted from* Prinzen *et al.* [6].)

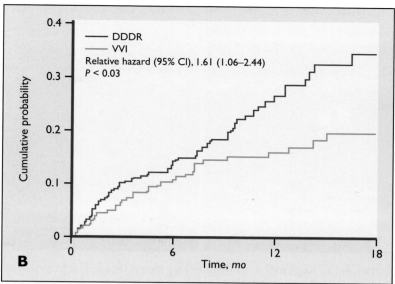

B

FIGURE 6-11. **A** and **B**, Clinical evidence of the adverse impact of generating discoordination in patients with underlying heart disease. The Dual Chamber and VVI Implantable Defibrillator (DAVID) trial was conducted to test two different modes of pacemaker therapy (ventricular pacing at a low backup rate of 40 min^{-1} [VVI] or dual-chamber rate-responsive pacing at a rate of 70 min^{-1} [DDDR]) in patients who had a clinical indication for an implantable cardioverter-defibrillator (ICD). There was a significant increased risk of death or new or worsened cardiac failure in the DDDR group. Importantly, of the differences between the study groups, a major one was the number of beats that were actually paced. Those at the higher backup rate had nearly 65% of their beats paced—*ie*, their hearts were made to contract dyssynchronously. In contrast, those with the lower rate had very few beats paced. CHF—congestive heart failure; EF—ejection fraction; HF—heart failure. (*Adapted from* Wilkoff *et al.* [7].)

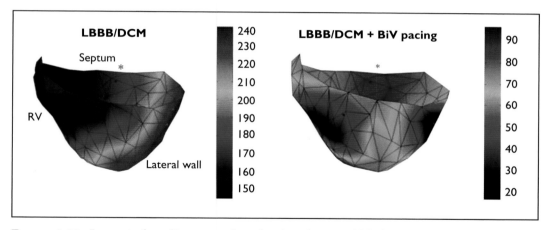

FIGURE 6-12. Impact of cardiac resynchronization therapy (CRT) on epicardial electrical activation in the failing heart. Data shown were generated in an animal model of heart failure and dyssynchrony, with the epicardium surrounded by a multi-electrode array to record activation times. With an underlying left bundle branch block (LBBB), activation starts early throughout most of the right ventricle (RV), then spreads gradually to the lateral wall. CRT is instituted using biventricular (BiV) pacing. There is initial stimulation at two opposing sites, and although conduction still must proceed intramyocardially and is therefore slower, there is less delay in activation between regions of the heart and importantly, the heart is no longer as polarized into two opposing regions (Leclercq *et al.*, Unpublished data). DCM—dilated cardiomyopathy.

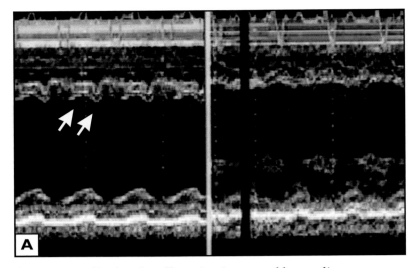

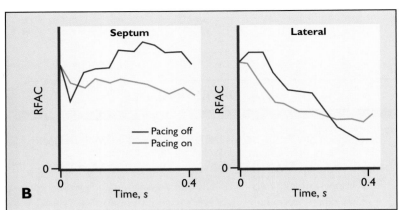

FIGURE 6-13. Regional wall motion improved by cardiac resynchronization therapy (CRT). M-mode echocardiographic images (**A**) show dyssynchrony and effects of CRT in a human subject. The primary observation is in the septal motion that contracts toward the opposing wall twice during each systole (*arrows*)—so-called paradoxic septal motion. As demonstrated by the stress-strain loop, this is caused by the opposing forces applied by the late-activated wall. CRT can remove this abnormal motion. This is better viewed by the radial motion plots derived by contrast echo imaging in a human subject (**B**). In the dyssynchronous condition, the initial inward septal motion is followed by late rightward motion (radial motion is positive—*ie*, a stretch). CRT changes this to inward motion throughout systole. The effects in the lateral wall are less marked, with the primary influence being on the phase of contraction, not its magnitude or qualitative appearance. RFAC— regional fractional area change.

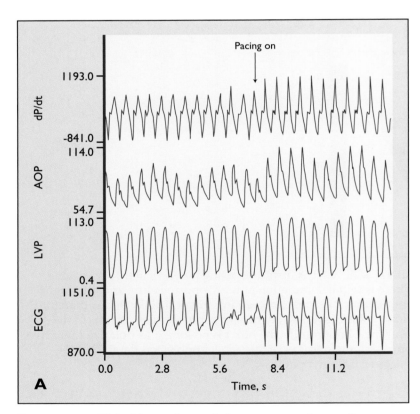

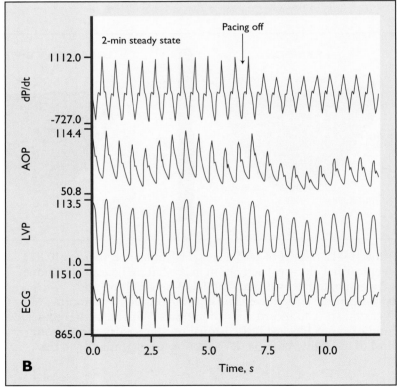

FIGURE 6-14. Global hemodynamic improvement by cardiac resynchronization therapy (CRT) in a human patient with dilated heart failure and a left bundle branch block–type conduction defect. With the institution of CRT (pacing on) (**A**), there is an abrupt rise in the rate of pressure rise (maximal dP/dt) and the arterial pulse (difference between systole and diastole, which reflects cardiac output), and a slight increase in left ventricular pressure (LVP). This is sustained with minimal change until pacing is discontinued (**B**) and the underlying dyssynchronous state is restored. With pacing termination, there is an abrupt decline in function back to baseline. AOP—aortic pressure.

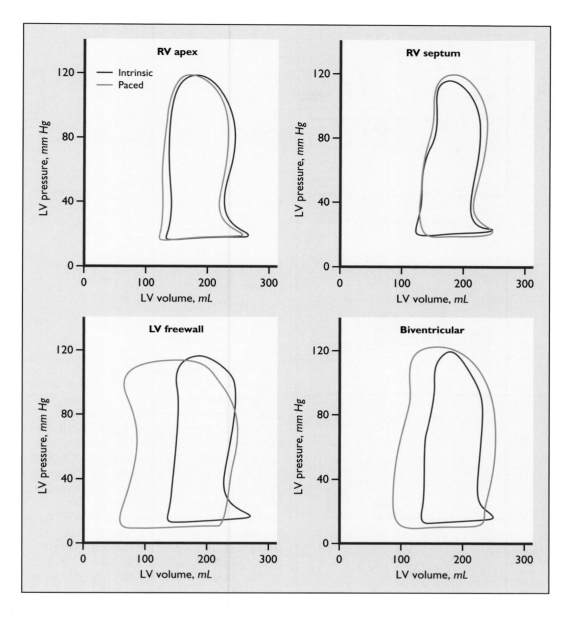

FIGURE 6-15. The effect of cardiac resynchronization therapy on global chamber function viewed as pressure-volume (PV) loops. Steady-state (intrinsic) loops are shown by *solid lines* from a patient with dilated cardiac failure and left bundle branch–type conduction delay. Paced beats are shown by the *dotted lines*. With stimulation at the right ventricular (RV) apex or septum, there is no improvement in cardiac function, whereas with both left ventricular (LV)-only and biventricular stimulation, the loop width increases, the area increases, and the end-systolic pressure-volume point shifts to the left (reduced stress, improved systolic function). (*Adapted from* Kass *et al.* [8].)

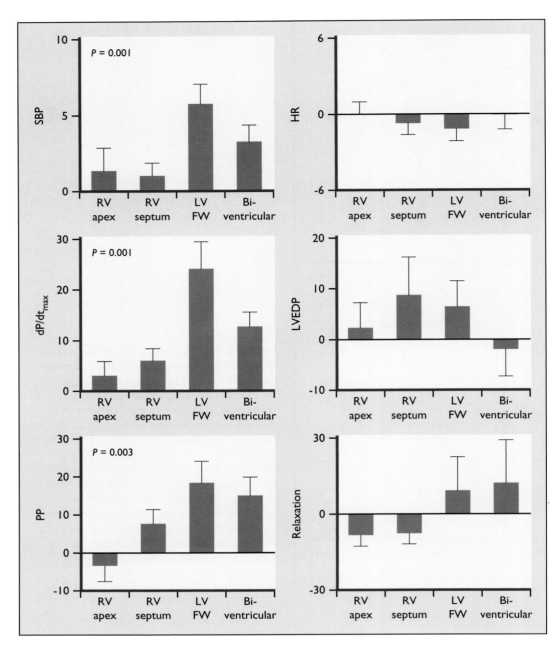

FIGURE 6-16. Mean hemodynamic responses to pacing stimulation in patients with dilated heart failure and left bundle branch block–type conduction delay. Pacing site varied among right ventricular (RV) apex versus RV (mid-upper) septum, left ventricular (LV) free (lateral) wall (FW), and biventricular (LV free wall + RV apex). Both of the latter resulted in improvement in systolic function, as shown by the changes in systolic blood pressure (SBP), maximal rate of pressure rise (dP/dt$_{max}$), and pulse pressure (PP)—although there was a slightly greater benefit from LV pacing alone. There was no change in heart rate (HR) by study design or in diastolic properties (LV end-diastolic pressure [LVEDP], or relaxation time constant). (*Adapted from* Kass *et al.* [8].)

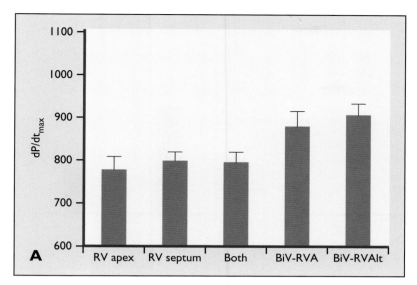

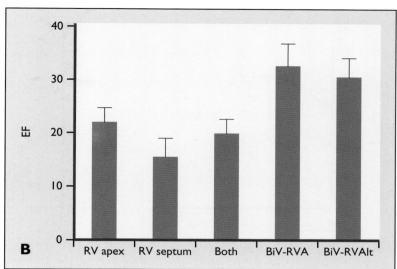

FIGURE 6-17. Relative effect of altering right ventricular (RV) pacing site on biventricular (BiV) pacing benefit of systolic function. Studies were performed in patients with chronic atrial fibrillation either with marked nodal delay or status post atrioventricular (AV) node ablation (pacer dependent). Systolic function indexed by either maximal rate of pressure rise (dP/dt_{max}) (**A**) or ejection fraction (EF) (**B**) increased in both BiV modes similarly, suggesting that the site of RV pacing did not have a major impact. Combining two sites of RV stimulation (*ie*, both apex and septum at the same time) showed no benefit over either RV site alone. Thus, it is essential that the left ventricle (LV) be stimulated prematurely to offset discoordination, but the site of RV stimulation may be less important. Afib—atrial fibrillation; RVA—RV apex; RVAlt—RV altering.

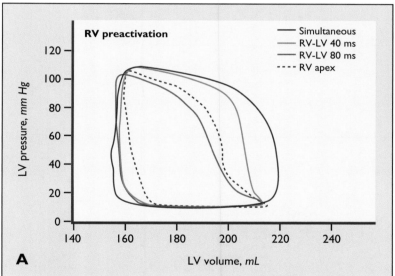

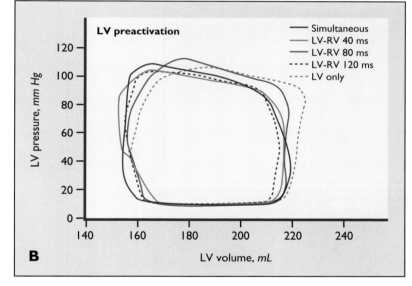

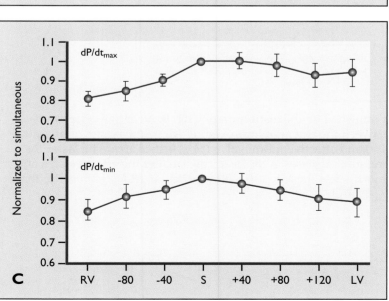

FIGURE 6-18. Effect of varying the right ventricular (RV)–left ventricular (LV) stimulation time on the systolic benefit of cardiac resynchronization therapy. Studies were performed in patients with atrial fibrillation with profound atrioventricular (AV) delay (or ablated AV node conduction) so that supraventricular excitation was not present. **A** and **B**, Pressure-volume loop examples with different delay times between RV and LV stimulation. **C**, Summary results for maximal rate of pressure rise (dP/dt_{max}) and minimal rate of pressure rise (dP/dt_{min}) at varying delay times. Early RV activation was consistently worse than earlier LV activation, and simultaneous stimulation was optimal on average for the nine subjects—particularly for improving both systolic and diastolic properties.

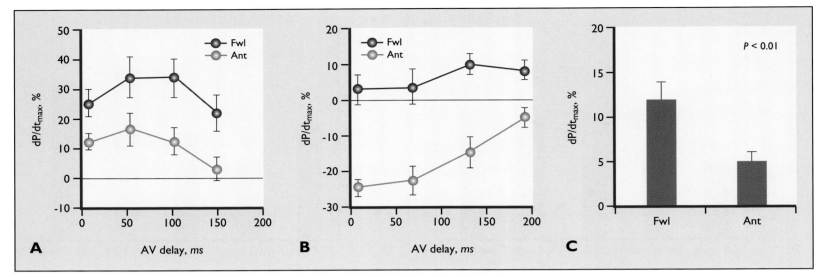

FIGURE 6-19. Effect of varying pacing site on cardiac resynchronization therapy (CRT) benefit. Data show comparison of pacing either the anterior wall (Ant) or lateral free wall (Fwl) in two subjects (**A** and **B**), and summary data (**C**). There was generally less than 50% of systolic functional improvement with more anterior pacing, with some individuals (**B**) displaying an actual decline in function if left ventricular (LV) pacing was instituted too anteriorly. This finding is important as it indicates that optimal placement of the LV lead is important for obtaining CRT benefit and that one can make a subject's cardiac function worse by pacing too close to the already prematurely stimulated territory. AV—atrioventricular; dP/dt_{max}—maximal rate of pressure rise. (*Adapted from* Butter *et al.* [9].)

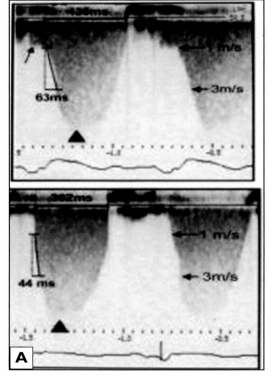

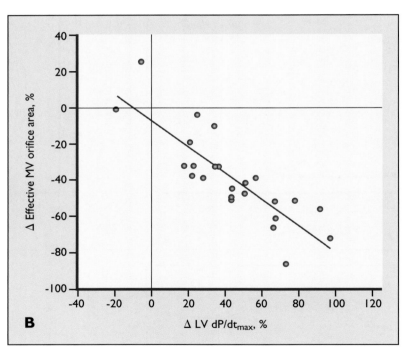

FIGURE 6-20. Cardiac resynchronization therapy (CRT) may reduce mitral regurgitation (MR). By increasing the speed of ventricular pressure rise, improving coordination between the papillary muscles, and possibly reducing chamber size (reverse remodeling), MR may be diminished by CRT. **A**, Doppler tracings for MR demonstrating significant presystolic MR that is diminished by the institution of CRT. **B**, Negative correlation between the extent of improved dP/dt_{max} (peak rate of pressure rise) and effective mitral valve (MV) orifice area. The faster the pressure increases in the heart, the smaller the effective area and thus the less the MR. LV—left ventricular. (*Adapted from* Breithardt *et al.* [10].)

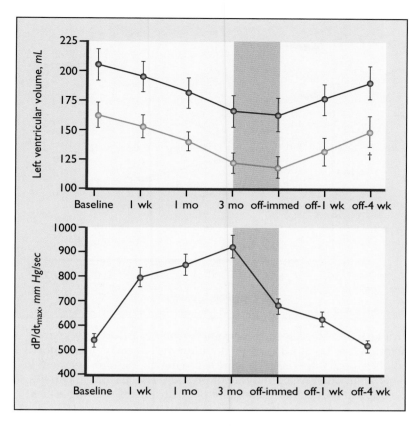

FIGURE 6-21. Reverse remodeling from chronic cardiac resynchronization therapy (CRT) in human subjects. Data are based on echocardiographic measurements of end-systolic and end-diastolic volume (*top*) and maximal rate of pressure rise (dP/dt$_{max}$; Doppler derived, *bottom*). Over a period of 3 months, there was a gradual fall in chamber volumes whereas the systolic improvement as indexed by dP/dt$_{max}$ was fast and sustained. At this time, the investigators turned pacing off and there was an immediate fall in dP/dt$_{max}$, much as shown previously in the acute catheterization laboratory study. However, chamber volumes did not rise, but were unaltered, which supports true remodeling. Over the next month, with pacing still turned off, there was a gradual rise in volume and further return of systolic function to original baseline. (*Adapted from* Yu *et al.* [11].)

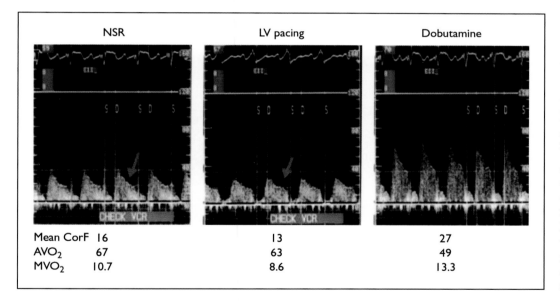

	NSR	LV pacing	Dobutamine
Mean CorF	16	13	27
AVO$_2$	67	63	49
MVO$_2$	10.7	8.6	13.3

FIGURE 6-22. Coronary blood flow measured during cardiac resynchronization therapy (CRT) (left ventricular [LV] pacing in this example) is minimally altered or even reduced despite improved function. Data are from a human subject with dilated heart failure and left bundle branch block. With CRT, there was a fall in mean coronary flow (CorF) and the arteriovenous oxygen difference (AVO$_2$) across the coronary circulation, and thus a net fall in myocardial oxygen consumption (MVO$_2$). In contrast, enhancing contractile function to the same extent, but using dobutamine, resulted in a marked rise in coronary flow and importantly MVO$_2$. NSR—normal sinus rhythm.

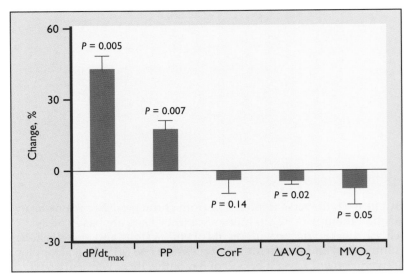

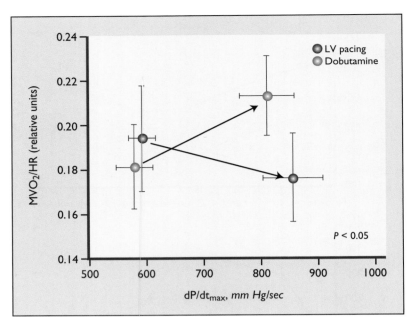

FIGURE 6-23. Mean data for the mechanoenergetics of cardiac resynchronization therapy. Data are from 10 patients and are all similar to the example shown in Figure 6-21. Despite near 45% increases in maximal rate of pressure rise (dP/dt_max) and improved arterial pulse pressure (PP), there was a significant net decline in arteriovenous oxygen difference (AVO₂) and myocardial oxygen consumption (MVO₂) from biventricular pacing. CorF—coronary flow. (*Adapted from* Nelson *et al.* [12].)

FIGURE 6-24. Mean results for comparison of cardiac resynchronization therapy (CRT) versus dobutamine effects on mechanoenergetics. Both interventions were set to match the improvement in systolic function (maximal rate of pressure rise [dP/dt_max] on the x-axis), but they had directionally opposite effects on the per-beat myocardial oxygen consumption (MVO₂). CRT improved myocardial efficiency, whereas dobutamine reduced it. HR—heart rate; LV—left ventricular. (*Adapted from* Nelson *et al.* [12].)

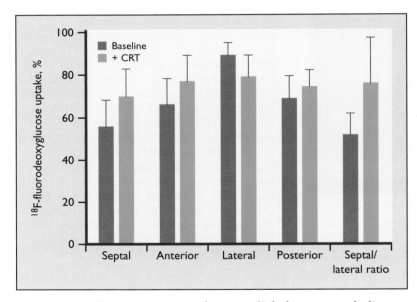

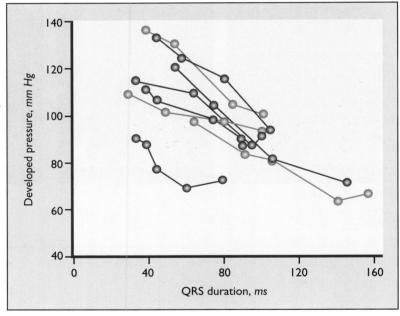

FIGURE 6-25. Homogenization of myocardial glucose metabolism due to chronic cardiac resynchronization therapy (CRT). Baseline data in dyssynchronous heart failure (*solid bars*) shows enhanced glucose uptake (positron emission tomography [PET] scan methodology) in the lateral wall compared with the anterior septum. With chronic CRT, there is improved homogeneity of metabolism across the ventricular regions. The most *rightward bars* show the ratio of septal/lateral wall for glucose metabolism, which rises closer to 1.0 with chronic CRT. (*Adapted from* Nowak *et al.* [13].)

FIGURE 6-26. Inverse correlation between QRS duration and mechanical function in isolated canine heart. Data are from an early publication in which varying ventricular pacing sites or a combination of sites were used to widen the QRS duration and then the developed pressure of the heart was measured [15]. The authors found that the wider the QRS, the worse the net systolic function. Data such as these helped fuel the initial expectation that QRS duration could be used to identify cardiac resynchronization therapy subjects and to help monitor treatment efficacy. However, this has not born out in subsequent trials. (*Adapted from* Burkhoff *et al.* [14].)

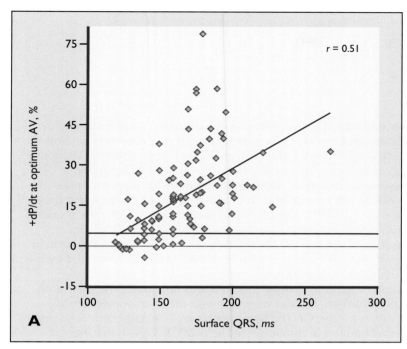

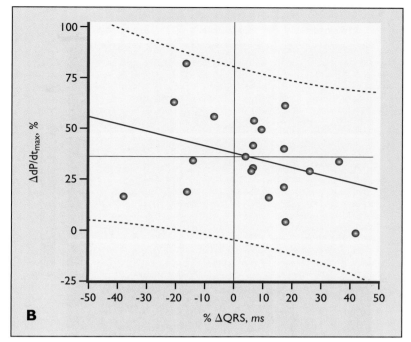

FIGURE 6-27. Correlation of cardiac resynchronization therapy (CRT) systolic effects to QRS duration at baseline, and the change in QRS duration during CRT. Data are from human subjects with dilated heart failure and conduction delay (primarily left bundle branch–type). Results are from acute hemodynamic studies, with pressures measured by micromanometer. There is an overall positive correlation between the acute chamber-level mechanical benefit from CRT and the duration of the QRS, but this regression relation is scattered, with a poor predictive value of QRS duration for acute response (**A**). Chronic response to CRT has been found to correlate with QRS duration very poorly or not at all [2,15]. **B**, The lack of correlation between the change in systolic function during CRT and QRS duration—again highlighting the disconnect that may exist between the electrical and mechanical behaviors in this disorder [2]. AV—atrioventricular; dP/dt$_{max}$—maximal rate of pressure rise.

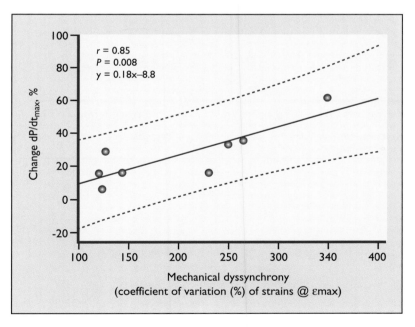

FIGURE 6-28. Correlation between the extent of mechanical dyssynchrony and the acute response to cardiac resynchronization therapy. These data were among the first to suggest that direct assessment of mechanical dyssynchrony would better correlate with functional improvement than would QRS duration. The index of dyssynchrony is based on a variance of the strain values taken at the time of maximal negative shortening (strain). dP/dt$_{max}$—maximal rate of pressure rise. (*Adapted from* Nelson [2].)

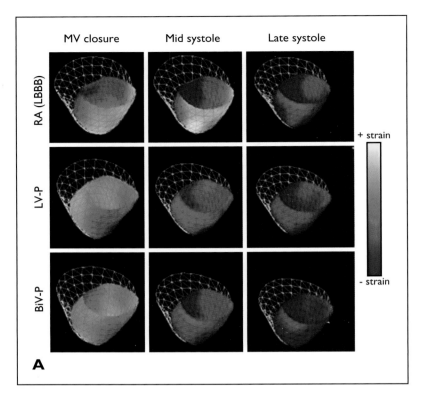

MV closure   Mid systole   Late systole

RA (LBBB)

LV-P

BiV-P

+ strain

− strain

A

FIGURE 6-29. Dissociation of mechanical from electrical dyssynchrony/synchrony in an animal model by comparison between left ventricular (LV) only and biventricular (BiV) modes of cardiac resynchronization therapy (CRT). **A,** Magnetic resonance images at different time points for three modes—baseline left bundle branch block (right atrial pacing), and then LV free wall and BiV stimulation of the same heart. Despite marked differences in electrical stimulation (*ie,* the LV-only mode produced substantial electric dyssynchrony), mechanical synchronization was improved with both pacing modes (reflected by the circumferential uniformity ratio index [CURE]) (**B**). The improvement in systolic function was not at all correlated with QRS duration, but did correlate with the level of mechanical dyssynchrony (**C**). The latter observation is consistent with prior data obtained in humans (*see* Fig. 6-28). BiV-p—biventricular pacing; dP/dt$_{max}$—maximal rate of pressure rise; FW—free wall; LBBB—left bundle branch block; LV-p—left ventricular pacing; MV—mitral valve; RA—right atrium; RAP—right atrial pacing.

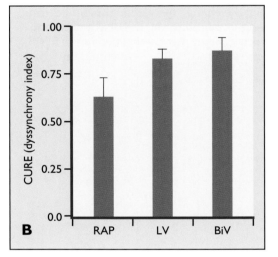

B

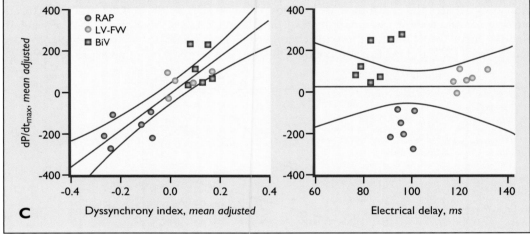

C

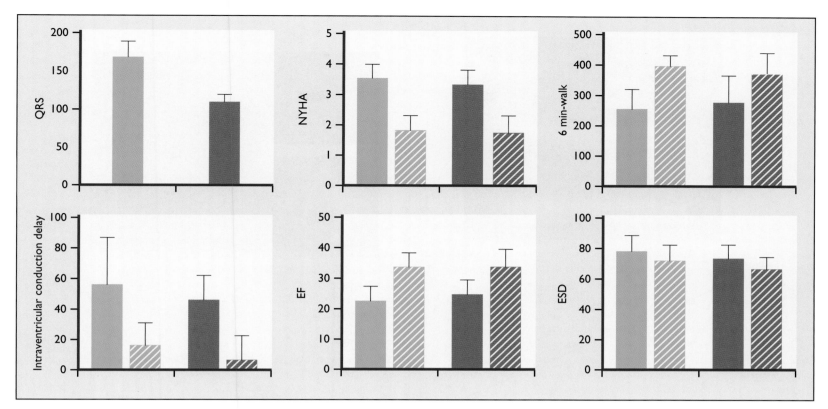

FIGURE 6-30. Efficacy of cardiac resynchronization therapy (CRT) in patients with a narrow QRS complex. Patients with discoordinate wall motion (*yellow*) and congestive heart failure (CHF) (*red*) were divided into two groups: those with widened QRS durations (*hatched*) and those with normal durations (*solid*). Both groups had similar levels of discoordinate wall motion detected by Doppler analysis. Both groups also had similar baseline severity of CHF—marked by similar New York Heart Association (NYHA) class, 6-minute walk, ejection fraction (EF), and end-systolic dimension (ESD). Furthermore, both groups displayed improvement in coordinate wall motion, symptoms, exercise capacity, and cardiac function with chronic CRT. These data add further support to the notion that mechanical dyssynchrony is the primary variable identifying patients most likely to benefit from CRT. (*Adapted from* Achilli *et al.* [16].)

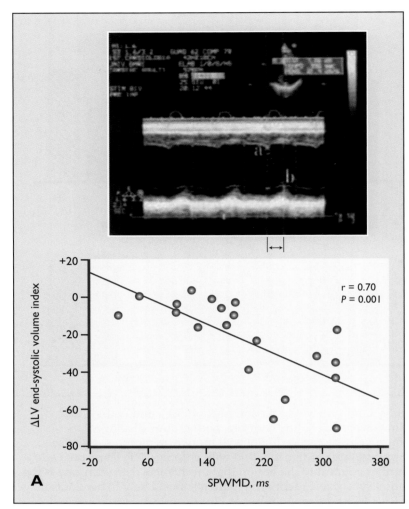

A

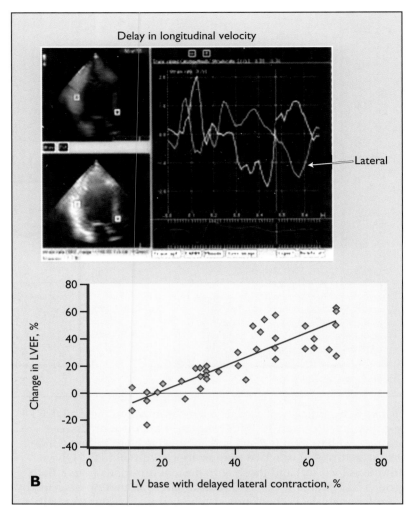

Delay in longitudinal velocity

Lateral

B

FIGURE 6-31. Assessment of cardiac dyssynchrony using M-mode echo (**A**) or tissue Doppler (**B**) in patients with congestive heart failure and dyssynchrony. With the echo approach, the timing delay between inward septal motion and inferolateral wall motion is determined. This delay was then shown to inversely correlate to chronic improvement from cardiac resynchronization therapy (CRT), as reflected by the reversal of chamber remodeling (end-systolic volume index is shown). Analogously, tissue Doppler is used to identify the regions of the heart with delayed longitudinal motion. The extent of segments with delayed motion is then determined and also correlates to chronic improvement in heart function (ejection fraction) as a result of CRT. LV—left ventricular; LVEF—LV ejection fraction; SPWMD—septal posterior wall motion delay. (**A** *adapted from* Pitzalis *et al.* [17]; **B** *adapted from* Sogaard *et al.* [18].)

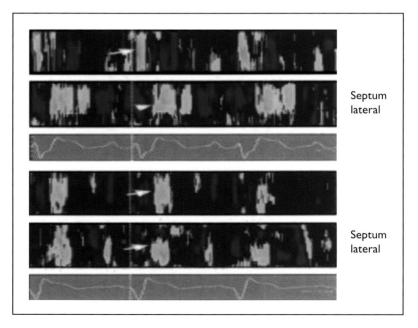

Septum
lateral

Septum
lateral

FIGURE 6-32. Strain-rate Doppler imaging for assessment of cardiac dyssynchrony. This analysis examines the relative difference in motion from two local myocardial samples in various regions of the heart to determine strain rate. Timing delay between septum and lateral motion is easily observed and can be measured. Improvement with cardiac resynchronization therapy is also clearly demonstrated (*arrows*). Newer software provides tissue velocity–based images in real time, with color coding of these images to assess relative contraction time in various cardiac regions. (*Adapted from* Breithardt *et al.* [19].)

REFERENCES

1. Curry CW, Nelson GS, Wyman BT, *et al.*: Mechanical dyssynchrony in dilated cardiomyopathy with intraventricular conduction delay as depicted by 3D tagged magnetic resonance imaging. *Circulation* 2000, 101(1):E2.

2. Nelson GS, Curry CW, Wyman BT, *et al.*: Predictors of systolic augmentation from left ventricular preexcitation in patients with dilated cardiomyopathy and intraventricular conduction delay. *Circulation* 2000, 101:2703–2709.

3. Askenazi J, Alexander JH, Koenigsberg DI, *et al.*: Alteration of left ventricular performance by left bundle branch block simulated with atrioventricular sequential pacing. *Am J Cardiol* 1984, 53:99–104.

4. Xiao HB, Brecker SJ, Gibson DG: Differing effects of right ventricular pacing and left bundle branch block on left ventricular function. *Br Heart J* 1993, 69:166–173.

5. Spragg DD, Leclercq C, Loghmani M, *et al.*: Regional alterations in protein expression in the dyssynchronous failing heart. *Circulation* 2003, 108:929–932.

6. Prinzen Hunter WC, Wyman BT, McVeigh ER. Mapping of regional myocardial strain and work during ventricular pacing: experimental study using magnetic resonance imaging tagging. *J Am Coll Cardiol* 1999, 33:1735–1742.

7. Wilkoff BL, Cook JR, Epstein AE, *et al.*: Dual-chamber pacing or ventricular backup pacing in patients with an implantable defibrillator: the Dual Chamber and VVI Implantable Defibrillator (DAVID) Trial. *JAMA* 2002, 288:3115–3123.

8. Kass DA, Chen C-H, Curry C, *et al.*: Improved left ventricular mechanics from acute VDD pacing in patients with dilated cardiomyopathy and ventricular conduction delay. *Circulation* 1999, 99:1567–1573.

9. Butter C, Auricchio A, Stellbrink C, *et al.*: Effect of resynchronization therapy stimulation site on the systolic function of heart failure patients. *Circulation* 2001, 104:3026–3029.

10. Breithardt OA, Sinha AM, Schwammenthal E, *et al.*: Acute effects of cardiac resynchronization therapy on functional mitral regurgitation in advanced systolic heart failure. *J Am Coll Cardiol* 2003, 41:765–770.

11. Yu C-M, Chau E, Sanderson JE, *et al.*: Tissue Doppler echocardiographic evidence of reverse remodeling and improved synchronicity by simultaneously delaying regional contraction after biventricular pacing therapy in heart failure. *Circulation* 2002, 105:438–445.

12. Nelson GS, Berger RD, Fetics BJ, *et al.*: Left ventricular or biventricular pacing improves cardiac function at diminished energy cost in patients with dilated cardiomyopathy and left bundle-branch block. *Circulation* 2000, 102:3053–3059.

13. Nowak B, Sinha AM, Schaefer WM, *et al.*: Cardiac resynchronization therapy homogenizes myocardial glucose metabolism and perfusion in dilated cardiomyopathy and left bundle branch block. *J Am Coll Cardiol* 2003, 41:1523–1538.

14. Burkhoff D, Oikawa RY, Sagawa K: Influence of pacing site on canine left ventricular contraction. *Am J Physiol* 1986, 251:H428–H435.

15. Kadhiresan V, Vogt J, Auricchio A, *et al.* Sensitivity and specificity of QRS duration to predict acute benefit in heart failure patients with cardiac resynchronization [abstract]. *Pacing Clin Electrophysiol* 2000, 23:555.

16. Achilli A, Sassara M, Ficili S, *et al.*: Long-term effectiveness of cardiac resynchronization therapy in patients with refractory heart failure and "narrow" QRS. *J Am Coll Cardiol* 2003, 42:2117–2124.

17. Pitzalis MV, Iacoviello M, Romito R, *et al.*: Cardiac resynchronization therapy tailored by echocardiographic evaluation of ventricular asynchrony. *J Am Coll Cardiol* 2002, 40:1615–1622.

18. Sogaard P, Egeblad H, Kim WY, *et al.*: Tissue Doppler imaging predicts improved systolic performance and reversed left ventricular remodeling during long-term cardiac resynchronization therapy. *J Am Coll Cardiol* 2002, 40:723–730.

19. Breithardt OA, Stellbrink C, Herbots L, *et al.* Cardiac resynchronization therapy can reverse abnormal myocardial strain distribution in patients with heart failure and left bundle branch block. *J Am Coll Cardiol* 2003, 42:486–494.

CARDIAC RESYNCHRONIZATION THERAPY

G. William Dec, Rakesh K. Pai, Kalyanam Shivkumar, and Isaac Wiener

Biventricular pacing has emerged as a meaningful nonpharmacologic therapy for patients with symptomatic congestive heart failure and dyssynchrony. Prolongation of the QRS complex, as a surrogate for electromechanical dyssynchrony, has been associated with reduced cardiac function, more advanced cardiomyopathy, and increased mortality. Approximately 30% to 40% of patients with New York Heart Association (NYHA) class III or IV heart failure will have significant QRS prolongation and may be candidates for resynchronization therapy.

Implantation of a resynchronization device can be accomplished with a high level of success via an endocardial approach utilizing the cardiac venous system. However, because of either technical limitations or diffuse anatomic remodeling that distorts the intracardiac anatomy, alternative approaches are occasionally utilized. The most common complication of biventricular pacing is coronary sinus lead dislodgement, which is reported to occur in up to 10% of cases.

Many patients have now been enrolled in cardiac resynchronization device trials. In the most recent American College of Cardiology/American Heart Association/North American Society of Pacing and Electrophysiology 2002 guideline update for implantation of cardiac pacemakers and antiarrhythmia devices, cardiac resynchronization therapy (CRT) is considered a class IIa indication for medically refractory, symptomatic NYHA class III or IV patients with idiopathic dilated or ischemic cardiomyopathy, prolonged QRS interval, left ventricular end-diastolic diameter greater than or equal to 55 mm, and an ejection fraction less than or equal to 35%. The majority of patients who undergo ventricular resynchronization will experience a reduction in heart failure symptoms, a decrease in hospitalizations for heart failure, improvements in well-being, and an increase in exercise performance. Recently, CRT has been shown to improve all-cause mortality when combined with defibrillation capability.

As discussed in a previous chapter, resynchronization therapy is associated acutely with improved contractility measured by rate of pressure rise (dP/dt), decreased mitral regurgitation, reduction in left ventricular end-systolic and -diastolic volumes, and lower left ventricular filling pressures. However, evidence from clinical trials suggests that approximately 30% of patients who receive resynchronization therapy do not respond favorably. Doppler echocardiography and tissue Doppler imaging are important tools to confirm hemodynamic improvement with left ventricular resynchronization following device therapy. This chapter describes CRT implantation techniques in detail, reviews pivotal CRT clinical trials, and discusses optimization of device function and future directions for this evolving therapy.

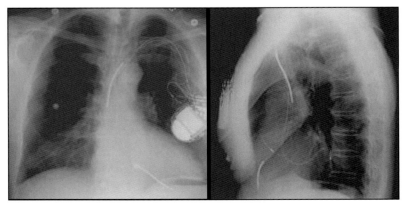

FIGURE 7-1. Left ventricular pacing. In the vast majority of patients, left ventricular stimulation is achieved with endocardial placement via the coronary venous system. Depicted is the posteroanterior chest radiograph of a patient with dilated, nonischemic cardiomyopathy and a cardiac resynchronization therapy (CRT) device. Three transvenous leads are present: a right atrial

appendage lead, a dual defibrillation coil right ventricular apical lead, and a left ventricular (LV) epicardial lead placed via the coronary sinus and positioned in a posterolateral coronary vein. The reported success rate with this approach in experienced centers exceeds 90%. However, implantation of the LV lead may be limited by difficult coronary sinus access or inability to stabilize the lead within a coronary vein. Thus, in some patients, a direct epicardial approach may be utilized by which the LV lead is placed thoracoscopically on the lateral left ventricular myocardium. The implantation of a CRT device includes the techniques utilized in implanting dual-chamber pacemakers and defibrillators, with the addition of coronary sinus cannulation for LV stimulation. The implantation of LV pacing leads to deliver resynchronization therapy involves obtaining venous access most commonly from subclavian or axillary venipuncture. The LV lead is advanced through a guide sheath over a guidewire to the targeted vein, and LV capture and sensing are tested to ensure an appropriate capture threshold and the absence of diaphragmatic stimulation. After the lead is stabilized, the guidewire and coronary sinus cannulation sheath are removed.

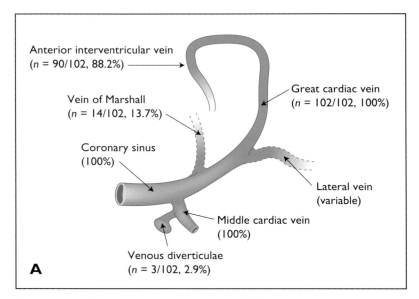

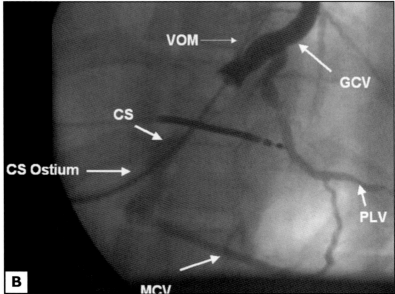

FIGURE 7-2. Coronary venous anatomy. The coronary venous system typically has the following components: the coronary sinus ostium; the middle cardiac vein (MCV); the first venous branch off of the coronary sinus, which courses adjacent to the dominant coronary artery (usually the posterior descending artery); the true coronary sinus, which runs from the ostium to the vein (or ligament) of Marshall (VOM), after which it is referred to as the great

cardiac vein (GCV); the lateral and/or posterolateral cardiac vein(s) (PLV); and the anterior interventricular vein, which courses adjacent to the left anterior descending artery. **A,** Venous anatomy of the heart, left anterior oblique (LAO) view. The prevalence of various coronary venous anatomy structures in 102 consecutive study patients. **B,** Representative view of the coronary venous anatomy demonstrating the pertinent structures.

Continued on next page

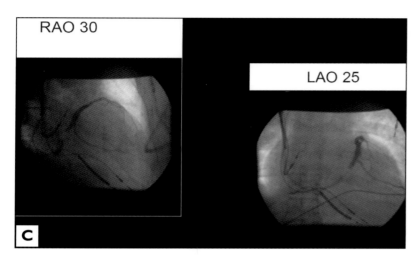

C

FIGURE 7-2. *(Continued)* **C**, Occlusive coronary sinus venography—coronary sinus (CS) and ventricular vein anatomy ideally are visualized in orthogonal fluoroscopic views. In the right anterior oblique (RAO), the CS is viewed on end. The body of the CS and the great cardiac vein proceed end-on, separating the ventricles from the atria. In this view, the ventricular veins proceed toward the sternum. In the LAO projection, the ostium of the CS is in the plane of the interatrial septum. The vein proceeds posteriorly from the right to left, wrapping around the lateral wall of the heart. The LAO projection is ideal for distinguishing lateral and septal locations of veins. Also present are a right ventricular apical pacing and defibrillation lead, as well as a lead in the right atrial appendage. The optimal target for left ventricular stimulation is the lateral (posterolateral) cardiac veins on the midlateral epicardium. Left ventricular lead placement in the anterior interventricular or middle cardiac veins does not correct ventricular dyssynchrony unless an appropriately lateral branch vein of these vessels can be targeted. (*Part B from* Cesario et al. [1]; with permission.)

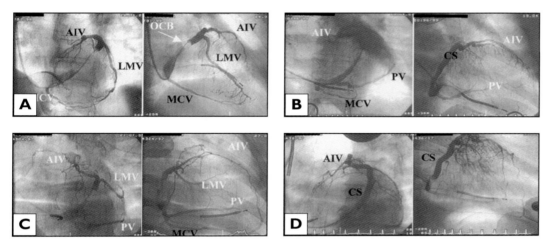

FIGURE 7-3. Variations in coronary venous anatomy. The coronary venous anatomy is highly variable among patients. Depicted are representative venograms showing different types of venous anatomy. Left and right columns show fluoroscopy images in left anterior oblique (LAO) and right anterior oblique (RAO) views, respectively. **A**, One additional vessel left marginal vein (LMV) between the middle cardiac vein (MCV) and the anterior interventricular vein (AIV). **B**, One additional vessel posterior vein (PV) between the MCV and AIV. **C**, Two additional vessels (PV and LMV) between the MCV and AIV. **D**, Multiple additional vessels between the MCV and AIV. The great cardiac vein and branch veins may differ in terms of number of vessels, vessel diameter, course, and tortuosity. The anatomic process of remodeling occurs in both the atria and ventricles. Left ventricular remodeling contributes to mitral annular dilatation, which in turn alters the angulation of the coronary sinus (CS) ostium, making the cannulation of this structure challenging in some patients. However, with the use of standard diagnostic coronary artery catheters, such as the Amplatz (AL 1 or AL 2) or a Judkins right coronary artery catheter (JR 4), the coronary sinus can be successfully accessed in the majority of patients. (*From* Meisel et al. [2]; with permission.)

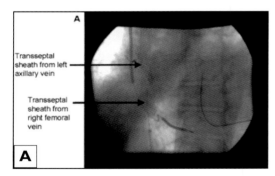 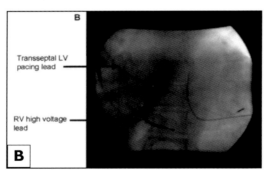 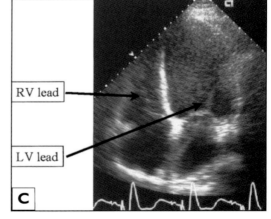

FIGURE 7-4. Alternative approaches to achieve left ventricular (LV) pacing. In rare cases, LV lead implantation can be performed via a modified transseptal approach to directly pace the LV endocardium. **A** and **B**, Fluoroscopy (left anterior oblique view). **A**, Transseptal wire placed through the right femoral vein as a marker to guide the transseptal sheath placed superiorly via the left axillary vein. **B**, LV and right ventricular (RV) leads after successful positioning and anchoring. **C**, Apical four-chamber view echocardiogram showing right RV and LV endocardial pacing leads. (*From* Ji et al. [3]; with permission.)

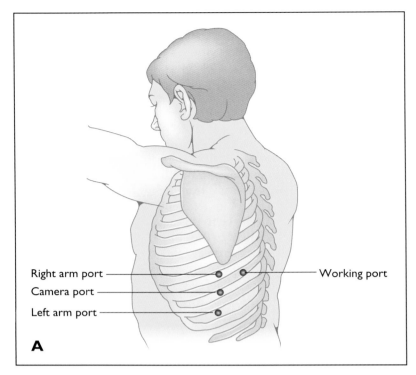

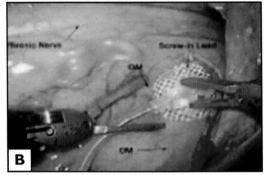

A

B

FIGURE 7-5. Epicardial approaches to achieve left ventricular (LV) pacing. If technical or anatomic limitations are present that prohibit successful placement of a coronary sinus vein lead, then consideration should be given to a direct epicardial approach. The LV lead can usually be placed with a limited thoracotomy or thoracoscopy. Robotically assisted thoracoscopic LV lead placement is also feasible. **A,** Port placement for totally endoscopic, robotic LV epicardial lead placement. The ports are placed in line with the tip of the scapula, allowing for posterior access to the LV surface. **B,** Operative photograph of robotic LV lead placement.

The pericardium is divided posterior to the phrenic nerve, exposing the obtuse marginal branch (OM) vessels on the posterolateral wall of the left ventricle. A two-turn, helical screw-in lead is being placed by a surgeon at a console. However, the long-term stability of epicardial capture thresholds with either an active fixation or steroid-eluting epicardial electrode is inferior when compared with a transvenous system. The advantage of direct epicardial placement is the ability to deliver lateral LV myocardial stimulation independent of the venous anatomy. (*From* DeRose *et al.* [4]; with permission.)

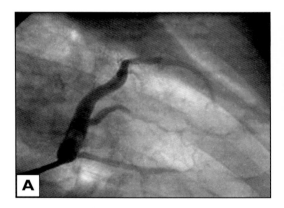

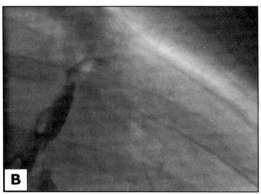

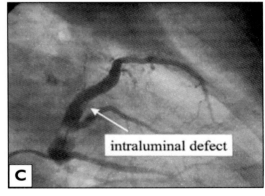

A

B

C intraluminal defect

FIGURE 7-6. Complications associated with biventricular implantation. The complications related to cardiac device implantation may include pneumothorax, hemothorax, cardiac perforation, pocket hematoma, and infection. Complications specific to resynchronization device implantation include those associated with coronary sinus (CS) cannulation and left ventricular lead placement, such as CS dissection. Pictured is a retrograde venogram before implantation (**A**), at the time of dissection (**B**), and after follow-up (**C**).

At the time of dissection, slow retrograde flow is visible in the midportion of the CS, with occlusion of the (posterolateral) side branch. Other complications include CS or cardiac vein perforation, extracardiac (diaphragmatic) stimulation, and acute decompensated congestive heart failure. Perhaps the most common complication of biventricular pacing is CS lead dislodgement; this complication is reported to occur in 4% to 10% of cases. (*From* de Cock *et al.* [5]; with permission.)

CONTROLLED TRIALS OF CARDIAC RESYNCHRONIZATION THERAPY

PATH-CHF I and II—Pacing Therapies in Congestive Heart Failure

MUSTIC SR and AF—Multisite Stimulation in Cardiomyopathies Sinus Rhythm and Atrial Fibrillation

MIRACLE and MIRACLE ICD—Multicenter InSync Randomized Clinical Evaluation Trial and Multicenter InSync Randomized Clinical Evaluation Implantable Cardioverter-Defibrillator Trial

COMPANION—Comparison of Medical Therapy, Pacing, and Defibrillation in Heart Failure

CARE-HF—Cardiac Resynchronization in Heart Failure

FIGURE 7-7. Controlled trials of cardiac resynchronization therapy.

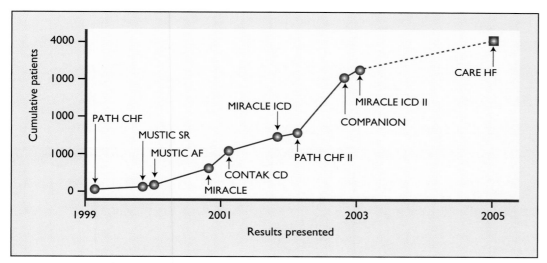

New York Heart Association (NYHA) class II to IV heart failure (with predominantly class III and IV patients), left ventricular ejection fraction equal to or less than 0.35, and varying degrees of QRS prolongation ($\geq$120, $\geq$130, or $\geq$150 ms). Excluded have been patients requiring permanent pacing and those in permanent atrial fibrillation, with the exception of subjects in the Multisite Stimulation in Cardiomyopathy-Atrial Fibrillation (MUSTIC-AF) study. The early trials of biventricular pacing enrolled small numbers of patients and thus assessed only "soft" end points, such as quality of life, 6-minute walk distance, improvement in NYHA functional class, and peak V_{O_2}, comparing resynchronization therapy to placebo (VVI backup rate, 40 bpm).

FIGURE 7-8. Timeline and cumulative enrollment of cardiac resynchronization therapy (CRT) trials. Presently, more than 3500 patients have been included in CRT clinical trials. In general, most of these clinical trials have had similar inclusion criteria: symptomatic

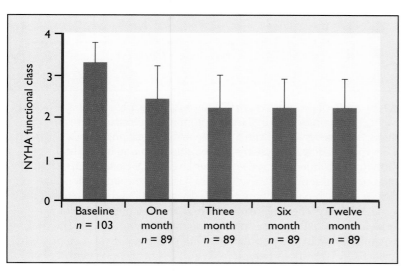

FIGURE 7-9. The effect of cardiac resynchronization therapy (CRT) on New York Heart Association (NYHA) functional class. CRT trials have evolved; the early trials demonstrated proof of the concept for left ventricular resynchronization and the safety of biventricular pacing. Subsequent trials have identified CRT as an adjunctive nonpharmacologic therapy for the treatment of congestive heart failure by showing acute and long-term improvements in cardiac hemodynamics, echocardiographic parameters, and functional status. The results of the InSync trial demonstrated a sustained decrease in NYHA functional class in the resynchronization therapy patients; this effect persists up to 1 year compared with baseline ($P < 0.001$). More recent studies have demonstrated the efficacy and safety of CRT when combined with defibrillator capability, and the ability of this therapy to favorably impact all-cause mortality. (*Adapted from* Gras *et al.* [6].)

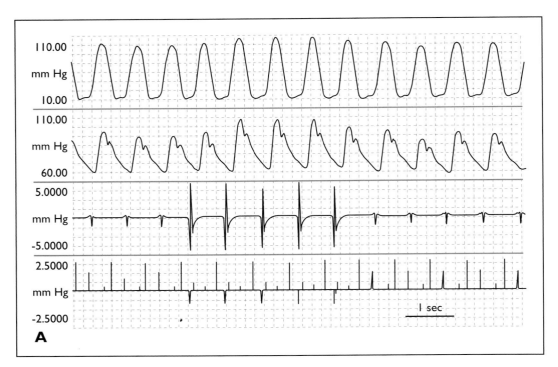

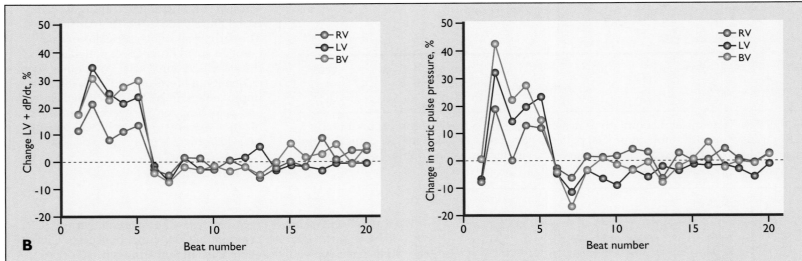

FIGURE 7-10. Hemodynamic benefit of cardiac resynchronization therapy as demonstrated in the Pacing Therapies in Congestive Heart Failure (PATH-CHF) trial. PATH-CHF investigated the effect of pacing chamber and atrioventricular (AV) delay with atrial-synchronous ventricular pacing on hemodynamic function in class III and IV congestive heart failure (CHF) patients with severe left ventricular (LV) systolic dysfunction, QRS duration greater than or equal to 120 ms, and PR interval greater than or equal to 150 ms. Twenty-seven patients were enrolled and were paced right ventricular (RV) only, LV only, or with biventricular (BV) stimulation. One third of patients had ischemia as the etiology of their cardiomyopathy. LV pacing leads were placed via an epicardial approach through a limited thoracotomy. The LV pacing site was most commonly the apex but could also be on the midlateral LV myocardium. **A,** Simultaneous recording of LV pressure waveforms and electrogram during a transient LV pacing sequence in VDD mode. Immediate changes in LV pressure, LV-positive rate of pressure rise (dP/dt), and aortic pressure occur when pacing starts (indicated by larger potentials in electrogram); all changes are reversed within a few beats when pacing ceases.
B, Hemodynamic impulse response plots from one individual showing an immediate percentage change in LV-positive dP/dt (*left*) and aortic pulse pressure (*right*) from baseline. Separate plots are shown for each pacing chamber (RV, LV, and BV) when pacing at the same AV delay. The first beat number is the first paced beat of a sequence; the sixth beat number is the first nonpaced beat. The trial concluded that in this population, CHF patients with sufficiently wide surface QRS durations benefit from atrial-synchronous ventricular pacing and that LV stimulation is necessary for maximum acute hemodynamic benefit. The PATH-CHF trial also acknowledged the important contribution of the patient-specific AV delay (regardless of ventricular pacing site) to maximize the hemodynamic benefit of pacing therapy. (*Adapted from* Auricchio *et al.* [7].)

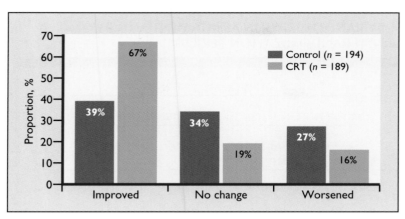

FIGURE 7-11. Multicenter InSync Randomized Clinical Evaluation (MIRACLE) trial. The MIRACLE trial randomized 453 patients with moderate to severe heart failure symptoms and QRS duration greater than or equal to 130 ms to cardiac resynchronization (N = 228) or continued medical therapy for 6 months (N = 225). At the end of 6 months, the control patients were given the opportunity to cross over to active pacing, and all patients were followed at 3- to 6-month intervals. Compared with the control group, patients randomized to cardiac resynchronization demonstrated significant improvement in quality-of-life assessment, 6-minute walk distance (+39 m vs +10 m; $P = 0.005$), New York Heart Association (NYHA) functional class ranking, treadmill exercise time (+81 seconds vs +19 seconds; $P = 0.01$), peak Vo_2 (+1.1 mL/kg/min vs +0.2 mL/kg/min; $P < 0.01$), and left ventricular ejection fraction (+4.6% vs -0.2%; $P < 0.001$). Patients randomized to active therapy were much more likely to be improved and much less likely to have worsened or to have remained unchanged, according to the definitions set forth by the composite response instrument. The effect of cardiac resynchronization therapy (CRT) on a composite clinical heart failure response end point in the MIRACLE trial is shown on the graph. The "worsened" category includes patients who died or were hospitalized because of worsening heart failure, or who demonstrated worsening in NYHA class at the last observation carried forward (LOCF) or moderate-marked worsening at patient global assessment at LOCF. The "improved" category includes patients who did not worsen (as defined above) and who demonstrated improvement in NYHA class at LOCF and/or moderate-marked improvement in patient global assessment score at LOCF. The "unchanged" category includes patients who neither improved nor worsened. $P < 0.01 \times 2$ analysis. (*Adapted from* Abraham [8].)

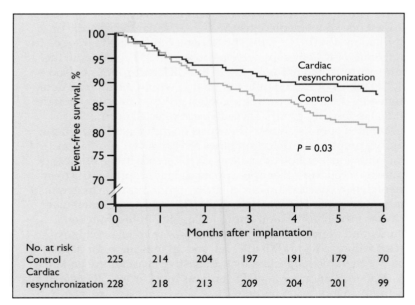

FIGURE 7-12. Time to death or hospitalization for worsening heart failure in the control and cardiac resynchronization therapy (CRT) groups of the Multicenter InSync Randomized Clinical Evaluation (MIRACLE) trial. MIRACLE was the first CRT clinical trial to demonstrate that resynchronization therapy could decrease the time to death or hospitalization for worsening heart failure. In this study, death from any cause was reduced by 27% ($P = $ not significant [NS]). The MIRACLE trial was neither designed nor adequately powered to evaluate the effect of CRT on all-cause mortality. However, the composite end point of death or worsening heart failure requiring hospitalization was significantly reduced by 40% ($P = 0.03$). By intention to treat, there were 16 deaths in the control group and 12 deaths in the resynchronization therapy arm ($P = $ NS). When compared with the control group, fewer patients in the CRT group required hospitalization (8% vs 15%) and intravenous heart failure therapy (7% vs 15%). Finally, in the control group, there were 50 hospitalizations in 34 patients for a total of 363 heart failure hospital days, which was significantly more when compared with the CRT group, which had 25 hospitalizations for congestive heart failure in 18 patients for a total of 83 heart failure hospital days ($P = 0.015$). (*Adapted from* Abraham *et al.* [9].)

APPROPRIATE AND INAPPROPRIATE ICD TREATMENT BY RANDOMIZATION ASSIGNMENT AND BY CRT TREATMENT RECEIVED DURING 6-MONTH RANDOMIZATION PERIOD*

	RANDOMIZATION ASSIGNMENT					CRT TREATMENT RECEIVED				
	CONTROL (N = 182)		CRT (N = 187)			NO CRT (N = 180)		CRT (N = 189)		
CATEGORY	EVENTS, N	PATIENTS, N (%)	EVENTS, N	PATIENTS, N (%)	P VALUE	EVENTS, N	PATIENTS, N (%)	EVENTS, N	PATIENTS, N (%)	P VALUE
Appropriate ICD shocks	154	26 (14)	89	24 (13)	.76	155	26 (14)	88	24 (13)	.65
Inappropriate ICD shocks	59	13 (7)	18	8 (4)	.27	49	13 (7)	28	8 (4)	.26
Appropriate: only ATP used	229	31 (17)	608	33 (18)	.89	618	32 (18)	219	32 (17)	.89
Inappropriate: only ATP used	32	8 (4)	35	13 (7)	.37	21	7 (4)	46	14 (7)	.18

*Note that the difference in numbers between the patients randomized to CRT and CRT received is the result of crossovers.

FIGURE 7-13. Appropriate and inappropriate implantable cardioverter-defibrillator (ICD) treatment by randomization assignment and by cardiac resynchronization therapy (CRT) received during a 6-month randomization period in the Multicenter InSync Randomized Clinical Evaluation (MIRACLE) ICD trial. The MIRACLE ICD trial investigated the efficacy and safety of combined CRT and ICD therapy in patients with New York Heart Association (NYHA) class III or IV congestive heart failure despite appropriate medical management. All patients also had an indication for defibrillator implantation. The study was a randomized, double-blind, parallel-controlled trial. A total of 369 patients were enrolled with a left ventricular ejection fraction of 35% or less, QRS duration of 130 ms or greater, a high risk of life-threatening ventricular arrhythmias (70% of all patients had ischemic cardiomyopathy), and NYHA class III (n = 328) or IV (n = 41) symptoms. Of the patients randomized to receive devices with combined CRT and ICD capabilities, 182 were controls (ICD activated, CRT off) and 187 were in the CRT group (ICD activated, CRT on).

The primary study end points were changes between baseline and 6 months in quality of life, functional class, and distance covered during a 6-minute walk test. Additional outcome measures included changes in exercise capacity, plasma neurohormones, left ventricular function, and overall heart failure status. Survival, incidence of ventricular arrhythmias, and rates of hospitalization were also compared. At 6 months, patients assigned to CRT had a greater improvement in median quality-of-life score ($P = 0.02$) and functional class ($P = 0.007$) than controls but did not differ in 6-minute walk distance (55 m [44–79 m] vs 53 m [43–75 m]; $P = 0.36$). Peak oxygen consumption increased by 1.1 mL/kg/min (0.7–1.6) in the CRT group versus 0.1 mL/kg/min (-0.1–0.8 mL/kg/min) in the control group ($P = 0.04$); after treadmill exercise, duration increased by 56 seconds (30–79 seconds) in the CRT group but decreased by 11 seconds (-55–12 seconds) in controls ($P < 0.001$). No significant differences were observed in left ventricular size or function, overall heart failure status, survival, or rates of hospitalization. No proarrhythmic events were observed. As presented in the table, during the 6-month randomization period, 47 patients (26%) in the control group and 42 patients (22%) in the CRT group experienced at least one spontaneous episode of ventricular tachycardia or fibrillation ($P = 0.47$). Of the spontaneous and treated episodes, outcomes of ICD therapy were recorded for 233 episodes in the control group and 678 episodes in the CRT group. Four episodes (1.7%) were not successfully terminated within the interval determined by device criteria in the control group versus one episode (0.1%) in the CRT group. These five episodes all eventually terminated spontaneously. There was no difference between the study groups in the detection times of ventricular fibrillation episodes. Furthermore, there was no difference in the number of patients receiving either appropriate or inappropriate ICD treatment, when comparisons are made by randomization assignment and by whether CRT was activated. The study concluded that cardiac resynchronization improved quality of life, functional status, and exercise capacity in patients with moderate to severe heart failure, a wide QRS interval, and an indication for defibrillator therapy, suggesting that congestive heart failure patients with an indication for an ICD derive as much from CRT as patients without an indication for an ICD. ATP—antitachycardia pacing. (*Adapted from* Young *et al.* [10].)

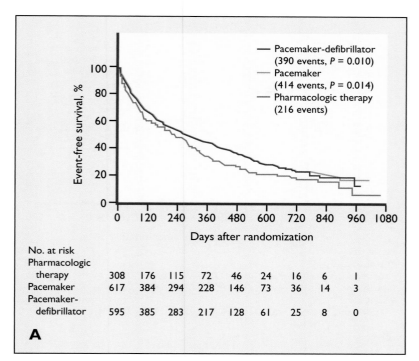

A

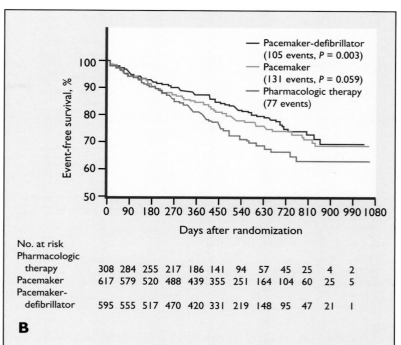

B

FIGURE 7-14. Comparison of Medical Therapy, Pacing, and Defibrillation in Heart Failure (COMPANION) trial. The figure shows Kaplan-Meier estimates of time to the primary end point of death from or hospitalization for any cause (**A**), time to the secondary end point of death from any cause (**B**), time to death from or hospitalization for cardiovascular causes (**C**), and time to death from or hospitalization for heart failure (**D**) from the COMPANION trial.

A, The 12-month rates of death from or hospitalization for any cause—the primary end point—were 68% in the pharmacologic-therapy group, 56% in the group that received a pacemaker as part of cardiac resynchronization therapy (CRT), and 56% in the group that received a pacemaker–defibrillator as part of CRT. **B,** The 12-month rates of death from any cause—the secondary end point—were 19% in the pharmacologic-therapy group, 15% in the pacemaker group, and 12% in the pacemaker–defibrillator group.

Continued on next page

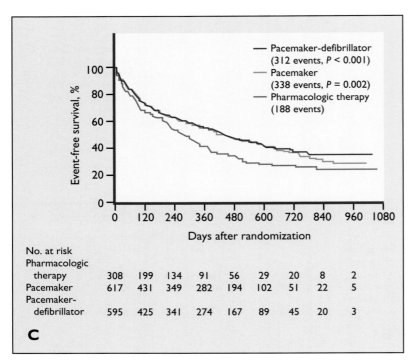

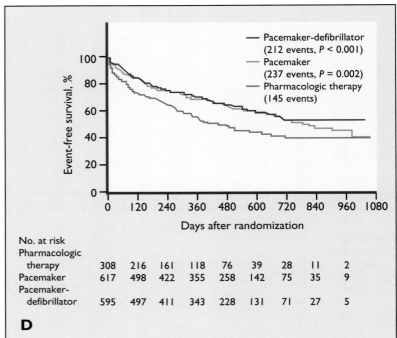

No. at risk									
Pharmacologic therapy	308	199	134	91	56	29	20	8	2
Pacemaker	617	431	349	282	194	102	51	22	5
Pacemaker-defibrillator	595	425	341	274	167	89	45	20	3

C

No. at risk									
Pharmacologic therapy	308	216	161	118	76	39	28	11	2
Pacemaker	617	498	422	355	258	142	75	35	9
Pacemaker-defibrillator	595	497	411	343	228	131	71	27	5

D

FIGURE 7-14. *(Continued)* **C,** The 12-month rates of death from or hospitalization for cardiovascular causes were 60% in the pharmacologic-therapy group, 45% in the pacemaker group, and 44% in the pacemaker–defibrillator group. **D,** The 12-month rates of death from or hospitalization for heart failure were 45% in the pharmacologic-therapy group, 31% in the pacemaker group, and 29% in the pacemaker–defibrillator group. In the pharmacologic-therapy group, death from heart failure made up 24% of the events; hospitalization for heart failure, 72% of events; and the intravenous administration of inotropes or vasoactive drugs for more than 4 hours, 4% of events. *P* values are for the comparisons of device-based treatment to optimal pharmacologic therapy.

The COMPANION trial investigated whether prophylactic CRT with or without a defibrillator would reduce the risk of death and hospitalization among patients with advanced heart failure and QRS prolongation. COMPANION was a large multicenter, nonblinded, prospective, randomized, controlled trial adequately powered to detect differences in mortality between optimal medical therapy and resynchronization therapy arms. The trial was not adequately powered to detect a mortality difference between CRT alone versus CRT plus defibrillator. The patients were randomized in a 1:2:2 fashion: medical therapy, medical therapy plus CRT, and medical therapy plus CRT plus defibrillator (CRT-D). A total of 1520 patients who had advanced heart failure (New York Heart Association class III or IV) due to ischemic (55%) or nonischemic cardiomyopathies and a QRS interval of at least 120 ms were randomized. The primary composite end point was the time to death from or hospitalization for any cause.

As depicted, when compared with optimal pharmacologic therapy alone, CRT with a pacemaker decreased the risk of the primary end

point (hazard ratio, 0.81; *P* = 0.014), as did CRT-D (hazard ratio, 0.80; *P* = 0.01). The risk of the combined end point of death from or hospitalization for heart failure was reduced by 34% in the pacemaker group (*P* < 0.002) and by 40% in the pacemaker–defibrillator group (*P* < 0.001 for the comparison with the pharmacologic-therapy group). A pacemaker reduced the risk of the secondary end point (death from any cause) by 24% (*P* = 0.059), and a pacemaker–defibrillator reduced the risk by 36% (*P* = 0.003).

The authors concluded that in patients with advanced heart failure and a prolonged QRS interval, CRT decreases the combined risk of death from any cause or first hospitalization and when combined with an implantable defibrillator, significantly reduces mortality. In selected patients, CRT or CRT-D can improve the clinical course of chronic heart failure patients. The pacemaker is associated with a reduction in hospitalizations and an improvement in symptoms, exercise performance, and quality of life; the addition of a defibrillator to CRT further reduces mortality. The decision of which of these two therapeutic options is most appropriate in a particular clinical setting is best determined on an individual basis by patients and their physicians. Additional trials are under way to confirm whether biventricular pacing alone will provide a long-term survival benefit. With regard to device selection, the indications for implantable cardioverter-defibrillator therapy continue to expand, with the results of the recently reported Sudden Cardiac Death in Heart Failure Trial (SCD-HeFT), demonstrating the benefit of defibrillator therapy for reducing sudden death risk in the nonischemic cardiomyopathy population. Thus, it is likely that the majority of resynchronization devices implanted will have defibrillation capability (CRT-D). (*Adapted from* Bristow *et al.* [11].)

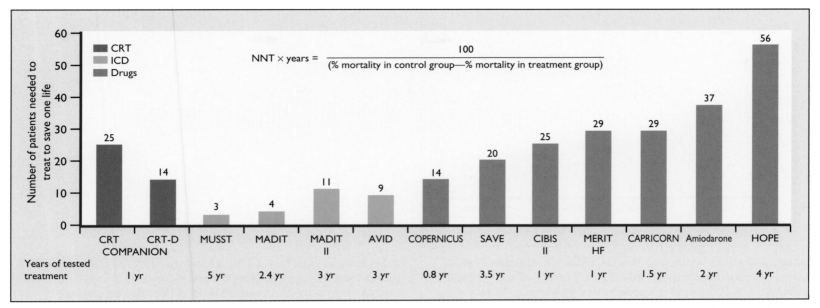

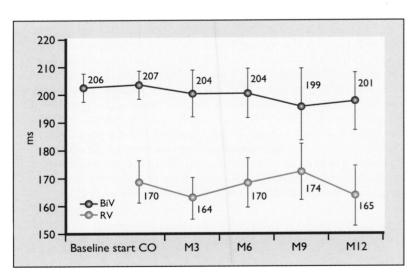

FIGURE 7-15. Comparison of different pharmacologic and device therapies, demonstrating the number of patients who need to be treated to save one life (NNTx). The NNTx is 25 with cardiac resynchronization therapy (CRT) and 14 with a CRT plus defibrillator (CRT-D) device. The formula used is presented at the top. Different studies had largely variable follow-up times; therefore, the mean follow-up is also presented. ICD—implantable cardioverter-defibrillator; MUSTT—Multicenter Unsustained Tachycardia Trial; MADIT and MADIT II—Multicenter Automatic Defibrillator Implantation Trial; AVID—Antiarrhythmics Versus Implantable Defibrillators Trial; COPERNICUS—Carvedilol Prospective Randomized Cumulative Survival Study; SAVE—Survival and Ventricular Enlargement Trial; CIBIS II—Cardiac Insufficiency Bisoprolol Study II; MERIT HF—Metoprolol Succinate Controlled-Release/Extended-Release Randomized Intervention Trial in Heart Failure; CAPRICORN—Carvedilol Post-Infarct Survival Control in Left Ventricular Dysfunction Study; HOPE—Heart Outcomes Prevention Evaluation Trial. (*Adapted from* Auricchio and Abraham [12].)

CARDIAC RESYNCHRONIZATION THERAPY AND ATRIAL FIBRILLATION

FIGURE 7-16. The Multisite Stimulation in Cardiomyopathies in Atrial Fibrillation (MUSTIC AF) trial. Many patients with severe congestive heart failure (CHF) develop permanent atrial fibrillation (AF). AF occurs in about 10% of patients with New York Heart Association (NYHA) functional class I and II heart failure and in approximately half of patients with NYHA class IV heart failure. The onset of AF eliminates regular atrioventricular (AV) transport and worsens cardiac performance in patients with already-reduced ventricular function. Radiofrequency catheter ablation of the AV junction and right ventricular (RV) apical pacing improve symptoms and quality of life in patients with AF refractory to pharmacotherapy. However, some patients may have persistent or pro-

gressive CHF symptoms after AV junction ablation and conventional RV apical pacing. The abnormal left ventricular activation sequence produced by cardiac pacing from the RV apex contributes to the lack of improvement observed in some patients after ablate-pace therapy. Chronic RV apical pacing produces geometric changes that appear similar on echocardiography to changes associated with intrinsic left bundle branch block. RV apical pacing may worsen symptoms and functional status when used in the patient with preexisting ventricular dysfunction.

The MUSTIC AF trial was a single-blind, randomized, controlled, crossover study that assessed for differences during two 3-month treatment periods of conventional RV versus biventricular (BiV) pacing. The trial enrolled 59 patients with NYHA class III heart failure, permanent AF, and symptomatic bradycardia requiring a permanent pacemaker (paced QRS duration > 200 ms). Unfortunately, because of a higher-than-expected drop-out rate, only 37 patients completed both crossover phases. Six-minute walk distance increased by 9.3% ($P = 0.05$); peak oxygen uptake increased by 13% ($P = 0.04$); importantly, hospitalizations decreased by 70%; and the majority of patients (85%) preferred BiV pacing when compared with RV apical pacing. As presented in the figure, for the AF group, *yellow lines* represent QRS durations during RV pacing at a rate of 70 bpm and *orange lines* those during BiV pacing. Despite the small number of patients completing both phases of the trial, MUSTIC-AF demonstrated that BiV pacing improves exercise tolerance in NYHA class III heart failure patients with permanent AF and paced QRS complexes. CO—cardiac output; M3—3 months; M6—6 months; M9—9 months; M12—12 months. (*Adapted from* Linde et al. [13].)

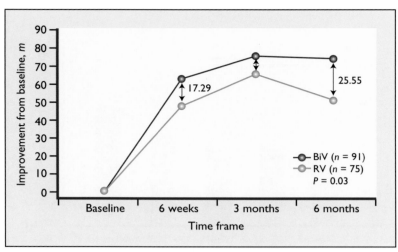

Figure 7-17. Left Ventricular Based Cardiac Stimulation Post AV Nodal Ablation Evaluation Study (PAVE): results of the 6-minute walk test. The PAVE trial is a prospective, randomized study evaluating biventricular (BiV) pacing after atrioventricular (AV) nodal ablation for patients with atrial fibrillation (AF) regardless of left ventricular systolic function or New York Heart Association (NYHA) functional class. The results of this study were presented at the annual scientific sessions of the American College of Cardiology in 2004 [14]. Patients were included in the study as follows: chronic AF for at least 1 month, electively undergoing AV node ablation procedure and permanent pacemaker implantation, NYHA class I to III symptoms, ability to ambulate less than 450 m during the 6-minute walk test, and receiving stable cardiovascular medication regimen for five drug half-lives prior to enrollment. The primary

end point was exercise capacity as measured by the distance walked during the 6-minute walk test; the secondary end points were functional capacity as measured by peak Vo_2 during cardiopulmonary exercise testing, and quality-of-life assessment. A total of 184 patients were included in the final analysis, right ventricular (RV) pacing ($n = 82$) and chronic resynchronization therapy pacing ($n = 102$). There were no significant baseline differences between the groups—mean left ventricular ejection fraction was 45%, mean QRS duration was 102 ms, and 34% had coronary artery disease. This trial suggests that in patients with chronic AF treated with AV nodal ablation, BiV pacing produces a statistically significant improvement in functional capacity over RV pacing as measured by the 6-minute walk test, peak Vo_2, and exercise duration. (*Adapted from* Doshi *et al.* [14].)

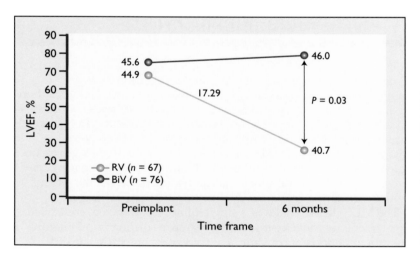

Figure 7-18. Left Ventricular Based Cardiac Stimulation Post AV Nodal Ablation Evaluation Study (PAVE): left ventricular ejection fraction (LVEF) assessment at 6 months between the biventricular (BiV) and right ventricular (RV) apical pacing groups. This improvement reflects a sustained benefit in the BiV group as compared with deterioration of ejection fraction in the RV pacing group ($P = 0.03$). The PAVE study infers that BiV pacing should be the preferred mode of therapy in patients undergoing atrioventricular nodal ablation for control of permanent atrial fibrillation secondary to improved functional status, and short-term preservation of left ventricular systolic function. (*Adapted from* Doshi *et al.* [14].)

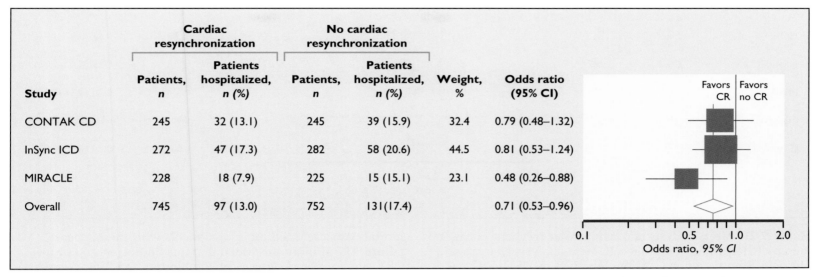

Study	Cardiac resynchronization		No cardiac resynchronization		Weight, %	Odds ratio (95% CI)
	Patients, n	Patients hospitalized, n (%)	Patients, n	Patients hospitalized, n (%)		
CONTAK CD	245	32 (13.1)	245	39 (15.9)	32.4	0.79 (0.48–1.32)
InSync ICD	272	47 (17.3)	282	58 (20.6)	44.5	0.81 (0.53–1.24)
MIRACLE	228	18 (7.9)	225	15 (15.1)	23.1	0.48 (0.26–0.88)
Overall	745	97 (13.0)	752	131(17.4)		0.71 (0.53–0.96)

FIGURE 7-19. Heart failure hospitalizations among patients randomized to cardiac resynchronization (CR) therapy or continued medical therapy. Cardiac resynchronization has been shown to reduce hospitalizations for heart failure in the CONTAK-CD, InSync ICD, and Multicenter InSynch Randomized Clinical Evaluation (MIRACLE) trials. Odds ratio refers to the odds ratio of heart failure hospitalization among patients randomized to resynchronization or no resynchronization. Weight refers to the value given each trial in statistical modeling. *Boxed area* is proportional to assigned weight. A meta-analysis of these three pivotal studies demonstrated a reduction in heart failure hospitalizations by 29% (odds ratio 0.71; 95% CI, 0.53 to 0.96). (*Adapted from* Bradley *et al.* [15].)

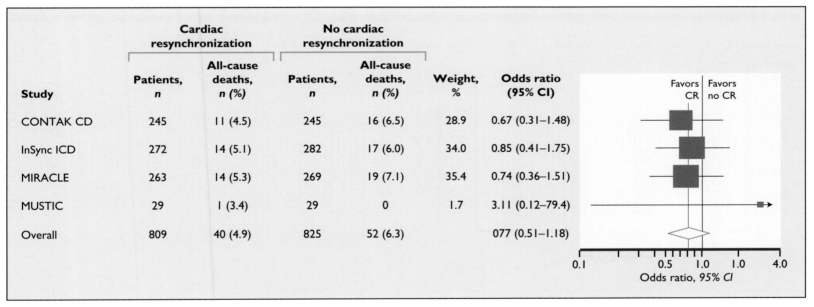

Study	Cardiac resynchronization		No cardiac resynchronization		Weight, %	Odds ratio (95% CI)
	Patients, n	All-cause deaths, n (%)	Patients, n	All-cause deaths, n (%)		
CONTAK CD	245	11 (4.5)	245	16 (6.5)	28.9	0.67 (0.31–1.48)
InSync ICD	272	14 (5.1)	282	17 (6.0)	34.0	0.85 (0.41–1.75)
MIRACLE	263	14 (5.3)	269	19 (7.1)	35.4	0.74 (0.36–1.51)
MUSTIC	29	1 (3.4)	29	0	1.7	3.11 (0.12–79.4)
Overall	809	40 (4.9)	825	52 (6.3)		077 (0.51–1.18)

FIGURE 7-20. Death among patients randomized to cardiac resynchronization therapy (CRT) versus no CRT. This meta-analysis of four reported CRT trials was associated with a trend toward reduction in all-cause mortality (odds ratio, 0.77; 95% CI, 0.51–1.18). Absolute rates of all-cause mortality, based on pooled data over 3 to 6 months of follow-up were 4.9% in the resynchronization group versus 6.3% in the control group. Meta-analysis of all-cause mortality among patients randomized to CRT or no resynchronization therapy. Odds ratio refers to the odds ratio of heart failure hospitalization among patients randomized to resynchronization or no resynchronization. Weight refers to weight given each trial in statistical modeling. *Boxed area* is proportional to weight. MIRACLE— Multicenter InSync Randomized Clinical Evaluation; MUSTIC— Multisite Stimulation in Cardiomyopathies. (*Adapted from* Bradley *et al.* [15].)

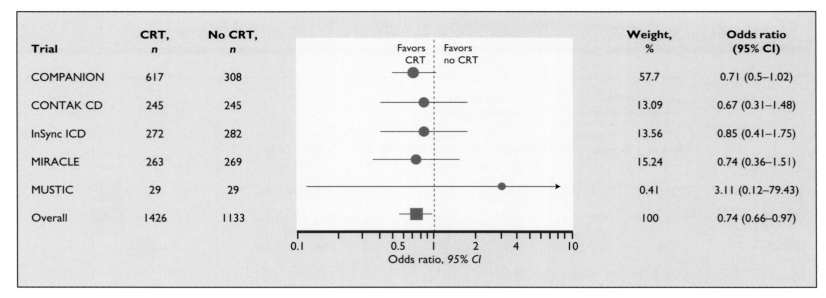

Trial	CRT, n	No CRT, n		Weight, %	Odds ratio (95% CI)
COMPANION	617	308		57.7	0.71 (0.5–1.02)
CONTAK CD	245	245		13.09	0.67 (0.31–1.48)
InSync ICD	272	282		13.56	0.85 (0.41–1.75)
MIRACLE	263	269		15.24	0.74 (0.36–1.51)
MUSTIC	29	29		0.41	3.11 (0.12–79.43)
Overall	1426	1133		100	0.74 (0.66–0.97)

FIGURE 7-21. Meta-analysis of recent cardiac resynchronization therapy (CRT) trials. A more recent meta-analysis assessing the Multisite Stimulation in Cardiomyopathies (MUSTIC), Comparison of Medical Therapy, Pacing and Defibrillation in Heart Failure (COMPANION), InSync ICD, Multicenter InSync Randomized Clinical Evaluation (MIRACLE), and CONTAK CD trials suggested that biventricular pacing may reduce all-cause mortality in a selected group of patients with chronic heart failure. The authors concluded that this finding should propel CRT into a similar league as ACE inhibitors and β-blockers as standard therapy in appropriately selected patients with heart failure and dyssynchrony. The odds ratios of all-cause mortality among patients randomized to CRT or no CRT. (*Adapted from* Salukhe *et al.* [16].)

OPTIMIZATION OF CARDIAC RESYNCHRONIZATION THERAPY

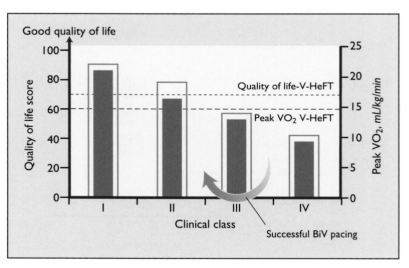

FIGURE 7-22. Estimated impact of biventricular (BiV) pacing in patients typical of those enrolled in heart failure clinical trials. Cardiac resynchronization therapy device optimization requires a multidisciplinary approach involving the patient, electrophysiologist, referring cardiologist, and echocardiography laboratory and cardiac device technicians. Successful biventricular pacing typically results in an improvement in symptoms by one New York Heart Association functional class and at least 20% improvement in Minnesota Living with Heart Failure Questionnaire scores. Quality-of-life score, calculated as 105 minus the Minnesota Living with Heart Failure Questionnaire score (thus, a higher score is better functional capacity), is shown in *open bars*. *Solid bars* are peak oxygen consumption (VO_2) during exercise testing. V-HeFT refers to the average values for these parameters for patients enrolled in the Vasodilator in Heart Failure Trials. However, evidence from clinical trials suggests that approximately 30% of patients who receive resynchronization therapy do not respond favorably; reasons for failure to respond include insufficient baseline ventricular dyssynchrony, failure to resynchronize left ventricular (LV) function because of inadequate LV lead position, lack of viable lateral wall myocardium, and suboptimal device programming. In particular, improper programming of atrioventricular delay can worsen heart failure by decreasing LV filling time, thus reducing LV stroke volume and cardiac output. (*Adapted from* Stevenson [17].)

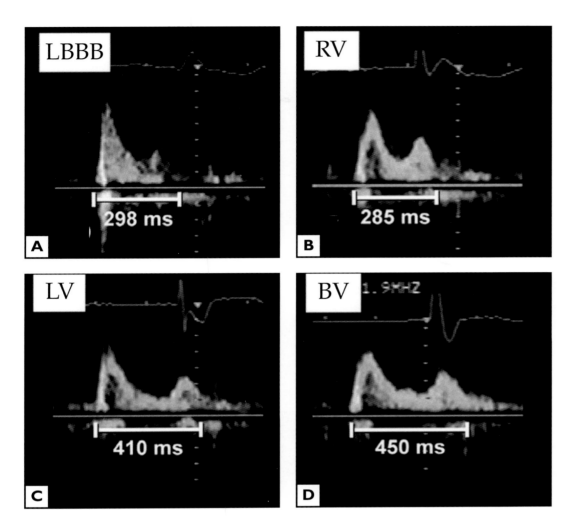

FIGURE 7-23. Doppler echocardiography: an important tool for proper atrioventricular (AV) delay selection. When the AV interval is too short, early mitral filling (E wave) tends to lengthen; however, the A wave is prematurely truncated, compromising LV filling. The effect of an optimized AV interval during three different pacing conditions on diastolic filling time as measured by pulsed wave Doppler. In this example, the longest diastolic filling time is achieved with left ventricular (LV) stimulation (**C**) and biventricular (BV) pacing (**D**), whereas right ventricular (RV) apical stimulation (**B**) and baseline left bundle branch block (**A**) had no significant effect on diastolic filling period. (*From* Breithardt *et al.* [18]; with permission.)

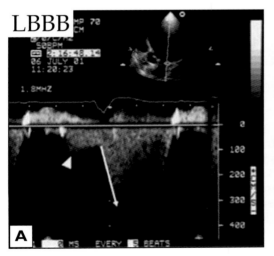
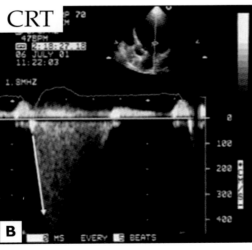

FIGURE 7-24. Use of Doppler echocardiography to assist device optimization. The use of Doppler echocardiography-assisted device programming is crucial to determine the shortest possible atrioventricular (AV) delay that allows for complete ventricular filling to optimize stroke volume while minimizing presystolic mitral regurgitation. The figure shows a regurgitant jet across the mitral valve by continuous-wave Doppler (**A**) at baseline left bundle branch block (LBBB) and (**B**) during biventricular resynchronization with optimized AV interval. The presence of first-degree AV block and LBBB leads to diastolic mitral regurgitation (*arrowhead*) and a lower rate of pressure rise, as elucidated by the slow increase in the regurgitation velocity. The presystolic component of mitral regurgitation can be completely eliminated by optimizing the AV delay. In addition, cardiac resynchronization significantly improves left ventricular systolic function, as demonstrated by the steeper regurgitant jet. Estimated left ventricular plus rate of pressure rise increases from 450 mm Hg/sec to 650 mm Hg/sec. CRT—cardiac resynchronization therapy. (*From* Breithardt *et al.* [18]; with permission.)

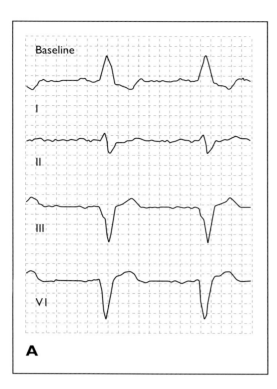

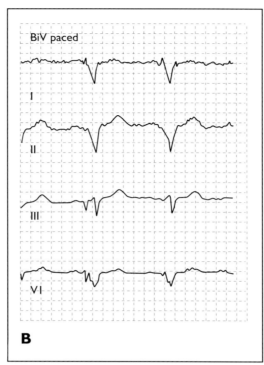

FIGURE 7-25. Typical ECG findings in a patient with a cardiac resynchronization therapy (CRT) device. Any change in a CRT patient's clinical course should prompt an evaluation that should include an ECG to ensure left ventricular capture, a chest radiograph to exclude lead dislodgement, and device interrogation to ensure appropriate sensing and capture. **A** and **B**, The figure shows a typical ECG tracing from a patient with a biventricular pacemaker. Note the negative QRS deflection in lead I, suggesting a lateral left ventricular (LV) stimulation site. Furthermore, the deeper S wave in lead II when compared with lead III suggests LV stimulation via a postero-lateral cardiac vein. Also notable is the narrowing of the QRS complex during biventricular (BiV) pacing (**B**) compared with the patient's intrinsic rhythm (**A**). Standard 12-lead ECGs are shown. Recording speed = 50 mm/s.

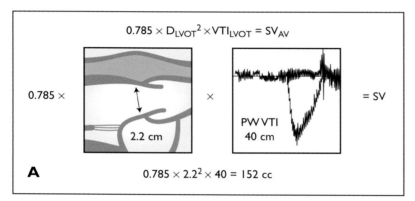

$$0.785 \times D_{LVOT}^2 \times VTI_{LVOT} = SV_{AV}$$

$0.785 \times$ 2.2 cm $\times$ PW VTI 40 cm $= SV$

A $0.785 \times 2.2^2 \times 40 = 152$ cc

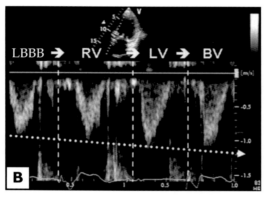

FIGURE 7-26. Hemodynamic assessment of stroke volume using the velocity time integral (VTI). In patients who fail to respond to resynchronization therapy, a thorough hemodynamic assessment of left ventricular (LV) performance should be performed with Doppler echocardiography interrogating mitral valve inflow, aortic VTI (as a surrogate for cardiac output), and tissue Doppler imaging. **A,** The VTI method to estimate the ventricular stroke volume (SV) uses two-dimensional echocardiography to measure the diameter (D) of the LV outflow tract (LVOT) and Doppler interrogation of the aortic interval to determine the stroke distance. Measuring the diameter of the LV outflow allows calculation of its cross-sectional area by assuming it is circular. The product of cross-sectional area and the stroke distance (the distance to the outer edge of the aortic outflow envelope) estimates SV. **B,** Pulsed-wave (PW) Doppler VTI from the LVOT as a surrogate for LV SV (taken with optimized atrioventricular delay in the pacing conditions and stable heart rate in all conditions). The VTI increase is dependent on the stimulation site: only a slight increase is observed in the aortic VTI during right ventricular (RV) apical pacing, whereas LV stimulation and biventricular (BV) pacing lead to significant increase in SV, as assessed by the aortic VTI. AV—atrioventricular. (*Part A from* Leon [19]; with permission. *Part B from* Breithardt *et al.* [18]; with permission.)

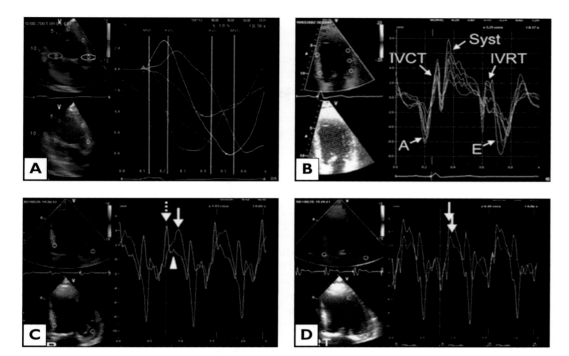

FIGURE 7-27. Tissue Doppler imaging (TDI). TDI is a newer technique that measures the velocity of myocardial wall motion. TDI allows for quantification of regional myocardial function. There are three main components of the TDI signal: systolic (Sm), early (Em), and late diastolic (Am). The diastolic components of myocardial velocities correlate with mitral inflow velocities. TDI myocardial velocities from apical views reflect longitudinal shortening and relaxation of the myocardium; the normal variation in TDI is greatest at the base and decreases toward the apex, which is relatively stationary. TDI is proving to be a useful tool not only to identify ventricular dyssynchrony, but also to confirm left ventricular (LV) resynchronization following cardiac device therapy. **A,** TDI strain analysis from a two-chamber view in a patient with left bundle branch block. The *solid lines* indicate mitral valve closure (MVC), aortic valve opening (AVO), aortic valve closure (AVC), and mitral valve opening (MVO). The *red and dark green cursors* are positioned on the inferior wall, which starts to contract on time whereas the anterior wall segments (*yellow and light green cursors*) are late activated and thus initially stretched before they start to contract late and reach their peak strain after AVC. Consequently, isovolumic contraction time (IVCT) is prolonged, ejection time is shortened, and isovolumic relaxation time (IVRT) is prolonged with impaired systolic and diastolic performance. **B,** TDI velocity curves from six LV segments (*circles, upper left*). The regional velocity-time profiles are well synchronized and display normal (rapid) conduction and synchronous contraction of all segments. The short isovolumic relaxation and contraction times can be distinguished from the systolic apical motion (Syst, positive velocity) and the early (E) and late (A) diastolic peaks. **C and D,** TDI curves from the basal septum and the basal lateral wall in a patient with nonischemic dilated cardiomyopathy and left bundle branch block. There is a large temporal delay between the regional velocity peaks (*dashed and solid arrow*) before stimulation (LSB), which is significantly reduced (synchronized) during cardiac resynchronization therapy (CRT; *solid arrows*). However, in some cases, the differentiation between isovolumic events and the systolic velocity peaks may be difficult and does not always allow a reliable assessment of CRT efficacy. In the present example, it remains unclear if the early peak velocity (*dashed arrow*) or the later and smaller systolic peak (*arrowhead*) in the septal velocity curve indicates peak systolic motion. The first peak (*dashed arrow*) might represent IVCT rather than systolic contraction. (*Part A from* Sogaard *et al.* [20]; with permission. *Parts B–D from* Breithardt *et al.* [18]; with permission.)

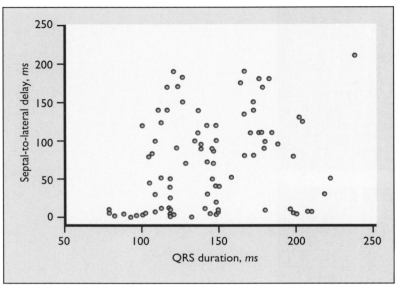

FIGURE 7-28. Future directions. Many subsets of patients are under-represented in clinical resynchronization trials, such as patients with permanent atrial fibrillation, New York Heart Association class I and II heart failure patients, children, congenital heart disease patients, and patients with left ventricular dysfunction undergoing cardiac surgery. Perhaps the largest patient population not included in resynchronization therapy trials are narrow QRS cardiomyopathy patients with evidence of ventricular dys-synchrony assessed by noninvasive imaging modalities (*eg*, tissue Doppler imaging, M-mode echocardiography, or MRI). As mentioned in a previous chapter, there is evidence to suggest that significant interventricular and intraventricular dyssynchrony may exist in cardiomyopathy patients despite normal QRS durations. The QRS duration is at best a "crude" surrogate for ventricular dyssynchrony. The graph shows normal QRS duration dyssynchrony and the relationship between septal-to-lateral delay and QRS duration. No significant relation existed between QRS duration and septal-to-lateral delay ($y = 0.44x + 9.1$, $n = 90$, $r = 0.26$, not significant). Extensive left ventricular dyssynchrony was defined as an electromechanical delay on tissue Doppler imaging between the septum and lateral wall, the so-called septal-to-lateral delay, of more than 60 ms. Severe dyssynchrony was observed in 27% of patients with narrow QRS complex (120 ms), 60% with intermediate QRS duration (120 to 150 ms), and 70% with wide QRS complex (>150 ms). Furthermore, little is known about bi-ventricular pacing in patients with heart failure due to diastolic dysfunction. Finally, the effectiveness of left ventricular stimulation alone in the absence of right ventricular pacing is under investigation. (*Adapted from* Bleeker *et al.* [21].)

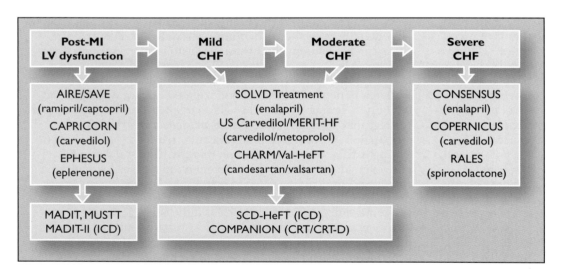

FIGURE 7-29. Union of pharmacotherapy and cardiac device therapy: optimal pharmacotherapy and device-based therapy across a spectrum of congestive heart failure (CHF), as well as the clinical trials that support the use of these various therapies. Biventricular pacing has proven beneficial in patients with ventricular dyssynchrony and symptomatic left ventricular (LV) dysfunction, regardless of the etiology of the cardiomyopathy. In the landmark Comparison of Medical Therapy, Pacing, and Defibrillation in Heart Failure (COMPANION) trial, resynchro-nization therapy in combination with an implantable cardioverter-defibrillator (ICD) has been shown to significantly reduce total mortality. Patient selection for resynchronization therapy remains an imperfect science. It is clear that identifying mechanically dyssynchronous ventricles with a high likelihood of being able to deliver site-specific resynchronization therapy is essential to selecting patients who are likely to benefit. Cardiac resynchro-nization therapy (CRT) has been studied largely among patients with advanced LV dysfunction and highly symptomatic heart failure; whether it should be extended to other subsets of patients requires further clinical investigation. Presently, CRT should be offered as an important nonpharmacologic and potentially life-saving intervention to eligible patients with ventricular dyssynchrony and symptomatic heart failure despite optimal phar-macotherapy. CRT-D—CRT plus defibrillator; MI—myocardial infarction; AIRE—Acute Infarction Ramipril Efficacy Trial; SAVE—Survival and Ventricular Enlargement; SOLVD—Studies of Left Ventricular Dysfunction; CONSENSUS—Cooperative North Scandinavian Enalapril Survival Study; CAPRICORN—Carvedilol Post-Infarct Survival Control in LV Dysfunction; COPERNICUS—Effect of Carvedilol on Survival in Severe Chronic Heart Failure; EPHESUS—Eplerenone Post-AMI Heart Failure Efficacy and Survival Study; MERIT-HF—Metroprolol XL/CR Randomized Intervention Trial in Chronic Heart Failure; CHARM—Candesartan in Heart Failure Assessment of Reduction in Mortality and Morbidity; Val-HeFT—Valsartan Heart Failure Trial; RALES—Randomized Aldactone Evaluation Study; MADIT—Multicenter Automatic Defibrillator Implantation Trial; MUSTT—Multicenter Unsustained Tachycardia Trial; SCD-HeFT—Sudden Cardiac Death in Heart Failure Trial. (*Adapted from* Abraham; Personal communication.)

REFERENCES

1. Cesario DA, Valderrabano M, Cai JJ, *et al.*: Electrophysiological characterization of cardiac veins in humans. *J Interv Card Electrophysiol* 2004, 10:241–247.

2. Meisel E, Pfeiffer D, Engelmann L, *et al.*: Investigation of coronary venous anatomy by retrograde venography in patients with malignant ventricular tachycardia. *Circulation* 2001, 104:442–447.

3. Ji S, Cesario DA, Swerdlow CD, Shivkumar K: Left ventricular endocardial lead placement using a modified transseptal approach. *J Cardiovasc Electrophysiol* 2004, 15:234–236.

4. DeRose JJ, Ashton RC, Belsley S, *et al.*: Robotically assisted left ventricular epicardial lead implantation for biventricular pacing. *J Am Coll Cardiol* 2003, 41:1414–1419.

5. de Cock CC, van Campen CM, Visser CA: Major dissection of the coronary sinus and its tributaries during lead implantation for biventricular stimulation: angiographic follow-up. *Europace* 2004, 6:43–47.

6. Gras D, Leclercq C, Tang AS, *et al.*: Cardiac resynchronization therapy in advanced heart failure: the multicenter InSync clinical study. *Eur J Heart Fail* 2002, 4:311–320.

7. Auricchio A, Stellbrink C, Block M, *et al.*: Effect of pacing chamber and atrioventricular delay on acute systolic function of paced patients with congestive heart failure. The Pacing Therapies for Congestive Heart Failure Study Group. The Guidant Congestive Heart Failure Research Group. *Circulation* 1999, 99:2993–3001.

8. Abraham WT: Cardiac resynchronization therapy: a review of clinical trials and criteria for identifying the appropriate patient. *Rev Cardiovasc Med* 2003, 4(Suppl 2):S30–S37.

9. Abraham WT, Fisher WG, Smith AL, *et al.*: Cardiac resynchronization in chronic heart failure. *N Eng J Med* 2002, 346:1845–1853.

10. Young JB, Abraham WT, Smith AL, *et al.*, Multicenter InSync ICD Randomized Clinical Evaluation (MIRACLE ICD) Trial Investigators: Combined cardiac resynchronization and implantable cardioversion defibrillation in advanced chronic heart failure: the MIRACLE ICD Trial. *JAMA* 2003, 289:2685–2694.

11. Bristow M, Saxon LA, Boehmer J, *et al.*: Cardiac-resynchronization therapy with or without an implantable defibrillator in advanced chronic heart failure. *N Engl J Med* 2004, 350:2140–2150.

12. Auricchio A, Abraham WT: Cardiac resynchronization therapy: current state of the art: cost versus benefit. *Circulation* 2004, 109:300–307.

13. Linde C, Leclercq C, Rex S, *et al.*: Long-term benefits of biventricular pacing in congestive heart failure: results from the MUltisite STimulation in cardiomyopathy (MUSTIC) study. *J Am Coll Cardiol* 2002, 40:111–118.

14. Doshi RN, Daoud E, Fellows C, *et al.*: The PAVE trial: the first prospective, randomized study evaluating BV pacing after ablate and pace therapy. Paper presented at the 53rd Annual Scientific Session of the American College of Cardiology. New Orleans, LA, March 7–10, 2004.

15. Bradley DJ, Bradley EA, Baughman KL, *et al.*: Cardiac resynchronization and death from progressive heart failure: a meta-analysis of randomized controlled trials. *JAMA* 2003, 289:730–740.

16. Salukhe TV, Dimopoulos K, Francis D: Cardiac resynchronisation may reduce all-cause mortality: meta-analysis of preliminary COMPANION data with CONTAK-CD, InSync ICD, MIRACLE and MUSTIC. *Int J Cardiol* 2004, 93:101–103.

17. Stevenson LW: The points for pacing. *J Am Coll Cardiol* 2003, 42:1460–1462.

18. Breithardt OA, Sinha AM, Franke A, *et al.*: Echocardiography in cardiac resynchronization therapy: identification of suitable patients, follow-up and therapy optimization [in German]. *Herz* 2003, 7:615–627.

19. Leon AR: Cardiac resynchronization therapy devices: patient management and follow-up strategies. *Rev Cardiovasc Med* 2003, 4(Suppl 2):S38–S46.

20. Sogaard P, Hassager C: Tissue Doppler imaging as a guide to resynchronization therapy in patients with congestive heart failure. *Curr Opin Cardiol* 2004, 5:447–451.

21. Bleeker GB, Schalij MJ, Molhoek SG, *et al.*: Relationship between QRS duration and left ventricular dyssynchrony in patients with end-stage heart failure. *J Cardiovasc Electrophysiol* 2004, 15:544–549.

Risk Stratification for Sudden Death in Patients With Heart Failure

William H. Sauer, Hemal M. Nayak, and Francis E. Marchlinski

Sudden cardiac death is a major public health problem affecting patients with congestive heart failure. Although it remains the most common cause of death in this population, significant progress has been made in the prevention and treatment of sudden death in patients with heart failure. The discovery of new medical therapies and the advent of the implantable cardioverter-defibrillator (ICD) have made a significant impact on reducing sudden death in patients with heart failure.

It is the use of the ICD for primary prevention of sudden cardiac death that provides the impetus for identification of individuals at highest risk of sudden death. Clinical trials investigating the efficacy of ICDs have used various methods for the identification of the high-risk patient, including left ventricular ejection fraction, ventricular ectopy, electrophysiologic studies, and markers for autonomic nervous system dysfunction. In addition, many observational studies and retrospective analyses of these trials have allowed for some insight into sudden death risk stratification using molecular markers, standard electrocardiography, and signal processing data.

Despite the myriad methods of assessing risk, there remains a lack of specificity for patients with congestive heart failure for predicting sudden death and uncertainty on the best approach for risk stratification. Nonetheless, important information pertaining to sudden death risk can be obtained from a patient's clinical presentation and measured electrophysiologic parameters. Studies evaluating myocardial function, the autonomic nervous system, and cardiac electrophysiology provide a wealth of information on the potential risk of sudden death. In addition, future risk assessment with newer serum and genetic assays may also assist in the identification of high-risk individuals and heart failure patients.

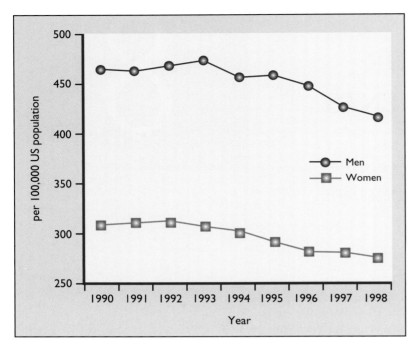

FIGURE 8-1. The incidence of sudden cardiac death in the US population. The incidence of sudden cardiac death in the US population has declined over the past decade, which is likely the result, in part, of improved identification of high-risk patients and the use of the implantable cardioverter-defibrillator for prevention of sudden death. Despite this decline, sudden death remains a major public health concern. Using US vital statistics mortality data, Zheng *et al.* [1] discovered that more than 450,000 people die from sudden death per year. These investigators also noted a higher death rate in the black population compared with whites and Hispanics, although race has not formally been assessed for risk of sudden death [2]. (*Data from* Zheng *et al.* [1].)

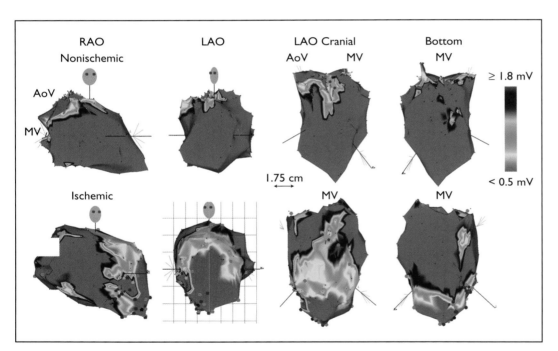

FIGURE 8-2. Electroanatomic voltage maps (CARTO images) of patients with ischemic and nonischemic cardiomyopathy and ventricular tachycardia. Electroanatomic mapping uses an external magnetic field and a magnetic field sensor at the tip of a catheter inside a cardiac chamber. The catheter tip records local electrogram voltage from within the cardiac chamber in addition to its precise location in three-dimensional space. As the electrogram voltages and spatial coordinates of the catheter are recorded and charted point by point within a cardiac chamber, the three-dimensional reconstruction of the local geometry is displayed as a color voltage map on a monitor. Here, the reconstructed voltage maps from two patients are displayed from multiple angles. The *top row* is the left ventricle of a patient with a nonischemic cardiomyopathy, and the *bottom row* is from a patient with a prior myocardial infarction. The patient with a nonischemic cardiomyopathy has perivalvular fibrosis and scarring (*red, low-voltage area*), which acts as the substrate for malignant ventricular arrhythmias. In the patient with coronary disease and ischemic cardiomyopathy, a large anterior wall scar was the substrate for frequent episodes of symptomatic ventricular tachycardia. Although both nonischemic and ischemic heart failure populations suffer from ventricular arrhythmias, the risk for sudden death has been observed to be higher in those with ischemic cardiomyopathy [3]. AoV—aortic valve; LAO—left anterior oblique; MV—mitral valve; RAO—right anterior oblique.

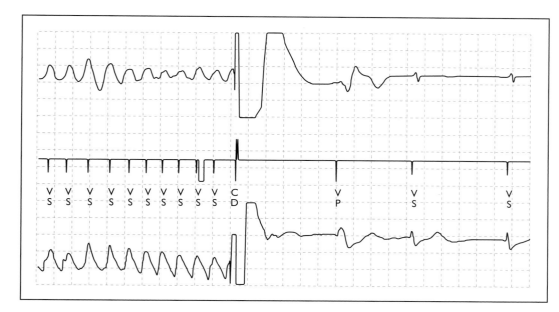

FIGURE 8-3. Intracardiac electrogram of implantable cardioverter-defibrillator (ICD) shock terminating ventricular fibrillation in patient with ischemic cardiomyopathy. The ICD is the most effective therapy for prevention of sudden death in patients with heart failure. The use of the ICD for primary prevention of sudden cardiac death has provided the impetus for identification of individuals at highest risk of sudden death. In this example, the ICD accurately recognized ventricular fibrillation and terminated the rhythm with a shock.

A. METHODS USED IN MAJOR TRIALS FOR RISK STRATIFICATION FOR SUDDEN DEATH

TRIAL NAME (ACRONYM)	METHODS FOR SUDDEN DEATH RISK STRATIFICATION USED AS INCLUSION CRITERIA
Multicenter Automatic Defibrillator Implantation Trial (MADIT-I)	Prior Q wave myocardial infarction, left ventricular ejection fraction < 0.35, nonsustained ventricular tachycardia, inducible ventricular tachycardia during invasive electrophysiologic testing that was not suppressible with procainamide
Multicenter Unsustained Tachycardia Trial (MUSTT)	Prior myocardial infarction, left ventricular ejection fraction < 0.40, inducible ventricular tachycardia during invasive electrophysiologic testing
Multicenter Automatic Defibrillator Implantation Trial (MADIT-II)	Prior myocardial infarction, left ventricular ejection fraction < 0.30
Coronary Artery Bypass Grafting Patch Trial (CABG Patch)	Coronary disease requiring surgical revascularization, left ventricular ejection fraction < 0.35, abnormal signal-averaged electrocardiogram
Defibrillators in Nonischemic Cardiomyopathy Treatment Evaluation (DEFINITE)	Nonischemic cardiomyopathy, left ventricular ejection fraction < 0.35, frequent premature ventricular complexes or nonsustained ventricular tachycardia
Defibrillators in Acute Myocardial Infarction Trial (DINAMIT)	Recent myocardial infarction (6–40 days), left ventricular ejection fraction < 0.35, depressed heart rate variability (standard deviation of normal RR intervals < 70 ms) or elevated heart rate (mean 24-hour RR < 750 ms)
Sudden Cardiac Death Heart Failure Trial (SCD-HeFT)	New York Heart Association functional class II or III, left ventricular ejection fraction < 0.35

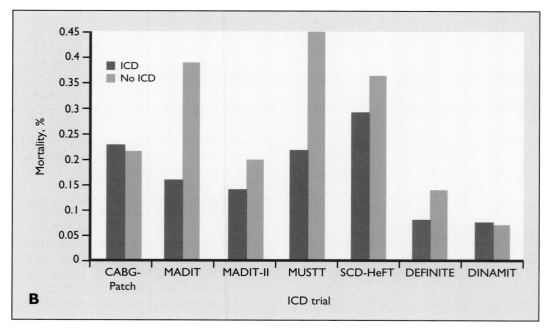

FIGURE 8-4. Risk stratification used in clinical trials investigating the efficacy of implantable cardioverter-defibrillators (ICDs) for prevention of sudden death. **A,** Various methods have been used for identifying patients at high risk for sudden death for the purpose of evaluating the efficacy of the ICD. All the major clinical trials listed here used reduced left ventricular ejection fraction as an inclusion criteria. In addition, the Multicenter Automatic Defibrillator Implantation Trial (MADIT-I) and Multicenter Unsustained Tachycardia Trial (MUSTT) used invasive electrophysiologic testing to identify the highest risk patients. The Coronary Artery Bypass Grafting Patch Trial (CABG Patch) used abnormal signal–averaged electrocardiography, and the Defibrillators in Acute Myocardial Infarction Trial (DINAMIT) used heart rate variability in addition to reduced ejection fraction for inclusion criteria. **B,** The main results of the trials showing improved mortality in subjects randomized to ICD therapy in all but two of the trials [4–6].

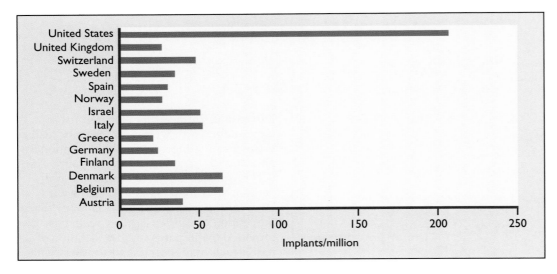

FIGURE 8-5. Annual implantable cardio-verter-defibrillator (ICD) implants per million people by country. There is an apparent discrepancy among nations in the worldwide implementation of screening for patients at high risk for sudden death, with the greatest number of ICD implants occurring in the United States. (*Data from* Huikuri *et al.* [2].)

ASSESSMENT OF CARDIAC FUNCTION

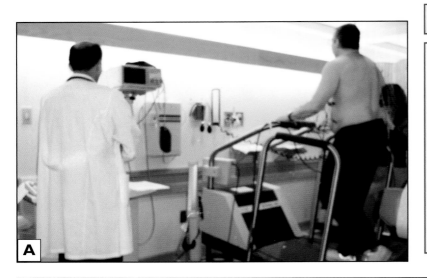

B. NAUGHTON PROTOCOL

NYHA CLASS	METS	STAGE	SPEED, MPH	GRADE, %
IV	2.5	1	1.0	0
IV	3.0	2	1.5	0
III	3.5	3	2.0	0
III	4.0	4	2.0	3.5
III	4.5	5	2.0	7.0
II	5.5	6	3.0	5.0
II	6.5	7	3.0	7.5
I	7.5	8	3.0	10.0

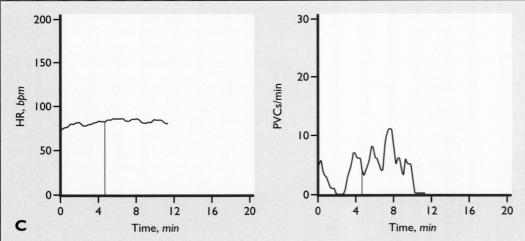

FIGURE 8-6. Exercise testing for assessment of functional status. Walking on a treadmill using the Naughton protocol (**A** and **B**), which gradually increases the demand for physical activity, quantifies physical activity in metabolic equivalents (METS). Each MET is equivalent to the myocardial oxygen consumption unit of 3.5 mL O_2/kg/min. The 6-minute walk test is also a measure of exercise capacity that is frequently used in patients with heart failure. Most of the data regarding the role of exercise stress testing for the prediction of sudden death are from studies investigating its role following myocardial infarction and are not specific to patients with heart failure. However, ischemic cardiomyopathy is the most common cause of heart failure, and stress test information including functional class, frequency of ventricular ectopy, and heart rate (HR) recovery may be applicable to this patient population for prediction of sudden death. In this example, the patient was able to achieve 3.5 METS before dyspnea limited further exercise. Frequent ventricular ectopy, a nonspecific marker for sudden cardiac death, was also noted (**C**). NYHA—New York Heart Association; PVCs—premature ventricular contractions.

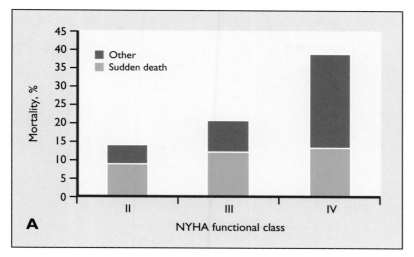

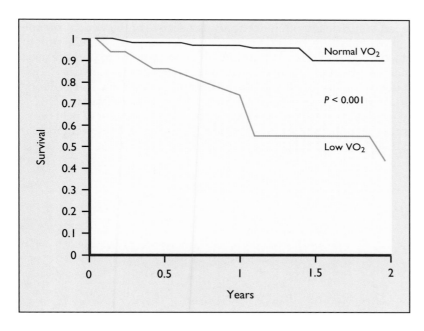

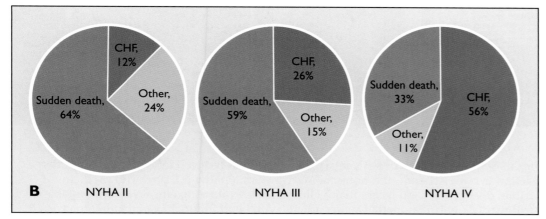

FIGURE 8-7. Mortality and prevalence of sudden cardiac death by New York Heart Association (NYHA) functional class. The NYHA functional classification system is a simple categorization describing a spectrum of symptom-limited activities that may affect patients with heart failure. Class I patients have structural heart disease but are asymptomatic and have no limitations. Class II patients have only modest limitations in their physical activity—they are comfortable at rest and can accomplish most ordinary activities of daily living but will be uncomfortable with any amount of exertion. Class III patients are comfortable at rest but are easily fatigued or dyspneic with ordinary activities of daily living. Finally, class IV patients are unable to carry out any physical activity without feeling uncomfortable. Clinical assessment of functional class is a simple and non-invasive method for determining mortality risk in patients with heart failure as described above. **A**, The mortality rate observed in the Metoprolol Randomized Intervention Trial in Congestive Heart Failure (MERIT-HF) over a 20-month period [7]. **B**, The proportion of sudden death is highest among those with mild to moderate congestive heart failure (CHF), thus the risk of sudden death is not as dramatic as this risk of total mortality with increasing severity of clinical heart failure.

FIGURE 8-8. Peak oxygen consumption and the risk of sudden death. Just as New York Heart Association (NYHA) functional class is associated with mortality, reduced myocardial oxygen consumption is also related to worse outcomes. Cardiopulmonary exercise testing is the most precise method for measuring exercise capacity because it accounts for pulmonary gas exchange, cardiac performance, and skeletal muscle metabolism. Exercise capacity can be quantified clinically by measurement of oxygen uptake (Vo_2), carbon dioxide production (Vco_2), and minute ventilation. These parameters are measured during exercise with rapidly responding gas analyzers capable of breath-by-breath determination of O_2 and CO_2 concentrations. The maximal oxygen uptake (Vo_2max) eventually reaches a plateau despite increasing workload. In one study evaluating the role of Vo_2max for risk stratification, patients with NYHA functional class II and III heart failure from either ischemic or nonischemic cardiomyopathy underwent cardiopulmonary exercise testing [8]. Patients who achieved less than 50% maximal predicted Vo_2 had a higher mortality rate compared with those with normal Vo_2 levels.

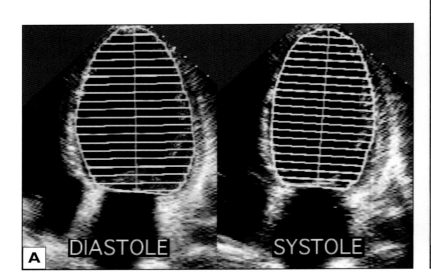

A DIASTOLE | SYSTOLE

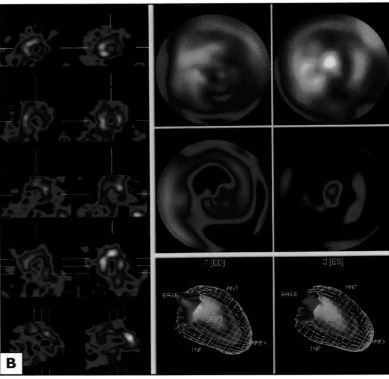

B

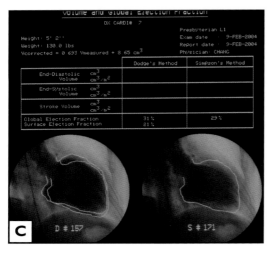

C

FIGURE 8-9. Assessment of left ventricular function. A reduced left ventricular ejection fraction in both ischemic and nonischemic cardiomyopathy is a powerful predictor of sudden death [9–11]. All recent major clinical trials evaluating efficacy of implantable cardioverter-defibrillators (ICDs) in patients with heart failure have included the use of ejection fraction for inclusion in the trial. Echocardiography is a common method for determining left ventricular function. Mathematical equations that assume a bullet or ellipsoid geometry of the left ventricle are often not accurate because of the variable shape and size of this chamber in patients with heart failure. For this reason, it is often helpful to use Simpson's rule, in which a series of discs in multiple ultrasonographic planes are used to calculate ejection fraction (**A**). Ejection fraction can also be assessed with nuclear imaging (**B**) and contrast ventriculography (**C**). In the Multicenter Automatic Defibrillator Implantation Trial II (MADIT-II), all three of these methods for assessment of left ventricular function were used. In this trial, a left ventricular ejection fraction of 0.30 or less was the only risk stratification method prior to randomization for ICD implantation for prevention of sudden death [12].

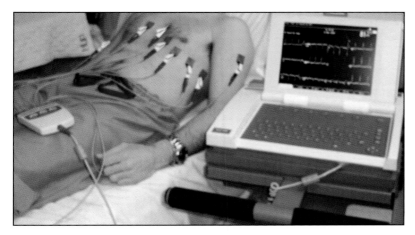

FIGURE 8-10. Standard 12-lead electrocardiography. Standard electrocardiography remains a widespread and powerful tool for risk stratification of sudden death. Electrocardiographic recordings of frequent ventricular ectopy and nonsustained ventricular tachycardia were used as inclusion criteria in the Multicenter Automatic Defibrillator Implantation Trial (MADIT-I), Defibrillators in Non-ischemic Cardiomyopathy Treatment Evaluation (DEFINITE), and Multicenter Unsustained Tachycardia Trial (MUSTT). In addition, abnormalities in intraventricular conduction and repolarization may be observed with standard electrocardiography and may play a role in sudden death risk assessment, as observed in other studies.

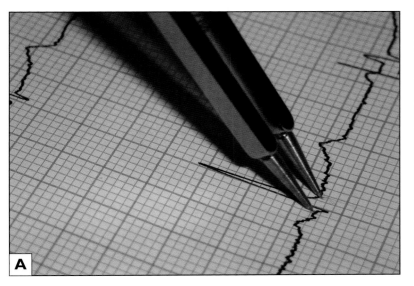

A

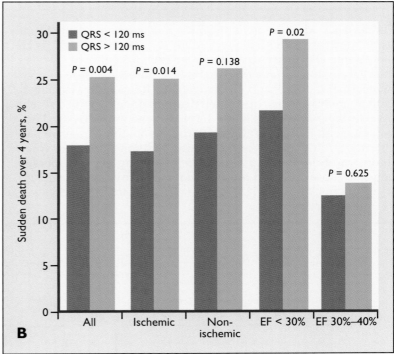

B

FIGURE 8-11. Assessment of QRS duration using standard 12-lead electrocardiography. **A,** QRS duration measurement on standard 12-lead ECGs is simple and inexpensive. In the Losartan Heart Failure Survival Study, QRS duration was significantly longer in patients who died from sudden cardiac death [13]. **B,** In the Survival Trial of Antiarrhythmic Therapy in Congestive Heart Failure (CHF-STAT), QRS prolongation (> 120 ms) was associated with a significant increase in mortality and sudden death in patients with low left ventricular ejection fraction (EF) [14]. In addition, retrospective analysis of the second Multicenter Automatic Defibrillator Implantation Trial (MADIT-II) suggested a greater benefit from prophylactic implantable cardioverter-defibrillator insertion in this group of patients [10]. (*Panel B adapted from* Iuliano *et al.* [14].)

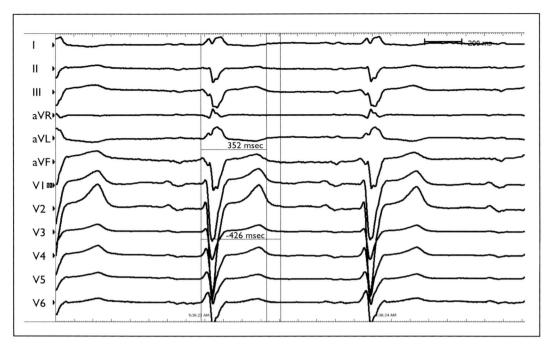

FIGURE 8-12. Measurement of QT dispersion. Another potentially useful measure provided by standard electrocardiography is QT dispersion. QT dispersion is the interlead variability of QT intervals on the surface ECG and is an indirect measure of myocardial repolarization heterogeneity. It has been associated with an increased risk of sudden death in patients with a recent myocardial infarction. Although QT dispersion is increased in patients with idiopathic dilated cardiomyopathy who have had an arrhythmic event, one study found that this parameter was of limited usefulness because of the large overlap of QT dispersion between those with and those without an arrhythmic event [15]. In addition, Gang *et al.* [13] found no significant differences in QT or JT dispersion in patients who died suddenly compared with survivors in the Losartan Heart Failure Survival Study (ELITE-II) [13]. In contrast, other investigations have reported a significant association with QT (or JTc) dispersion of more than 85 to 90 ms and sudden death in patients with ischemic or nonischemic cardiomyopathy [16,17]. In one study of patients with advanced heart failure, the 3-year mortality in those with QT dispersion greater than 90 ms was significantly higher than for those with QT dispersion of 90 ms or less (31% vs 17%) [18]. Shown in the figure is a measured QT dispersion of 73 ms, with 352 ms measured in lead I and 425 ms measured in lead V_2.

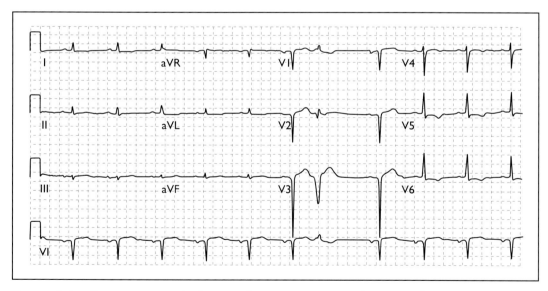

FIGURE 8-13. Premature ventricular complexes in a patient with ischemic cardiomyopathy. Although ventricular ectopy following myocardial infarction has been identified as a risk factor for sudden death, the utility of this marker in patients with congestive heart failure remains uncertain. In patients with heart failure enrolled in the Prospective Randomized Milrinone Survival Evaluation (PROMISE), ventricular ectopy did not predict sudden death [19]. However, analysis of recordings in patients with reduced left ventricular ejection fraction, which were obtained from implanted cardioverter-defibrillators, shows monomorphic ventricular tachycardia is most often initiated by multiple ventricular premature beats [20]. These complexes had a distinct morphology that is different from the ventricular tachycardia, suggesting their role in triggering ventricular arrhythmias. Shown here is a 12-lead ECG of sinus rhythm with a premature ventricular complex in a patient with a remote anterior wall myocardial infarction and ischemic cardiomyopathy.

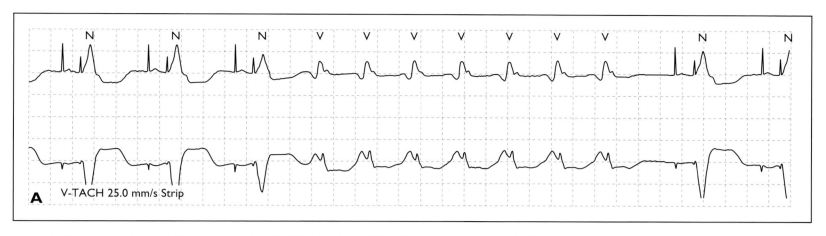

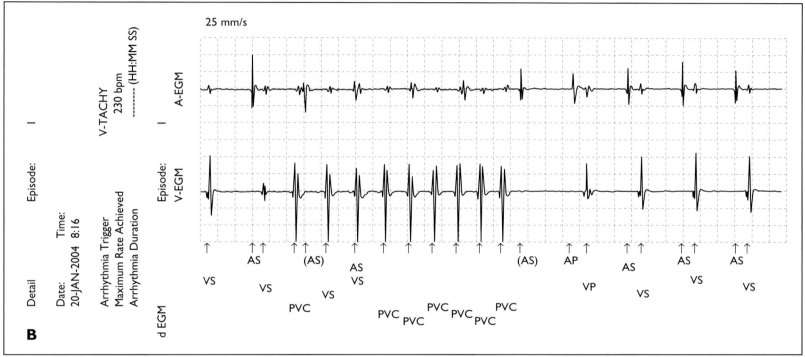

FIGURES 8-14. Nonsustained ventricular tachycardia (NSVT).
A, Asymptomatic episode of NSVT captured on Holter monitoring.
B, A similar patient with a dual-chamber pacemaker had an episode recorded by the device and retrieved during routine pacemaker interrogation. NSVT is a common asymptomatic finding in patients with heart failure. Its identification as a marker for sudden death in this population was validated with data analyzed from the Multicenter Post-Infarction Program [21]. In this study, patients with NSVT and left ventricular ejection fraction less than 0.40 had a fivefold higher risk of sudden death compared with other patients after myocardial infarction. NSVT as a marker for sudden death was used for identification of high-risk patients with coronary artery disease enrolled in the Multicenter Unsustained Tachycardia Trial (MUSTT) [22]. The association between NSVT and sudden

death is less clear in patients with nonischemic cardiomyopathy. Although a prospective cohort analysis from the Grupo de Estudio de la Sobrevida en la Insuficiencia Cardiaca en Argentina (GESICA) study demonstrated a significant association between NSVT and sudden death in patients with nonischemic cardiomyopathy, other investigations did not support this observation [9,23]. The Survival Trial of Antiarrhythmic Therapy in Congestive Heart Failure (CHF-STAT) observed a higher rate of sudden death in patients with nonischemic cardiomyopathy and NSVT, which was not apparent after adjustment for functional class and ejection fraction [24]. In addition, a meta-analysis of major studies evaluating the importance of NSVT in nonischemic cardiomyopathy concluded that its presence is not specific to subsequent sudden death [25]. EGM—electrogram; PVC—premature ventricular contraction.

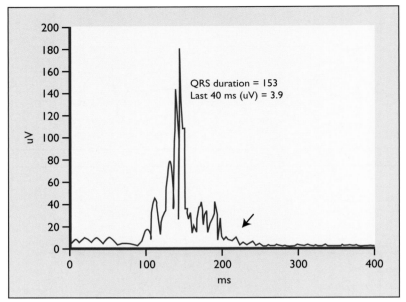

FIGURE 8-15. Signal-averaged electrocardiography (SAECG). SAECG is a noninvasive technique that can identify the presence of slow conduction through infracted or fibrosed myocardium, which may serve as the substrate for malignant ventricular arrhythmias. SAECG is used to identify low-amplitude signals at the end of the QRS complex, referred to as late potentials, that cannot be detected on standard ECGs and that represent regional delayed activation. The late potentials are seen after averaging hundreds of QRS complexes and processing the signals through digital filtering and spectral analysis. Late potentials are defined by the total filtered QRS duration (> 114 ms), the voltage in the terminal portion of the QRS (the last 40 ms), and the duration of the terminal QRS that is below a particular amplitude (40 microvolts). The use of the SAECG for prediction of sudden death in patients with low left ventricular ejection fraction (< 0.40) was evaluated in the Multicenter Unsustained Tachycardia Trial (MUSTT), in which an abnormal signal-averaged ECG was a powerful predictor of mortality [26]. In addition, SAECG was associated with a high negative predictive power when normal in an observational study of patients following myocardial infarction [27]. Shown here is an abnormal SAECG from a patient with nonischemic cardiomyopathy with the presence of a late potential (*arrow*).

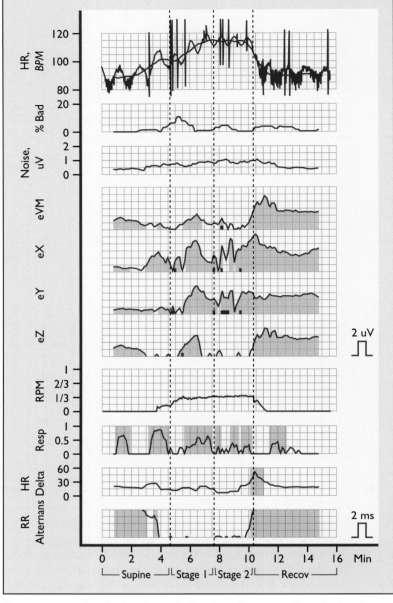

FIGURE 8-16. Analysis of repolarization alternans. Repolarization alternans, or T wave alternans, is the altered repolarization timing or morphology observed on alternating beats, reflecting repolarization heterogeneity. Detection of the microvolt alternans requires analysis of at least 128 electrograms (recorded during exercise) using the fast Fourier transformation spectral method. This method uses the signal recorded from three orthogonal leads and detects amplitude differences in beat-to-beat fluctuations. A test is determined to be positive when there is sustained alternans with an amplitude of at least 1.9 microvolts. Patients with heart failure and abnormal repolarization alternans are at significantly increased risk for sudden death [28,29]. In one study of 107 patients with New York Heart Association functional class II or III heart failure, 11 of 52 patients (21%) with an abnormal T wave alternans test suffered an arrhythmic death, compared with 0 of 33 patients with normal tests [28]. This suggests a possible role for microvolt T wave alternans in the identification of heart failure patients at low risk for sudden death. Shown here is an example of a positive microvolt T wave alternans test with the presence of sustained T wave alternans greater than 1.9 microvolts after the patient achieved a heart rate (HR) greater than 70% of the maximum predicted.

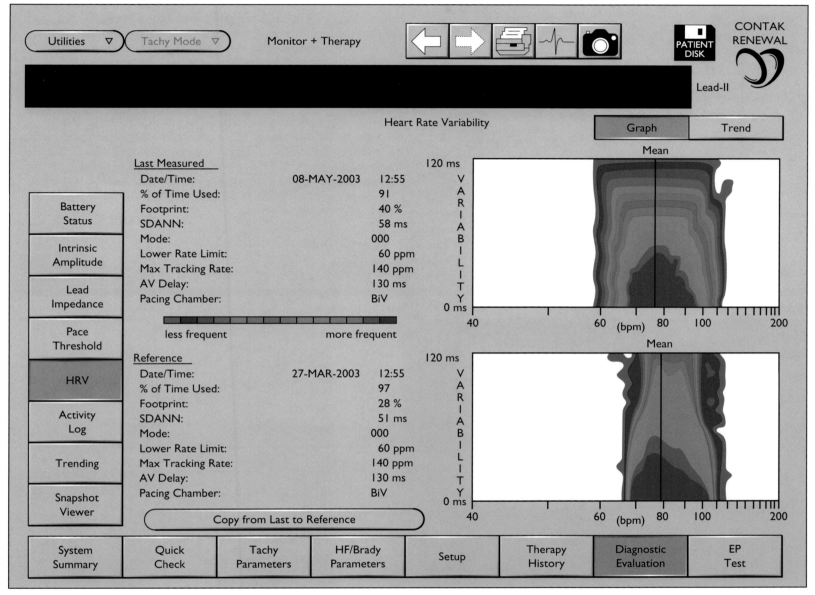

FIGURE 8-17. Heart rate variability (HRV) map in a patient with a biventricular (BiV) pacemaker. There is a growing body of evidence that the autonomic nervous system affects the triggering and maintenance of malignant ventricular tachyarrhythmias. Heart rate variability is an indirect measure of autonomic nervous system effects on the cardiovascular system. There are two separate methods for analysis of heart rate variability: time and frequency domain measurements. In a study examining heart rate variability in patients with congestive heart failure, individuals with a standard deviation of normal RR intervals (SDNN) less than 50 ms had a 51% mortality compared with a 5% mortality in those with an SDNN greater than 100 ms [30]. Another study of patients with ischemic cardiomyopathy showed that low heart rate variability (SDNN < 65.3 ms) was independently associated with risk for sudden death [31]. However, a substudy of the Danish Investigations of Arrhythmia and Mortality on Dofetilide (DIAMOND) found that measures of heart rate variability were predictive of mortality in patients with class II heart failure, but did not provide independent prognostic information in patients with the most severe functional impairment (class IV heart failure) [32]. The figure shows time-domain heart rate variability in a patient with an implanted biventricular defibrillator. In this example, the frequency of altered RR intervals is denoted by color and the degree of the altered RR interval is plotted on the two-dimensional array, with the mean RR interval represented by a *vertical line*. AV—atrioventricular; EP—electrophysiologic; HF—heart failure; ppm—pulses per minute.

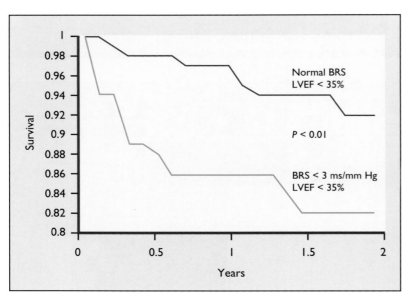

FIGURE 8-18. Assessment of baroreflex sensitivity (BRS). Similar to heart rate variability, baroreflex sensitivity is another measure of the autonomic nervous system's effect on the cardiovascular system. A normal baroreflex response is vagally mediated heart rate slowing in response to elevation in blood pressure. An abnormal baroreflex results from autonomic dysfunction and will lead to unchanged heart rate or minimal slowing with an acute rise in blood pressure. The accepted abnormal value for baroreflex sensitivity based on phenylephrine administration is less than 3 ms reduction in sinus rhythm cycle length per 1 mm Hg rise in mean arterial blood pressure. Although not specifically addressing arrhythmia mortality, the Autonomic Tone and Reflexes After Myocardial Infarction (ATRAMI) trial demonstrated a significantly increased mortality in patients with an ejection fraction less than 0.35 and an abnormal baroreflex sensitivity compared with those with similar ejection fractions but normal baroreflex sensitivity (8% vs 18%; $P < 0.01$) [11]. LVEF—left ventricular ejection fraction.

INVASIVE ELECTROPHYSIOLOGIC TESTING

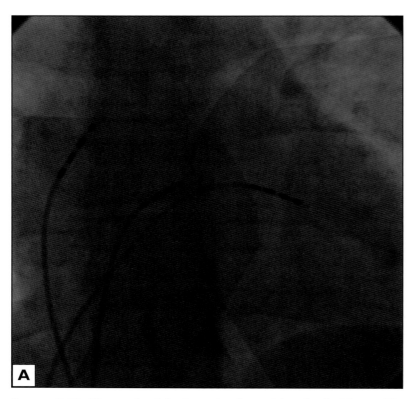

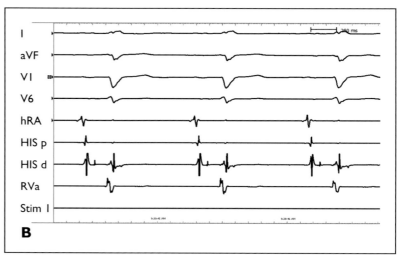

FIGURE 8-19. Electrophysiologic testing for sudden death risk stratification. The electrophysiologic (EP) study is an invasive test in which catheters are positioned in the heart to record intracardiac electrograms and deliver programmed electrical stimulation to induce arrhythmias. Early studies evaluating the usefulness of programmed stimulation for prediction of sudden death in patients with heart failure enrolled very few patients and had limited power for detecting increased risk of sudden death [33]. In the Multicenter Unsustained Tachycardia Trial (MUSTT), EP testing played an important role in identification of patients who would benefit from prophylactic implantable cardioverter-defibrillators (ICDs). Subjects with coronary disease, a left ventricular ejection fraction less than 0.40, nonsustained ventricular tachycardia, and inducible ventricular arrhythmias with EP testing benefited from ICD implantation. This study was the largest randomized trial using this technique for risk stratification and solidified its role in sudden death risk stratification in this population. Compared with those who were not inducible for ventricular tachycardia with EP testing, those who were had a significantly higher risk of sudden death [22]. A fluoroscopic image illustrates the positions of the high right atrial (hRA), His bundle, and right ventricular (RVa) catheters (**A**). The intracardiac recordings and surface electrograms are also seen in sinus rhythm (**B**)

Continued on next page

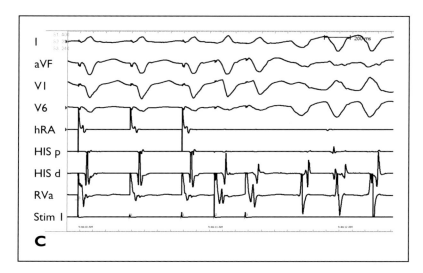

C

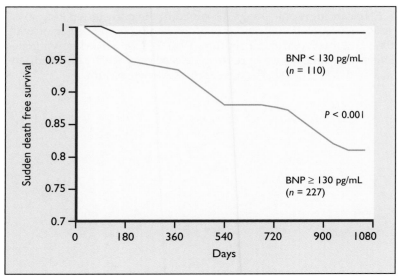

FIGURE 8-19. *(Continued)* and during the induction of ventricular tachycardia with double extrastimuli (**C**).

MOLECULAR MARKERS OF SUDDEN CARDIAC DEATH RISK

FIGURE 8-20. Serum B-type natriuretic peptide (BNP) and the risk of sudden cardiac death. BNP is a hormone secreted by myocardial cells in response to wall stress and elevated filling pressures. It may be elevated in patients with symptomatic and asymptomatic left ventricular dysfunction. Elevated BNP levels are associated with increased mortality [34] and, specifically, sudden death [35,36] in patients with a history of heart failure. Investigators evaluating the prognostic utility of serum BNP level for determining the risk of sudden death in patients with heart failure demonstrated a significant association between a level greater than 130 pg/mL and sudden death compared with those with lower BNP levels. Berger *et al.* [35] described a 19% rate (43 of 227 subjects) of sudden death over 3 years in patients with elevated BNP levels compared with a 1% rate (one of 110 subjects) in those with lower BNP levels. In this study of patients with left ejection fraction less than 35% and history of congestive heart failure, BNP level was the only independent predictor of sudden death in multivariable analyses. In a separate study of heart failure patients, Isnard *et al.* [36] observed a significant association between elevated BNP levels and risk of sudden cardiac death. In this study, BNP remained the only independent predictor of sudden death after adjustment for left ventricular ejection fraction and exercise capacity. (*Adapted from* Berger *et al.* [35].)

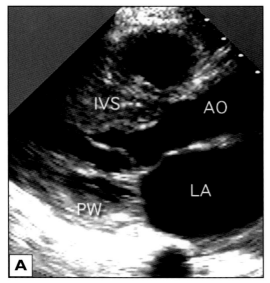

B. GENE DEFECTS ASSOCIATED WITH HYPERTROPHIC CARDIOMYOPATHY AND SUDDEN CARDIAC DEATH (SCD)

GENE PRODUCT	CHROMOSOME	SCD RISK
β-Myosin heavy chain	14q11.2-12	High
Troponin T	1q3	High
Troponin I	19q13.4	High
α-Tropomyosin	15q22	High
Myosin-binding protein C	11p11.2	Low
Myosin light chain-1	3p21	Low
Myosin light chain-2	12q23-24.3	Low
Actin	15q24	Low
AMP-activated protein kinase γ2	7q3	Low

FIGURE 8-21. Hypertrophic cardiomyopathy as the cause of both congestive heart failure and sudden cardiac death. Hypertrophic cardiomyopathy is characterized by hypertrophy of the left ventricle with variable morphologic and clinical manifestations. It is an autosomal dominant genetic disease caused by mutations in the cardiac sarcomere complex. Echocardiographic population studies suggest an incidence of approximately one in 500 people, with many asymptomatic individuals [37]. In symptomatic individuals, the most common complaint is dyspnea on exertion [38]. However, sudden death may occur in 2% to 3% of patients with hypertrophic cardiomyopathy [39]. An analysis of a cohort of 368 patients with hypertrophic cardiomyopathy followed for 6 years identified several risk factors for sudden death: non-sustained ventricular tachycardia, left ventricular wall thickness greater than 3 cm, history of syncope and/or family history of sudden death, and abnormal blood pressure response [40]. **A,** Echocardiographic image, obtained in the parasternal long-axis view, showing left ventricular wall thickening in the posterior wall (PW) and interventricular septum (IVS). **B,** List of the known gene defects associated with hypertrophic cardiomyopathy and sudden cardiac death (SCD) [41]. AO—aorta; LA—left atrium.

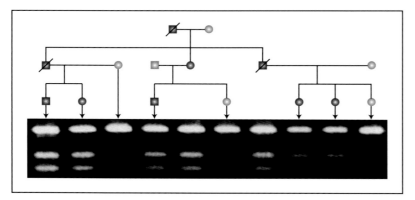

FIGURE 8-22. Analysis of genetic polymorphisms related to cardiac arrhythmias in patients with heart failure. Distinct genetic poly-morphisms attributed to sudden cardiac death in the heart failure population are rare. A more common scenario is genetic predis-position for the development of heart failure, which remains a risk factor for sudden death. Nonetheless, as we continue to have a better understanding of the human genome, genetic analysis may become an important tool for risk stratification. An example of this can be seen in the heart failure population with certain variants of hypertrophic cardiomyopathy and arrhythmogenic right vent-ricular cardiomyopathy that are associated with a higher risk of sudden death [41]. The figure shows restriction fragment length polymorphism (RFLP) analysis identifying affected family members at risk for sudden death. A single mutation in the β-myosin heavy chain causes differential migration of DNA through gel electrophoresis after enzymatic breakdown [42].

REFERENCES

1. Zheng ZJ, Croft JB, Giles WH, Mensah GA: Sudden cardiac death in the United States, 1989 to 1998. *Circulation* 2001, 104:2158–2163.
2. Huikuri HV, Makikallio TH, Raatikainen MJ, *et al.*: Prediction of sudden cardiac death: appraisal of the studies and methods assessing the risk of sudden arrhythmic death. *Circulation* 2003, 108:110–115.
3. Bart BA, Shaw LK, McCants CB, *et al.*: Clinical determinants of mortality in patients with angiographically diagnosed ischemic or nonischemic cardiomyopathy. *J Am Coll Cardiol* 1997, 30:1002–1008.
4. Ezekowitz JA, Armstrong PW, McAlister FA: Implantable cardioverter defibrillators in primary and secondary prevention: a systematic review of randomized, controlled trials. *Ann Intern Med* 2003, 138:445–452.
5. Bardy GH, Lee KL, Mark DB, *et al.*; Sudden Cardiac Death in Heart Failure Trial (SCD-HeFT) Investigators: Amiodarone or an implantable cardioverter-defibrillator for congestive heart failure. *N Engl J Med* 2005, 352:225–237.
6. Hohnloser SH, Kuck KH, Dorian P, *et al.*: Prophylactic use of an implantable cardioverter-defibrillator after acute myocardial infarction. *N Engl J Med* 2005, 351:2481–2488.
7. MERIT-HF Investigators: Effect of metoprolol CR/XL in chronic heart failure: Metoprolol CR/XL Randomised Intervention Trial in Congestive Heart Failure (MERIT-HF). *Lancet* 1999, 353:2001–2007.
8. Stelken AM, Younis LT, Jennison SH, *et al.*: Prognostic value of cardiopulmonary exercise testing using percent achieved of predicted peak oxygen uptake for patients with ischemic and dilated cardiomyopathy. *J Am Coll Cardiol* 1996, 27:345–352.
9. Grimm W, Christ M, Bach J, *et al.*: Noninvasive arrhythmia risk stratification in idiopathic dilated cardiomyopathy: results of the Marburg Cardiomyopathy Study. *Circulation* 2003, 108:2883–2891.
10. Bigger JT Jr, Fleiss JL, Kleiger R, *et al.*: The relationships among ventricular arrhythmias, left ventricular dysfunction, and mortality in the 2 years after myocardial infarction. *Circulation* 1984, 69:250–258.
11. La Rovere MT, Bigger JT Jr, Marcus FI, *et al.*: Baroreflex sensitivity and heart-rate variability in prediction of total cardiac mortality after myocardial infarction. ATRAMI (Autonomic Tone and Reflexes After Myocardial Infarction) Investigators. *Lancet* 1998, 351:478–484.
12. Moss AJ, Zareba W, Hall WJ, *et al.*; Multicenter Automatic Defibrillator Implantation Trial II Investigators: Prophylactic implantation of a defibrillator in patients with myocardial infarction and reduced ejection fraction. *N Engl J Med* 2002, 346:877–883.
13. Gang Y, Ono T, Hnatkova K, *et al.*; ELITE II Investigators: QT dispersion has no prognostic value in patients with symptomatic heart failure: an ELITE II substudy. *Pacing Clin Electrophysiol* 2003, 26:394–400.
14. Iuliano S, Fisher SG, Karasik PE, *et al.*; Department of Veterans Affairs Survival Trial of Antiarrhythmic Therapy in Congestive Heart Failure: QRS duration and mortality in patients with congestive heart failure. *Am Heart J* 2002, 143:1085–1091.
15. Statters DJ, Malik M, Ward DE, Camm AJ: QT dispersion: problems of methodology and clinical significance. *J Cardiovasc Electrophysiol* 1994, 5:672–685.
16. Galinier M, Vialette JC, Fourcade J, *et al.*: QT interval dispersion as a predictor of arrhythmic events in congestive heart failure. Importance of aetiology. *Eur Heart J* 1998, 19:1054–1062.

17. Fu GS, Meissner A, Simon R: Repolarization dispersion and sudden cardiac death in patients with impaired left ventricular function. *Eur Heart J* 1997, 18:281–289.
18. Anastasiou-Nana MI, Nanas JN, Karagounis LA, *et al.*: Relation of dispersion of QRS and QT in patients with advanced congestive heart failure to cardiac and sudden death mortality. *Am J Cardiol* 2000, 85:1212–1217.
19. Teerlink JR, Jalaluddin M, Anderson S, *et al.*: Ambulatory ventricular arrhythmias in patients with heart failure do not specifically predict an increased risk of sudden death. PROMISE (Prospective Randomized Milrinone Survival Evaluation) Investigators. *Circulation* 2000, 101:40–46.
20. Saeed M, Link MS, Mahapatra S, *et al.*: Analysis of intracardiac electrograms showing monomorphic ventricular tachycardia in patients with implantable cardioverter-defibrillators. *Am J Cardiol* 2000, 85:580–587.
21. Bigger JT Jr, Fleiss JL, Rolnitzky LM: Prevalence, characteristics and significance of ventricular tachycardia detected by 24-hour continuous electrocardiographic recordings in the late hospital phase of acute myocardial infarction. *Am J Cardiol* 1986, 58:1151–1160.
22. Buxton AE, Marchlinski FE, Waxman HL, *et al.*: Prognostic factors in nonsustained ventricular tachycardia. *Am J Cardiol* 1984, 53:1275–1279.
23. Doval HC, Nul DR, Grancelli HO, *et al.*: Nonsustained ventricular tachycardia in severe heart failure. Independent marker of increased mortality due to sudden death. GESICA-GEMA Investigators. *Circulation* 1996, 94:3198–3203.
24. Singh SN, Fisher SG, Carson PE, Fletcher RD: Prevalence and significance of nonsustained ventricular tachycardia in patients with premature ventricular contractions and heart failure treated with vasodilator therapy. Department of Veterans Affairs CHF STAT Investigators. *J Am Coll Cardiol* 1998, 32:942–947.
25. Larsen L, Markham J, Haffajee CI: Sudden death in idiopathic dilated cardiomyopathy: role of ventricular arrhythmias. *Pacing Clin Electrophysiol* 1993, 16:1051–1059.
26. Gomes JA, Cain ME, Buxton AE, *et al.*: Prediction of long-term outcomes by signal-averaged electrocardiography in patients with unsustained ventricular tachycardia, coronary artery disease, and left ventricular dysfunction. *Circulation* 2001, 104:436–441.
27. el Sherif N, Denes P, Katz R, *et al.*: Definition of the best prediction criteria of the time domain signal-averaged electrocardiogram for serious arrhythmic events in the postinfarction period. The Cardiac Arrhythmia Suppression Trial/Signal-Averaged Electrocardiogram (CAST/SAECG) Substudy Investigators. *J Am Coll Cardiol* 1995, 25:908–914.
28. Klingenheben T, Zabel M, D'Agostino RB, *et al.*: Predictive value of T-wave alternans for arrhythmic events in patients with congestive heart failure. *Lancet* 2000, 356:651–652.
29. Hohnloser SH, Ikeda T, Bloomfield DM, *et al.*: T-wave alternans negative coronary patients with low ejection and benefit from defibrillator implantation. *Lancet* 2003, 362:125–126.
30. Nolan J, Batin PD, Andrews R, *et al.*: Prospective study of heart rate variability and mortality in chronic heart failure: results of the United Kingdom heart failure evaluation and assessment of risk trial (UK-heart). *Circulation* 1998, 98:1510–1516.
31. Bilchick KC, Fetics B, Djoukeng R, *et al.*: Prognostic value of heart rate variability in chronic congestive heart failure (Veterans Affairs' Survival Trial of Antiarrhythmic Therapy in Congestive Heart Failure). *Am J Cardiol* 2002, 90:24–28.

32. Makikallio TH, Huikuri HV, Hintze U, *et al.*; DIAMOND Study Group (Danish Investigations of Arrhythmia and Mortality ON Dofetilide): Fractal analysis and time- and frequency-domain measures of heart rate variability as predictors of mortality in patients with heart failure. *Am J Cardiol* 2001, 87:178–182.

33. Poll DS, Marchlinski FE, Buxton AE, Josephson ME: Usefulness of programmed stimulation in idiopathic dilated cardiomyopathy. *Am J Cardiol* 1986, 58:992–997.

34. Tsutamoto T, Wada A, Maeda K, *et al.*: Attenuation of compensation of endogenous cardiac natriuretic peptide system in chronic heart failure: prognostic role of plasma brain natriuretic peptide concentration in patients with chronic symptomatic left ventricular dysfunction. *Circulation* 1997, 96:509–516.

35. Berger R, Huelsman M, Strecker K, *et al.*: B-type natriuretic peptide predicts sudden death in patients with chronic heart failure. *Circulation* 2002, 105:2392–2397.

36. Isnard R, Pousset F, Chafirovskaia O, *et al.*: Combination of B-type natriuretic peptide and peak oxygen consumption improves risk stratification in outpatients with chronic heart failure. *Am Heart J* 2003, 146:729–735.

37. Maron BJ, Gardin JM, Flack JM, *et al.*: Prevalence of hypertrophic cardiomyopathy in a general population of young adults. Echocardiographic analysis of 4111 subjects in the CARDIA Study. Coronary Artery Risk Development in (Young) Adults. *Circulation* 1995, 92:785–789.

38. Wigle ED, Rakowski H, Kimball BP, Williams WG: Hypertrophic cardiomyopathy. Clinical spectrum and treatment. *Circulation* 1995, 92:1680–1692.

39. McKenna WJ, Franklin RC, Nihoyannopoulos P, *et al.*: Arrhythmia and prognosis in infants, children and adolescents with hypertrophic cardiomyopathy. *J Am Coll Cardiol* 1988, 11:147–153.

40. Elliott PM, Poloniecki J, Dickie S, *et al.*: Sudden death in hypertrophic cardiomyopathy: identification of high risk patients. *J Am Coll Cardiol* 2000, 36:2212–2218.

41. Franz WM, Muller OJ, Katus HA: Cardiomyopathies: from genetics to the prospect of treatment. *Lancet* 2001, 358:1627–1637.

42. Ko YL, Chen JJ, Tang TK, *et al.*: Malignant familial hypertrophic cardiomyopathy in a family with a 453Arg—>Cys mutation in the beta-myosin heavy chain gene: coexistence of sudden death and end-stage heart failure. *Hum Genet* 1996, 97:585–590.

SUPRAVENTRICULAR ARRHYTHMIAS IN HEART FAILURE

Samuel J. Asirvatham and Paul A. Friedman

There is an intricate interplay, both in terms of pathogenesis and clinical course, between supraventricular arrhythmia and congestive heart failure (CHF). The most common arrhythmia, atrial fibrillation (AF), is more difficult to treat and more likely to be symptomatic, thus necessitating treatment in patients with CHF. Drugs with proarrhythmic potential need to be avoided in symptomatic AF in patients with structural heart disease. Nonpharmacologic options, particularly radiofrequency ablation, are especially useful in this population.

It is important to consider tachycardia-worsened or tachycardia-caused cardiomyopathy when supraventricular arrhythmia and reduced ventricular function coexist. Timely cure of AF or supraventricular tachycardia (SVT) with rapid ventricular rates may reverse cardiomyopathy and often normalize ventricular function. Post–cardiac transplant patients present specific challenges in identifying treatable atrial arrhythmias and in avoiding complex drug interactions and proarrhythmias. In all, a stepwise algorithmic approach to diagnosing and treating supraventricular arrhythmia in heart failure is required.

In patients with heart failure, the development of SVTs, and in particular AF, is a strong and independent prediction for death, stroke, and hospitalization for worsening CHF [1]. Moreover, CHF and AF frequently coexist [2]. Many of the conditions that predispose to CHF, *eg*, hypertension, diabetes, advancing age, valvular heart disease, are also risk factors for AF [3]. Mounting epidemiologic, hemodynamic, neurohormonal, clinical, and electrophysiologic observations suggest that beyond sharing common risk factors, the pathophysiologic changes induced by CHF facilitate the develop-

ment of AF. Conversely, the development of AF similarly leads to similar changes that favor the development and deterioration of CHF [4]. In addition to the complex interactions and adverse synergy resulting in progressive CHF and more entrenched AF, CHF and SVTs share two other points of intersection. First, patients with refractory heart failure who have undergone cardiac transplantation are at risk for atrial flutters related to incisional scars or rejection [5]. Second, specific syndromes such as Fabry's disease predispose to both cardiomyopathy and atrial arrhythmias.

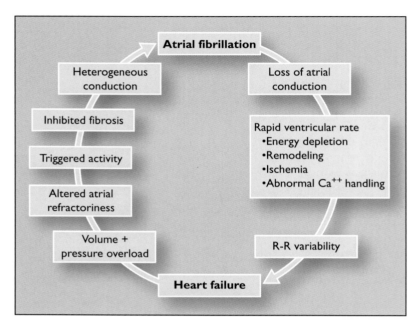

FIGURE 9-1. Complex interdependent relationship between atrial fibrillation (AF) and congestive heart failure. Development of AF impairs cardiac function via several mechanisms. Loss of atrioventricular synchrony impairs diastolic filling and may reduce cardiac output by up to 20%. Associated rapid ventricular rates lead to ventricular myocardial energy depletion, abnormal calcium handling, and cellular and extracellular remodeling. Irregularity of ventricular contraction variability itself adversely affects cardiac output. Similarly, the development of heart failure leads to fluid overload and atrial stretch, which increases triggered activity, slows atrial conduction, alters atrial refractory periods, and promotes heterogeneity of atrial repolarization. Neurohormonal activation of the renin-angiotensin-aldosterone system affects the extracellular matrix, promoting fibrosis and heterogeneity of electrical conduction. (*Adapted from* Maisel *et al.* [3].)

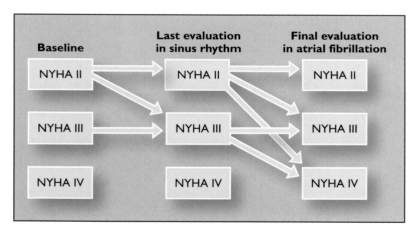

FIGURE 9-2. Deterioration of stable heart failure with atrial fibrillation (AF) development. In a study of 344 patients with congestive heart failure and sinus rhythm, the development of AF during a follow-up period of 19 ± 12 months was associated with clinical and hemodynamic deterioration. Independent risk factors for development of AF included lower transmitral flow at last sinus rhythm follow-up and previous reversible AF during the follow-up period [6]. NYHA—New York Heart Association (functional class). (*Adapted from* Pozzoli *et al.* [6].)

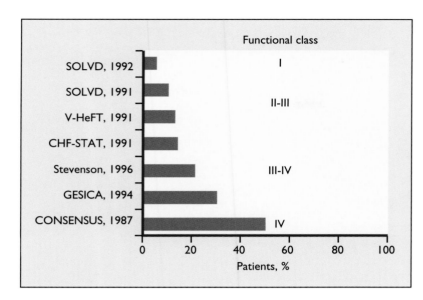

FIGURE 9-3. Incidence of atrial fibrillation (AF) in congestive heart failure (CHF) study populations, grouped by severity of heart failure. The strong association between CHF and AF is demonstrated by the increase in AF incidence in study populations as progressively more severe heart failure patients are included. CHF-STAT—Amiodarone in Patients With Congestive Heart Failure and Asymptomatic Ventricular Arrhythmia; CONSENSUS—The Effects of Enalapril on Mortality in Severe Congestive Heart Failure; GESICA—Randomized Trial of Low-Dose Amiodarone in Severe Congestive Heart Failure; SOLVD—Studies of Left Ventricular Dysfunction.

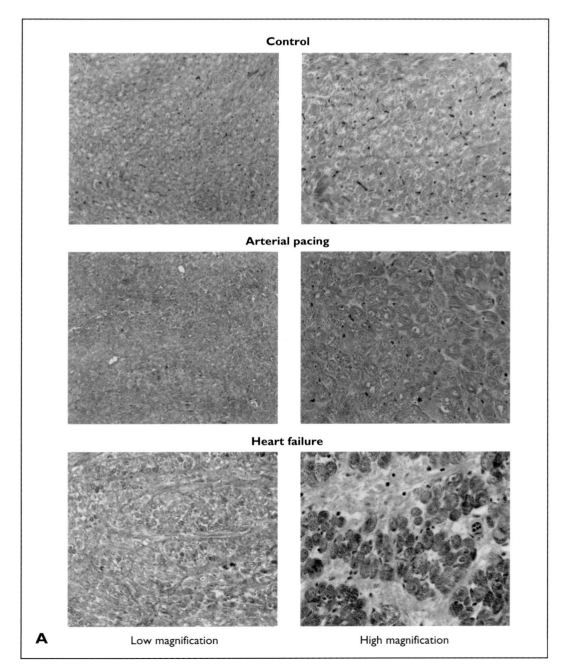

FIGURE 9-4. A and **B,** Chronic heart failure produces increased atrial electrical heterogeneity that predisposes to atrial fibrillation.

Continued on next page

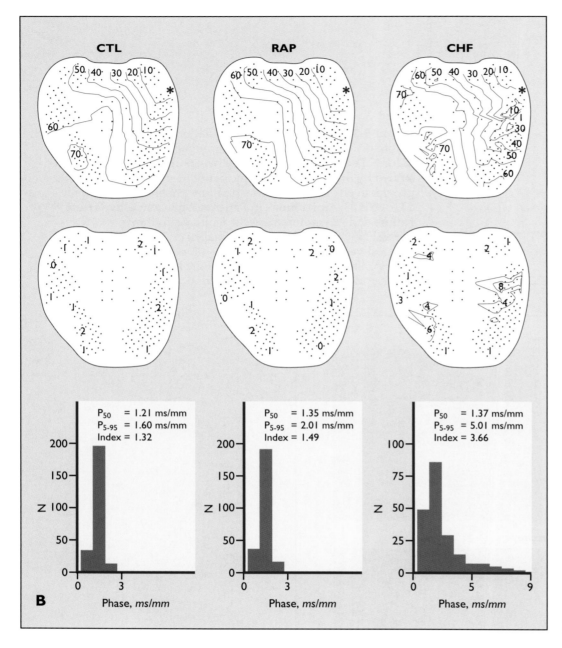

CTL

RAP

CHF

P_{50} = 1.21 ms/mm
P_{5-95} = 1.60 ms/mm
Index = 1.32

P_{50} = 1.35 ms/mm
P_{5-95} = 2.01 ms/mm
Index = 1.49

P_{50} = 1.37 ms/mm
P_{5-95} = 5.01 ms/mm
Index = 3.66

Phase, *ms/mm*

B

FIGURE 9-4. *(Continued)*

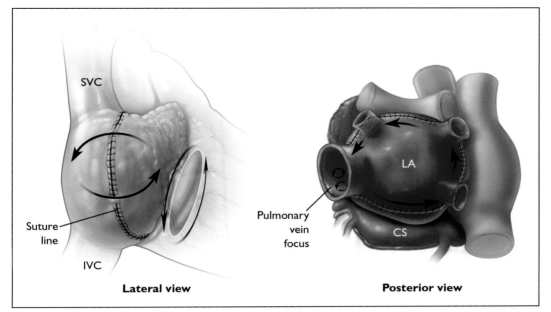

FIGURE 9-5. Post-transplant atrial arrhythmia. The post-transplant population is unique in that the pulmonary veins are electrically isolated from the left atrium and the suture line scar between the donor and recipient atria may act as an anatomic boundary for atrial flutters. Typical caval tricuspid isthmus–dependent atrial flutter is more common in this population and may be a marker for transplant rejection. Other scar-related atrial flutters and atrial flutter occurring between the donor and recipient atria have been described [7,8]. CS—coronary sinus; IVC—inferior vena cava; LA—left atrium; SVC—superior vena cava.

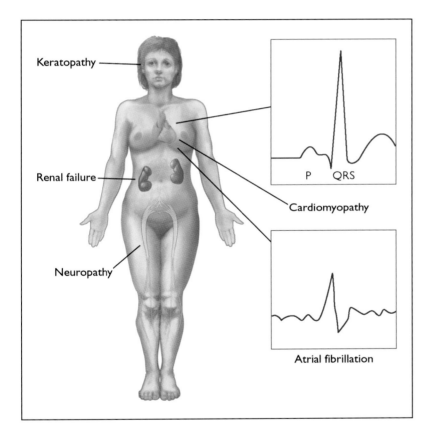

FIGURE 9-6. Cardiomyopathy and atrial arrhythmias. Although any type of cardiomyopathy may predispose to atrial arrhythmias, particularly atrial fibrillation (AF), some cardiomyopathies are associated with unique arrhythmia. In Fabry's disease and hypertrophic cardiomyopathy, an ECG pattern of preexcitation has been described. Interfascicular ventricular tachycardia giving rise to AF (tachycardia-induced cardiomyopathy) has been described in Friedreich's ataxia and some muscular dystrophies [9,10].

Anatomic and Physiologic Basis of Supraventricular Tachycardia in Heart Failure

Atrial fibrillation may arise from rapidly discharging foci emanating predominantly from sites of smooth muscle–cardiac muscle interface (most notably the pulmonary veins) or from substrate abnormalities that promote and accommodate reentrant waves [11–13]. Fluctuations in autonomic tone or abnormalities in electrolytes further favor arrhythmogenesis. Heart failure results in changes in substrate, triggers, and modulating factors resulting in a propensity toward atrial arrhythmias.

Anatomically distinct muscular sleeves extend from the left atrium into the pulmonary vein. These are universally circumferential at the ostium of the vein and extend for varying distances. There is a unique interface between syncytial cardiac muscle and venular smooth muscle at the site. Remnants of nodal tissue are found in various species at the sites of intersection between the veins and the atria. Distinct anatomic anomalies have been described in relation to specific arrhythmias, for example, anomalies of the cavotricuspid isthmus in atrial flutter. At times, primary electrical abnormalities may exist. These include increased capture latency for atrial tissue in CHF or prominent intra-atrial conduction defects that may predispose to arrhythmia.

Animal models of stretch-related AF demonstrate increased frequency of pulmonary vein discharge in association with increasing left atrial pressure [14]. The interplay between the neurohumoral systems and gross anatomical abnormalities is complex. For a given degree of atrial fibrosis, neurohumoral changes may predispose to unidirectional conduction block, inhomogeneous conduction, giving rise to the electrical heterogeneity necessary for substrate-mediated AF frequently seen in advanced stages of CHF. Bioenergetic abnormalities in CHF well described in the ventricular myocardium also occur in the atrial myocardium, further increasing the predisposition to arrhythmia.

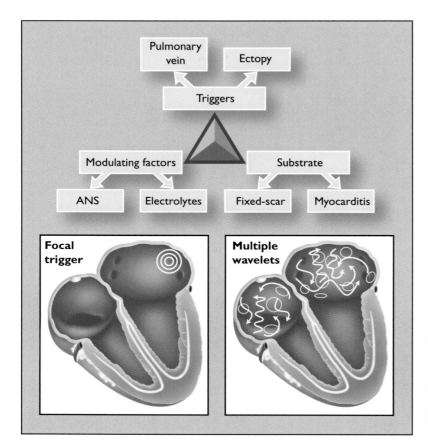

Figure 9-7. Pathophysiology of atrial arrhythmias in heart failure. The understanding of the pathophysiology of atrial fibrillation (AF) has changed markedly over the past 5 years. Substrate mediation due to multiple wavelets occurs with the diseased atria, often from congestive heart failure. The triggers to insight AF often, however, arise from the pulmonary veins, which also may be abnormally enlarged in heart failure [15]. ANS—autonomic nervous system.

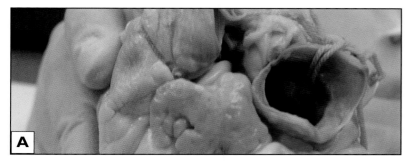

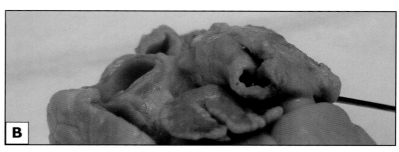

FIGURE 9-8. A and **B**, Anatomic distortions of the atrium in congestive heart failure. Increased left atrial pressures are common in patients with either systolic or diastolic ventricular dysfunction. In addition, valvular dysfunction seen with mitral annular dilation further causes atrial enlargement. The venous portions of the atrium (sinus venosus derivative) tend to enlarge the most [16]. Thus, left atrial enlargement may be severe in comparison with left atrial appendage enlargement. Pulmonary vein dilation seen along with atrial enlargement may predispose to atrial fibrillation.

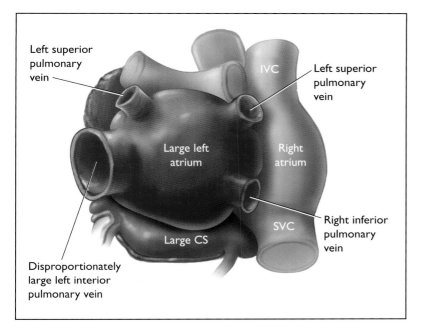

FIGURE 9-9. Congestive heart failure and atrial arrhythmia: gross anatomic changes (*see* Fig. 9-12). CS—coronary sinus; IVC—inferior vena cava; SVC—superior vena cava

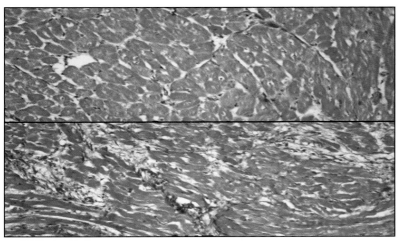

FIGURE 9-10. Histologic derangements in the atria observed in patients with congestive heart failure (CHF). Patchy areas of fibrosis and myocardial disarray are commonly seen in patients with CHF. To some extent, this is from atrial dilation alone, but the pathologic process that has affected the ventricle, *eg*, lupus myocarditis, Sjögren's syndrome, or viral myocarditis, may affect the atrium as well [17,18].

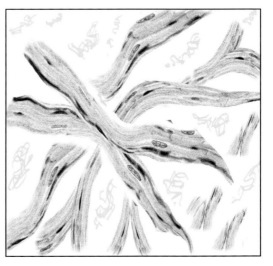

FIGURE 9-11. Histologic derangements in congestive heart failure.

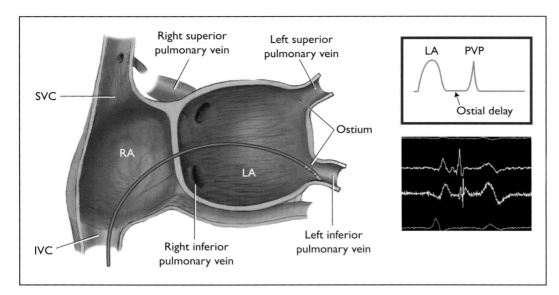

Figure 9-12. Electrophysiologic tracing of pulmonary vein potential (PVP) in patients with congestive heart failure. In this tracing, a prominent delay from the left atrial activation (*arrow*) and local activation of the pulmonary vein musculature can be seen [19]. This patient had a markedly enlarged left inferior pulmonary vein measuring 2.4 cm in diameter at the ostium [20]. The patient's ventricular function was 25%, and left atrial pressures were markedly elevated. IVC—inferior vena cava; LA—left atrium; RA—right atrium; SVC—superior vena cava.

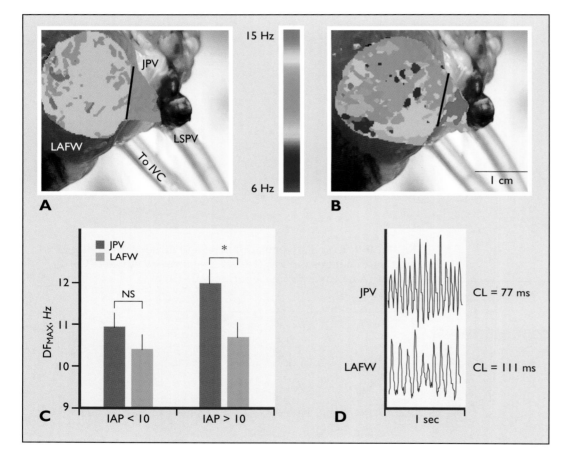

Figure 9-13. Association between left atrial pressure and dominant frequency at the left atrial free wall (LAFW) and left atrial superior pulmonary vein junction (JPV) in a stretch-related atrial fibrillation (AF) sheep model—stretch-induced venous discharge. The association between heart failure (with increased left atrial pressures) and AF may be the result of increased venous electrical discharge with elevated pressures. Dominant frequencies determined by optical voltage mapping are displayed at left atrial pressures of 5 cm H_2O (**A**) and 18 cm H_2O (**B**). Maps are superimposed on color photographs of the heart for illustrative purposes. With lower atrial pressure (*panel A*), the frequency of the LAFW and JPV are similar; with increased pressure (*panel B*), the JPV dominant venous frequency increases and is greater than that of the LAFW. The bar graph (**C**) shows maximum dominant frequency (DF_{max}) at intra-atrial pressure (IAP) less than 10 cm H_2O and IAP greater than 10 cm H_2O ($P < 0.001$). Also shown are single-pixel recordings from the JPV and LAFW at 30 cm H_2O (**D**). CL—cycle length; IVC—inferior vena cava; LSPV—left superior pulmonary vein. (*Adapted from Kalifa et al.* [14].)

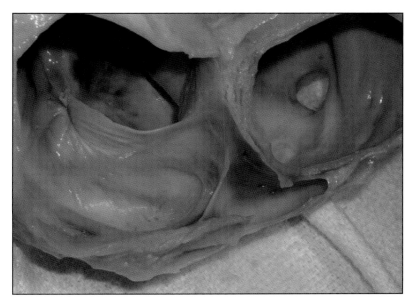

FIGURE 9-14. Anatomic specimen of the atrium from a patient with congestive heart failure (CHF) showing marked enlargement and dilation of the atrial tissue between the tricuspid annulus and the inferior vena cava. This "cavotricuspid" isthmus is the critical region for the usual atrial flutter circuit. Patients with CHF and morphologic abnormalities in this region of the atrium are predisposed to sustained atrial flutter.

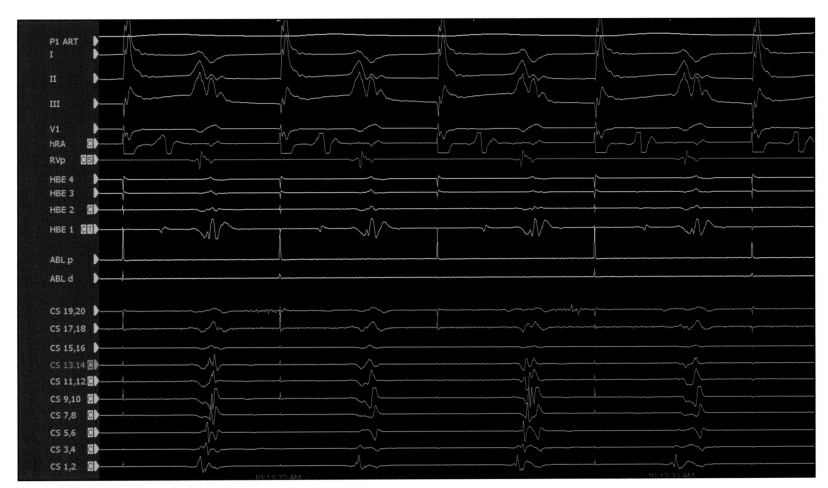

FIGURE 9-15. Increased capture latency: one of the electrical problems seen in the atrium in congestive heart failure (CHF). Atrial pacing performed from the right atrial appendage shows a marked delay prior to other electrogram or electrocardiographic criteria for capture. This abnormality, a sign of a diseased atrium, existed in this patient secondary to CHF and atrial enlargement [21].

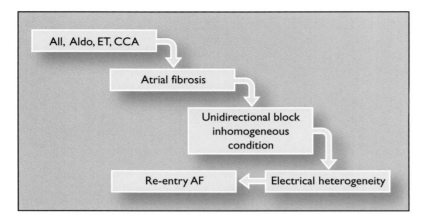

FIGURE 9-16. Neurohumoral influences, as well as atrial fibrosis, combine to create the ideal milieu for atrial fibrillation (AF). Congestive heart failure contributes to atrial stretch and fibrosis and to adverse neurohumoral effects [22]. AII—angiotensin II; Aldo—aldosterone; CCA—calcium channel antagonist; ET—endothelin.

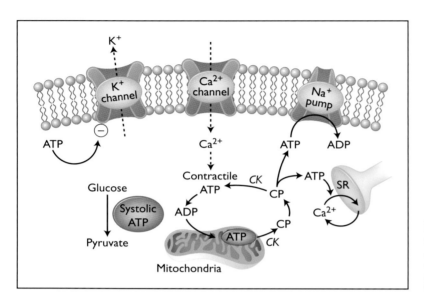

FIGURE 9-17. Various electrogenic dysfunctions occur as a result of abnormal energy utilization at the cellular level, which predisposes to arrhythmia and electrical inhomogeneity [23]. CK—creatine kinase; CP—creatine phosphokinase; SR—sarcoplasmic reticulum.

A broad number of symptoms and physical examination abnormalities may suggest the presence of heart failure and/or AF. On the electrocardiogram (ECG), the resting ventricular rate in patients with atrial tachyarrhythmias is particularly important; heart rates in excess of 100 beats per minute in an asymptomatic patient may suggest prolonged arrhythmia and tachycardia-induced cardiomyopathy. Alternatively, the presence of an atrial arrhythmia may account for deterioration in a patient with previously stable CHF. Any number of abnormalities may be seen on the ECG in association with heart failure. Although none is diagnostic, the presence of left bundle branch block and right axis deviation may suggest primary cardiomyopathy [24]. The combination of increased QRS voltage in the precordial leads with low voltage in the limb leads is characteristic of dilated cardiomyopathy [25]. Numerous abnormalities of electrolytes with characteristic ECG findings may develop in CHF and may predispose to SVTs.

It is not uncommon to observe ventricular ectopy in CHF; when AF is present, wide complexes of ventricular origin must be distinguished from aberrant conduction (Ashman's phenomenon). An ECG demonstrating AF and left bundle branch morphology paced ventricular complexes in the absence of native conduction suggest previous atrioventricular nodal ablation and right ventricular apical pacing. In the setting of refractory heart failure, upgrade to a biventricular pacing system may offer therapeutic benefit [26]. Numerous abnormalities of the chest radiograph may occur with CHF. The presence of AF may make assessment of ejection fraction and diagnosis of CHF difficult because of variations in cardiac filling associated with irregular activation and elevated rates. Elevations in circulating neurohormones such as B-type natriuretic peptide may facilitate diagnosis of heart failure under varying conditions [27,28].

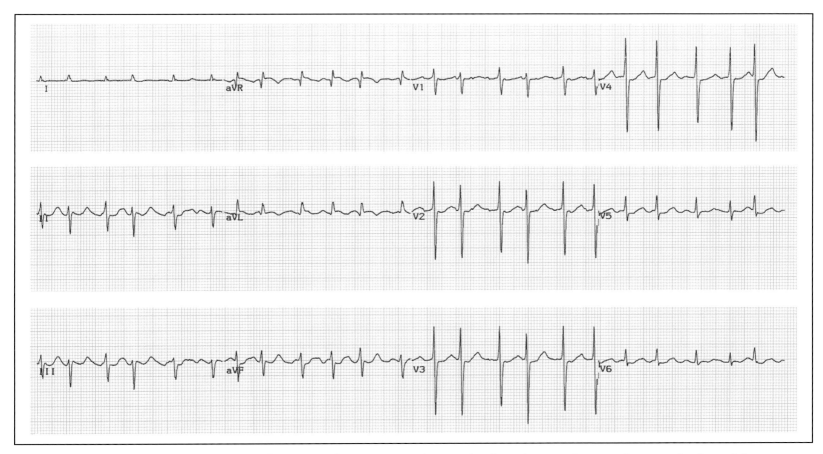

FIGURE 9-18. Electrocardiographic tracing of a sustained monomorphic atrial tachycardia seen in a 17-year-old female athlete that gave rise to severe ventricular dysfunction (tachycardia-mediated cardiomyopathy). Although congestive heart failure (CHF) frequently gives rise to an increased propensity for atrial arrhythmias, atrial arrhythmia itself may worsen or cause CHF. In this patient, following ablation of the tachycardia focus, ventricular function improved from 28% to 60% [29,30].

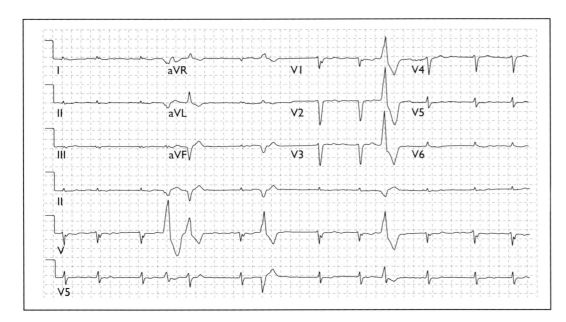

FIGURE 9-19. Electrocardiogram of digitalis toxicity. In this example, multiform ventricular bigeminy is seen. Here, the bigeminal premature ventricular contractions vary in morphology and may be an early marker for digitalis toxicity (Scherf phenomenon) [31].

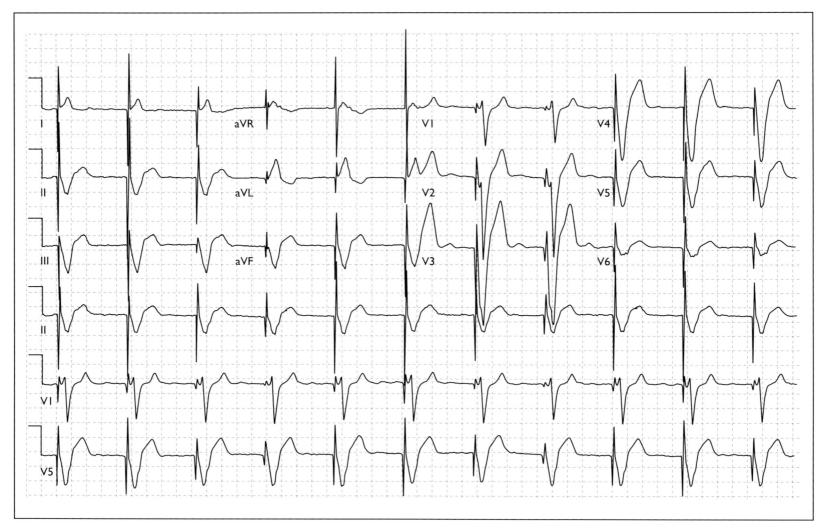

FIGURE 9-20. Atrial fibrillation and right ventricular apical pacing in a patient with congestive heart failure (CHF). The electrocardiogram demonstrates right ventricular apical (RVA) pacing, fine atrial fibrillation (fine, irregular baseline deflections), and no evidence of intrinsic (nonpaced) conduction. RVA pacing most commonly has left bundle branch block morphology because the right ventricle is activated before the left ventricle (as is the case with left bundle branch block). RVA pacing may introduce ventricular dyssynchrony, which may aggravate heart failure. Such patients may benefit from an upgrade to a pacing system with a left ventricular lead (cardiac resynchronization or biventricular pacing).

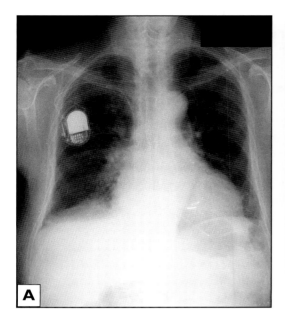
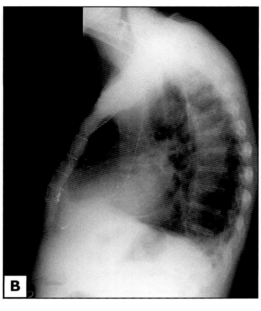

FIGURE 9-21. Chest radiograph of a patient with congestive heart failure. The radiograph demonstrates the cardiomegaly and pulmonary vascular congestion often seen in heart failure. A single-chamber pacemaker with tip in the right ventricular apex is seen (**A**). The lateral view (**B**) is particularly useful for identification of lead position, as the right ventricle is an anterior structure.

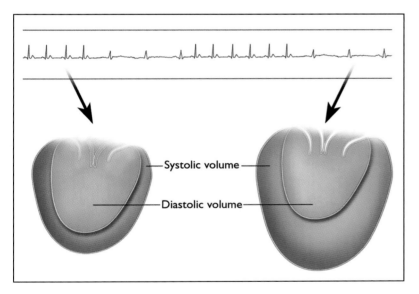

Systolic volume

Diastolic volume

FIGURE 9-22. Difficulty of ejection fraction assessment in congestive heart failure in patients with arrhythmias. The electrocardiogram is the most commonly used test to assess ventricular function. During rapidly conducted atrial arrhythmias (atrial fibrillation with rapid ventricular rates), it may be difficult to accurately assess ventricular function. End-diastolic volumes may be very low, particularly with the shorter cardiac cycle, giving rise to an underestimation of ventricular function. Fractional shortening, Doppler tissue velocity change, or the use of other radiologically gated techniques may optimize ejection fraction measurement in heart failure patients and atrial arrhythmias.

Physiologic and Clinical Consequences of Atrial Arrhythmias in Congestive Heart Failure

The onset of SVT in patients with heart failure predicts death, thromboembolism, and subsequent heart failure hospitalization. The presence of AF has been associated with an increased risk of pump failure mortality. The decrease in cardiac output in AF is multifactorial. Loss of atrial contraction and atrioventricular synchrony may impair diastolic filling, reduce stroke volume, increase atrial pressure, and diminish cardiac output by 20% [3]. Independent of changes in heart rate, the irregularity introduced by AF reduces cardiac output. Additionally, information from implantable cardioverter-defibrillator (ICD) recipients suggests the rapid rates and irregularities in ventricular activation may result in a propensity for ventricular arrhythmias.

PROGNOSTIC SIGNIFICANCE OF SUPRAVENTRICULAR TACHYCARDIA (SVT) IN CONGESTIVE HEART FAILURE (CHF)*

OUTCOMES	SVT EVENTS, N/TOTAL PATIENTS, N (%)	NO SVT EVENTS, N/TOTAL PATIENTS, N (%)	RR	95% CI	P VALUE
Total mortality	375/866 (43)	2231/6922 (32)	2.45	2.19–2.74	0.0001
Stroke	56/866 (6)	272/6922 (4)	2.35	1.68–3.29	0.0001
Hospitalization for CHF	502/866 (58)	1789/6922 (26)	3.00	2.71–3.33	0.0001

*From Cox proportional hazards model (n = 7788). RR for each outcome reflects SVT as a time-dependent variable.

Figure 9-23. Survival of patients with congestive heart failure (CHF) following the development of supraventricular tachycardia (SVT). The Digitalis Investigation Group trial prospectively randomized patients with CHF in sinus rhythm to digoxin (n = 3889) or placebo (n = 3889) and followed them for a mean of 37 months. The 11.1% of patients who developed SVT during follow-up had a greater risk of subsequent total mortality (RR 2.451; P = 0.0001) and hospitalization for worsening CHF (RR 3.004; P = 0.0001). (*Adapted from* Mathew *et al.* [1].)

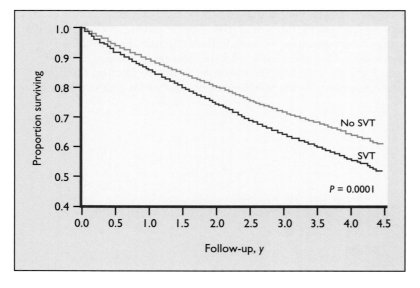

Figure 9-24. Effect of supraventricular tachycardia (SVT) on all-cause mortality in congestive heart failure patients. Although all SVTs were included, most were likely atrial fibrillation [1]. (*Adapted from* Mathew *et al.* [1].)

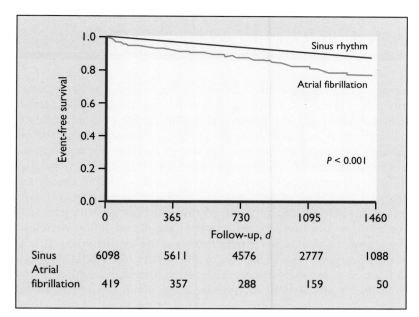

FIGURE 9-25. Pump failure mortality in atrial fibrillation (AF) patients with and without congestive heart failure. In this retrospective analysis of the Studies of Left Ventricular Dysfunction Prevention and Treatment (SOLVD), patients with AF and sinus rhythm at baseline were compared for all-cause mortality, progressive pump failure, and arrhythmic death. Patients with AF had higher all-cause mortality and higher pump failure mortality. There was no difference in arrhythmic deaths, suggesting that AF is associated with increased mortality in heart failure patients as a result of pump failure, because of progressive ventricular systolic dysfunction [32]. This concept is supported by acute hemodynamic studies. (*Adapted from* Dries *et al.* [32].)

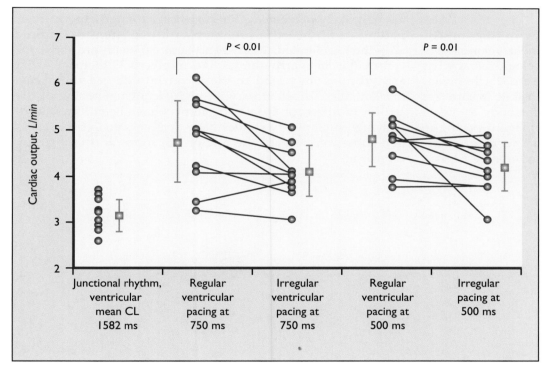

FIGURE 9-26. Adverse effect of an irregular ventricular rhythm on cardiac output. Fick cardiac outputs were measured in 11 patients undergoing catheter ablation of the atrioventricular junction for creation of complete heart block. The graph depicts the cardiac output during slow junctional rhythm following ablation and during regular and irregular pacing at a cycle length (CL) of 750 ms (80 bpm) and 500 ms (120 bpm). At both paced heart rates, the irregular pacing resulted in cardiac output lower than that obtained from regular pacing at the same rate. This observation suggests that an irregular ventricular rhythm, independent of rate, has a detrimental effect on cardiac performance, which may partly account for the increased pump failure mortality seen in heart failure patients with atrial fibrillation.

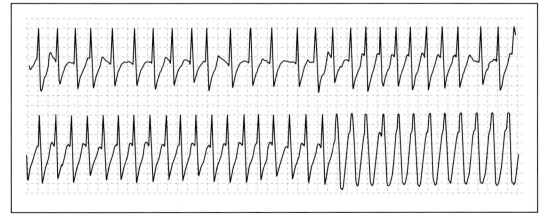

FIGURE 9-27. Intracardiac electrocardiogram recorded from an implantable cardioverter-defibrillator (ICD) demonstrating atrial fibrillation (AF) degenerating to ventricular tachycardia. The initial tracing (*top strip*) depicts a narrow complex, irregular rhythm AF. The complexes then become wide and regular (very fast ventricular tachycardia). A study in ICD recipients has suggested an increase in ventricular arrhythmias in association with atrial tachyarrhythmias [33]. The fast and irregular ventricular activation caused by AF may promote ventricular tachycardia and fibrillation. Irregular activation leads to variability in refractoriness and may promote reentry.

Drug therapy for atrial fibrillation in CHF patients is often challenging. The major limitations are the lack of universal efficacy and proarrhythmia. In most patients with cardiomyopathy, class I agents are typically contraindicated. This is particularly true in patients with ischemic cardiomyopathy and heart failure. The most commonly used drugs for AF in congestive heart failure patients are sotalol, amiodarone, and dofetilide. Frequently however, sotalol is difficult to use because of exacerbation of heart failure symptoms and/or worsening fatigue with the use of this drug at doses appropriate for AF. The long-term sequelae of amiodarone use make it quite unattractive, especially in younger patients with CHF. Finally, dofetilide, although safe to use in patients with heart failure, is difficult to monitor because of frequent changes in the creatinine clearance in patients with CHF, making frequent dose adjustments necessary and its use often impractical.

The limitation of pharmacologic therapy in treating AF, particularly in the setting of CHF, has led to the development of nonpharmacologic approaches. Nonpharmacologic therapy has been used to control the ventricular rate, while atrial arrhythmias persist, and to target atrial arrhythmogenic substrate to suppress arrhythmia. Ablation of the atrioventricular node to create complete heart block with concomitant permanent pacing to control the ventricular rate eliminates the need for pharmacologic rate control, and has been shown to improve a broad range of clinical outcomes, including quality of life, ventricular function, exercise duration, and health care use [34]. Long-term survival following the procedure is similar for patients treated with ablation and medications [35]. A significant minority of patients will experience improvement in ejection fraction due to the introduction of rate control [36]. However, pacing from the right ventricular apex may not be optimal, as it introduces an artificial activation of the ventricle, which itself may favor heart failure development, particularly in patients with depressed ventricular function. Stimulation of right and left ventricles, simultaneously or with a programmed interventricular delay, offers additional benefit following atrioventricular nodal ablation in selected patients by augmenting left ventricular function.

Catheter ablation of arrhythmogenic atrial tissue has been found effective in preventing recurrences of atrial flutter. More recently, isolation of rapidly discharging pulmonary vein foci has effectively prevented AF recurrence, although experience in patients with heart failure and with persistent or chronic arrhythmia is limited. Many heart failure patients are at risk for ventricular tachyarrhythmias and receive ICD therapy. Atrial arrhythmias may lead to inappropriate device therapies. Implantable defibrillators with high-frequency pacing of the atrium to interrupt atrial arrhythmias have been introduced. Although preliminary studies have demonstrated effectiveness in a subset of patients, the role of this form of atrial therapy is unclear.

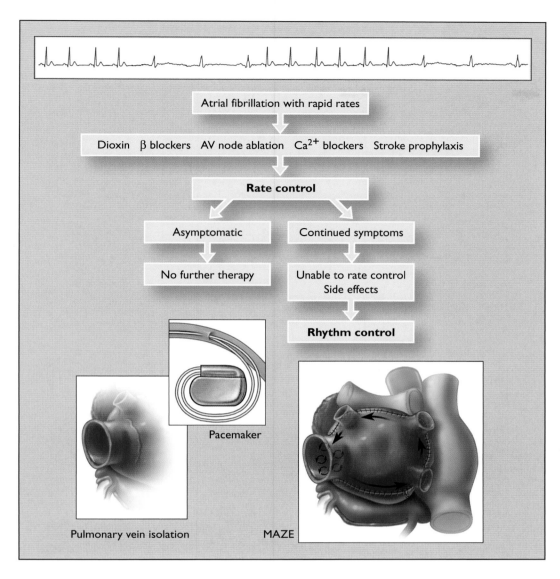

FIGURE 9-28. Drug therapy for atrial fibrillation in heart failure: rate versus rhythm control. In the AFFIRM (Atrial Fibrillation Follow-up Investigation of Rhythm Management) trial, patients were randomized to rate control (drugs or atrioventricular [AV] node ablation) versus rhythm control (majority with antiarrhythmic drug therapy). This important study demonstrated that there was no benefit to maintaining sinus rhythm over rate control [37]. There was a tendency for higher morbidity, primarily from stroke, in the rhythm control arm. It should be noted that the patients in this study were older, and many in the rhythm control arm were not receiving adequate warfarin anticoagulation [38].

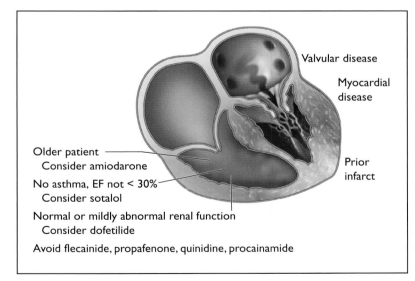

FIGURE 9-29. Drug therapy for atrial arrhythmia and heart failure: selecting the right drug. Risk–benefit assessment with drug therapy in patients with heart failure is critical. Certain antiarrhythmic drugs, such as flecainide and propafenone, are highly unlikely to cause proarrhythmic ventricular tachycardia when ventricular function is normal [39]. However, the risk of ventricular tachycardia with these drugs in patients with markedly depressed ventricular function is prohibitive [40]. Potassium channel–blocking agents such as sotalol and amiodarone may produce polymorphic ventricular tachycardia associated with QT interval prolongation (torsades de pointes) [41]. This proarrhythmic potential exists regardless of the presence or absence of ventricular dysfunction. Dofetilide has been shown to be safe (minimal risk of torsades) when adequate attention is paid to dosing, scrupulous attention is given to creatinine clearance, and serial QT interval measurements are made [42,43]. EF—ejection fraction.

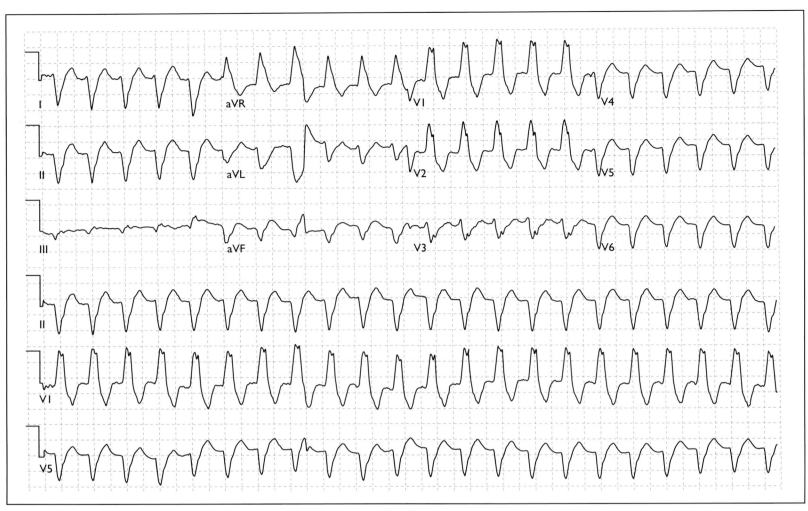

Figure 9-30. Electrocardiogram of flecainide toxicity. QRS prolongation and monomorphic ventricular tachycardia are seen in this patient with ambulation. Flecainide demonstrates use dependence. With this phenomenon, both a beneficial flecainide effect and predisposition to proarrhythmia are more likely to be seen with more rapid heart rates, such as those that occur with exercise.

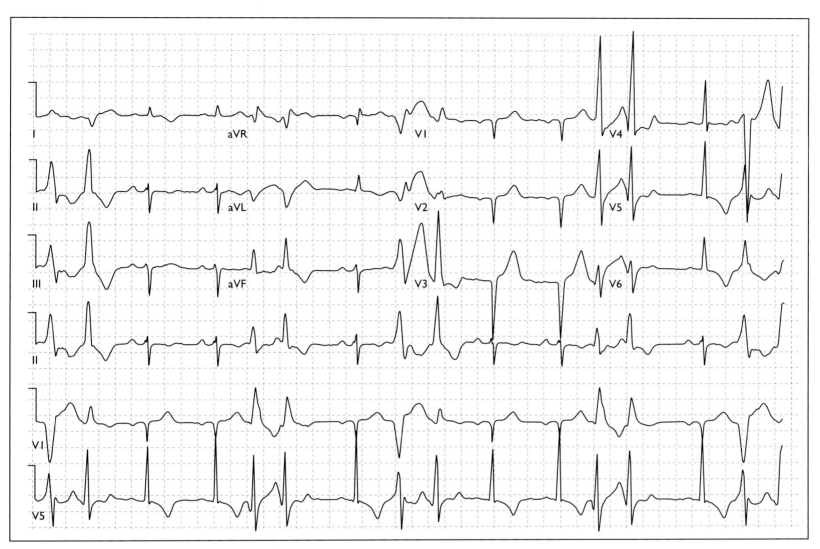

FIGURE 9-31. Coexistence of congestive heart failure (CHF) and arrhythmias. In this patient with CHF, digoxin was used to improve symptomatic heart failure. Because of paroxysmal atrial fibrillation, amiodarone was instituted and resulted in digitalis toxicity that gave rise to multiple morphologies of premature ventricular contractions and nonsustained polymorphic ventricular tachycardia. This case illustrates the difficult issues that arise when CHF and arrhythmias coexist [44].

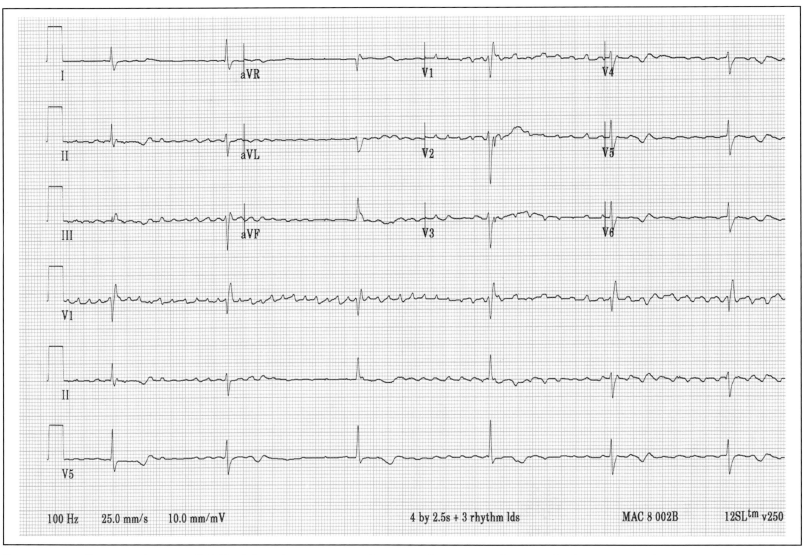

FIGURE 9-32. Electrocardiogram (ECG) of digitalis toxicity. In this ECG, a classic arrhythmia of atrial tachyarrhythmia (atrial fibrillation) associated with complete atrioventricular node block and a junctional escape rhythm is seen. The patient was also on a β-blocker, which may explain the relatively slow rate of the junctional escape.

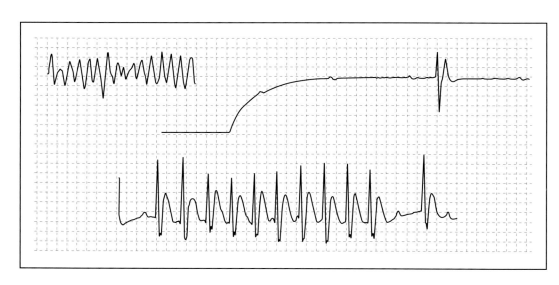

FIGURE 9-33. Electrocardiogram (ECG) of digitalis toxicity. The ECG shows multiple morphology ventricular tachycardias giving rise to frequent implantable cardioverter-defibrillator shocks in a patient with heart failure and digitalis toxicity.

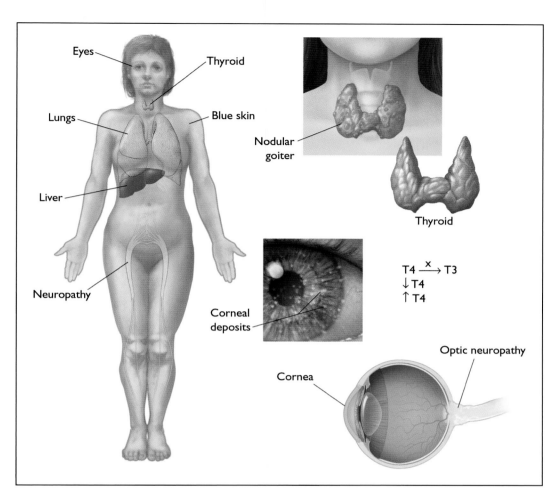

$$T4 \xrightarrow{\ x\ } T3$$
$$\downarrow T4$$
$$\uparrow T4$$

FIGURE 9-34. Amiodarone toxicity. Thyroid dysfunction, both hyperthyroidism and hypothyroidism, may be seen with amiodarone. In turn, these abnormalities may complicate management of congestive heart failure. Amiodarone containing an iodine moiety may suppress thyroxine formation (Wolff-Chaikoff effect), inhibit T_4 to T_3 conversion, or give rise to a sudden increase in thyroxine production and thyrotoxicosis in patients who are iodine deficient and have multinodular goiter (Jod-Basedow phenomenon) [45].

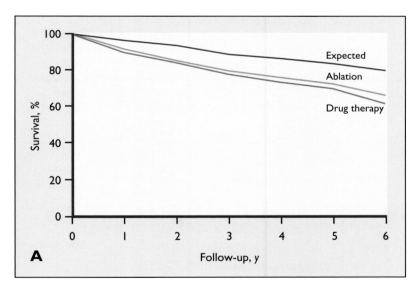

FIGURE 9-35. Long-term survival after ablation of the atrioventricular (AV) node and pacemaker implantation in patients with atrial fibrillation (AF). Ablation of the AV junction with pacemaker placement results in regularization and improvement in cardiac output and has been associated with improvements in clinical symptoms. The long-term survival in patients with refractory AF treated with AV junction ablation and permanent pacing is worse than the expected survival based on mortality among age- and gender-matched members of the Minnesota population; however, it is similar to the survival among controls treated with drugs for atrial fibrillation (**A**).

Continued on next page

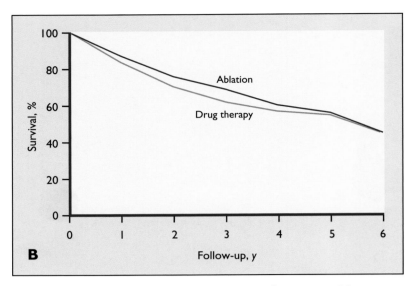

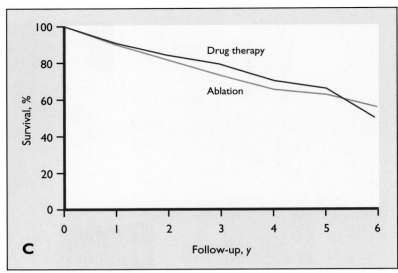

FIGURE 9-35. *(Continued)* In the subgroup of patients with congestive heart failure (CHF) (**B**) or coronary disease (**C**), survival among ablation patients was similar to survival among drug-treated controls. Biventricular pacing may add additional benefit to AV junction ablation outcomes in patients with CHF [35]. (*Adapted from* Ozcan *et al.* [35].)

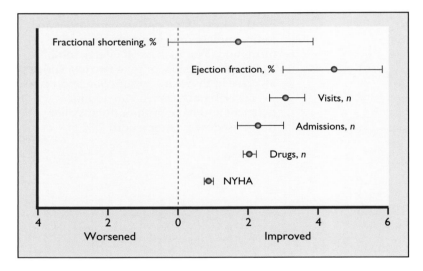

FIGURE 9-36. Clinical outcomes after atrioventricular (AV) node ablation and permanent pacemaker implantation. Meta-analysis has demonstrated that AV node ablation and permanent pacing results in clinical improvement as assessed by a number of measures. This improvement is likely the result of control and regularization of the ventricular response during atrial fibrillation (AF). Additionally, side effects associated with rate control medications are eliminated as these are no longer required following the ablation procedure. Because asymptomatic AF is expected following ablation, anticoagulation is typically continued [34]. NYHA—New York Heart Association (functional class). (*Adapted from* Wood *et al.* [34].)

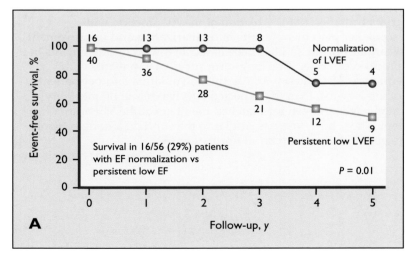

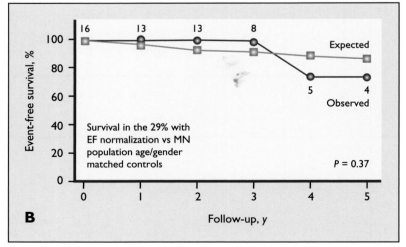

FIGURE 9-37. Change in ejection fraction (EF) and survival following atrioventricular node ablation and pacing: the importance of adequate rate control. In a Mayo Clinic population-based study of patients with atrial fibrillation (AF) and depressed ventricular function (EF < 40%), EF nearly normalized (to > 45%) in 16 of 56 patients (29%). The long-term survival in patients in whom the EF normalized was better than the survival in patients without normalization (**A**). Patients with a normalized EF experienced survival similar to the observed age- and gender-matched survival in the Minnesota population (**B**). These results suggest that a reversible tachycardia-induced cardiomyopathy is present in a significant proportion of patients with refractory AF [36]. LVEF—left ventricular ejection fraction. (*Adapted from* Ozcan *et al.* [36].)

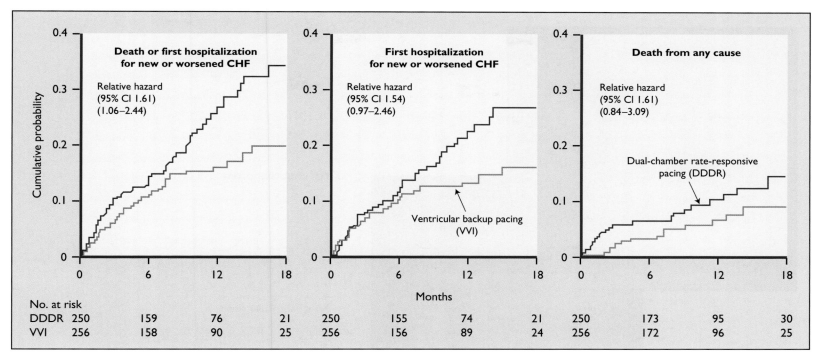

FIGURE 9-38. Detrimental effect of right ventricular apical (RVA) pacing in patients with depressed ventricular function. The DAVID (Dual Chamber and VVI Implantable Defibrillator) study randomized patients with left ventricular ejection fraction of 40% or less and no indication for bradycardia pacing to ventricular backup pacing (VVI-40) or dual-chamber rate-responsive pacing (DDDR) at 70 bpm. Patients randomized to DDDR pacing tended to be at greater risk for death or heart failure than were patients who were infrequently paced (VVI-40). This likely resulted because the RVA pacing intrinsic to the DDDR mode introduced ventricular dyssynchrony, which counteracted the anticipated benefit with atrioventricular synchrony [46]. CHF—congestive heart failure. (*Adapted from* DAVID Trial Investigators [46].)

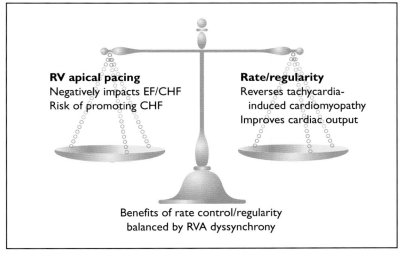

Benefits of rate control/regularity balanced by RVA dyssynchrony

FIGURE 9-39. Atrioventricular (AV) node ablation for atrial fibrillation (AF) and heart failure: balancing rate control and right ventricular apical (RVA) pacing. The improvement in symptoms seen with AV node ablation and pacing and improvement in ejection fraction (EF) observed in a subset of patients stems from rate control and regularization. Some of this benefit may be mitigated, however, by RVA pacing, which promotes dyssynchrony and heart failure. These effects suggest, at least for some patients with heart failure and AF undergoing AV node ablation, that use of biventricular pacing (which improves cardiac output by pacing both right and left ventricles) may be preferred. CHF—congestive heart failure.

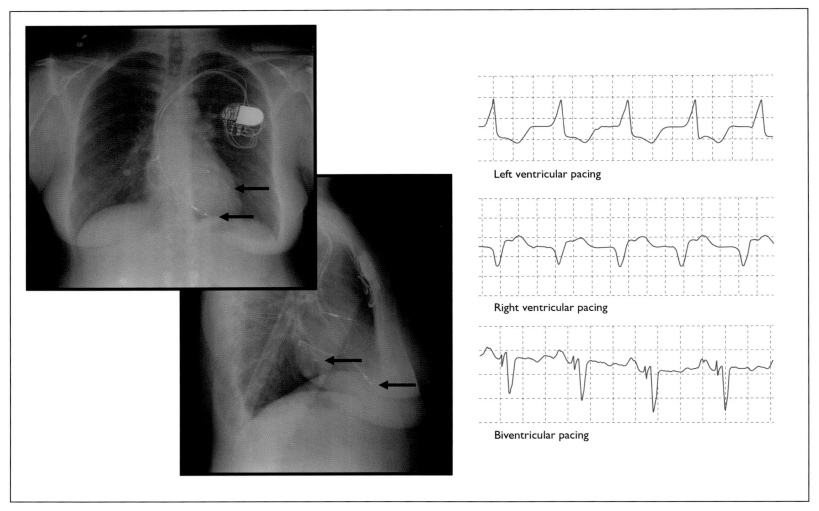

FIGURE 9-40. Cardiac resynchronization (biventricular pacing). In patients with congestive heart failure, depressed ventricular function, and ventricular dyssynchrony (manifest as a wide QRS, most commonly with left bundle branch block pattern), pacing from right and left ventricles simultaneously (or with a short programmed interventricular delay) improves cardiac output, ejection fraction, and heart failure symptoms. The chest radiograph demonstrates a biventricular system with lead tips in the right ventricular apex and left ventricular epicardium (*arrows*). Left ventricular leads are most commonly placed by cannulating the coronary sinus in the right atrium to access the coronary veins, avoiding the need for thoracotomy. The electrocardiographic strips show the dramatic changes in vector with pacing from the left and right ventricular leads and the narrowed QRS resulting from simultaneous biventricular pacing.

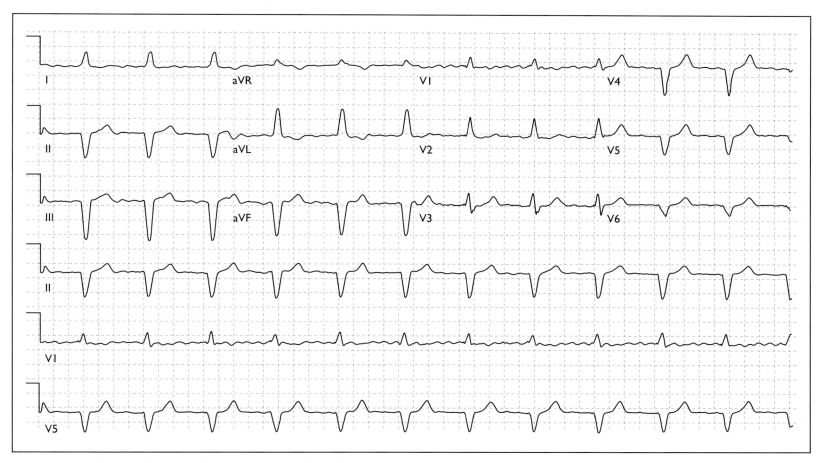

FIGURE 9-41. Electrocardiogram from a patient with atrial fibrillation and a biventricular pacing system. Note the right bundle branch block (RBBB) morphology in lead V_1, which suggests predominant activation of the left ventricle before the right ventricle (as is seen during RBBB). Although an RBBB pattern is occasionally seen with right ventricular apical pacing, it is common with biventricular pacing and expected with isolated left ventricular pacing. The patient also had an atrioventricular node ablation; the completely regular ventricular rate and lack of fusion are consistent with heart block and a paced rhythm.

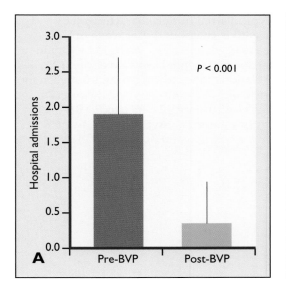

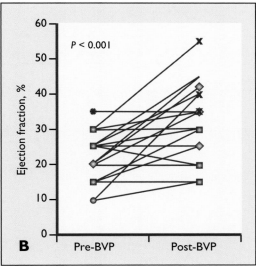

FIGURE 9-42. Effect of upgrading to biventricular pacing (BVP) after chronic right ventricular apical pacing in patients with atrial fibrillation, previous atrioventricular (AV) node ablation, and refractory congestive heart failure. This study enrolled 20 consecutive patients with severe heart failure (ejection fraction [EF] < 0.35, New York Heart Association class III or IV), prior AV node ablation, and right ventricular pacing for at least 6 months. Following upgrade to biventricular pacing, hospital admissions significantly declined (**A**) and EF improved (**B**). The study highlights the impact of ventricular synchrony in patients with heart failure, a low EF, and a high frequency of pacing [26]. (*Adapted from* Leon *et al.* [26].)

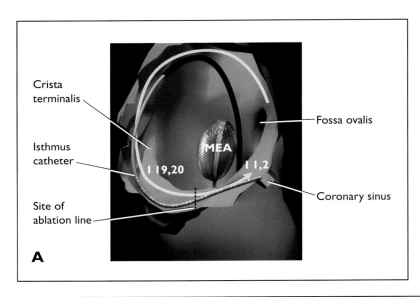

A

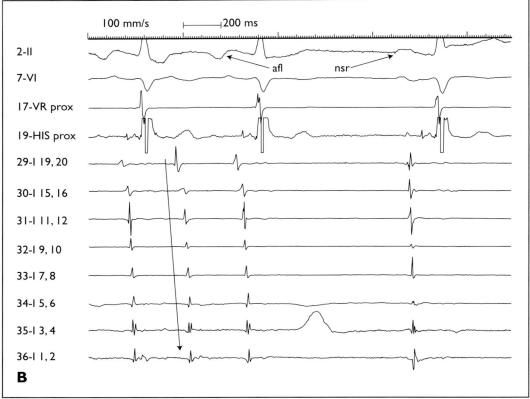

B

FIGURE 9-43. Catheter ablation of atrial flutter. Patients with congestive heart failure and atrial fibrillation may develop atrial flutter despite antiarrhythmic drug therapy, or they may develop atrial flutter in the absence of rhythm medication. Typical atrial flutter, characterized by negative sawtooth flutter wave in ECG leads II, III, and aVF, is caused by a counterclockwise right atrial wave front (**A**). Ablation of the critical isthmus between the tricuspid valve annulus and the inferior vena cava interrupts the circuit (**B**), restoring normal rhythm [47]. (*Adapted from* Friedman and Stanton [47].)

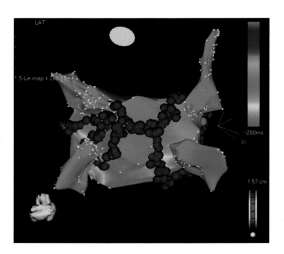

FIGURE 9-44. Pulmonary vein isolation ablation of atrial fibrillation (AF). The posterior left atrium is a critical structure for the initiation and likely for the maintenance of AF. This may stem from the interaction of venous smooth muscle (which is capable of very rapid electrical discharge) with left atrial endocardium, regional vagal nervous input, or anisotropic conduction. Catheter ablation to electrically isolate pulmonary veins (*shown*) or to modify the left atrial substrate has restored sinus rhythm in 70% to 90% of patients. In most series, however, the number of patients with heart failure or significant structural heart disease has been modest. The figure demonstrates a posteroanterior view of the left atrium as depicted by a computer mapping system used to guide ablation.

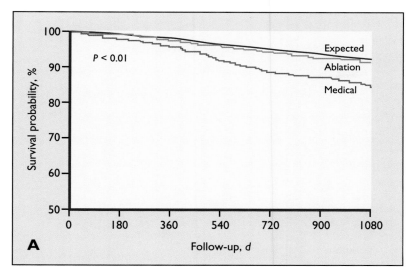

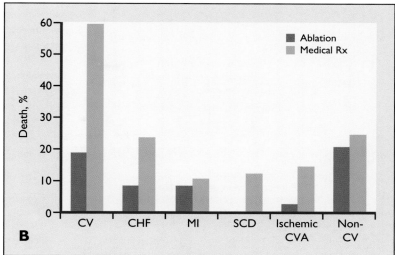

FIGURE 9-45. **A** and **B**, Survival in atrial fibrillation (AF) patients after medical therapy or ablation. This nonrandomized study of 1171 consecutive patients with symptomatic AF compared outcomes of patients treated medically with antiarrhythmic drugs with those treated with circumferential pulmonary vein transcatheter ablation. Patients treated with ablation had survival similar to age- and gender-matched persons in the Italian population. Patients treated with medical therapy had increased mortality due to cardiovascular (CV) events (**B**). The study suggests that ablation improves mortality, morbidity, and (not shown) quality of life compared with medical therapy. It is important to note, however, that patients were not randomized [48]. CHF—congestive heart failure; CVA—cerebrovascular accident; MI—mycardial infarction; SCD—sudden cardiac death. (*Adapted from* Pappone *et al.* [48].)

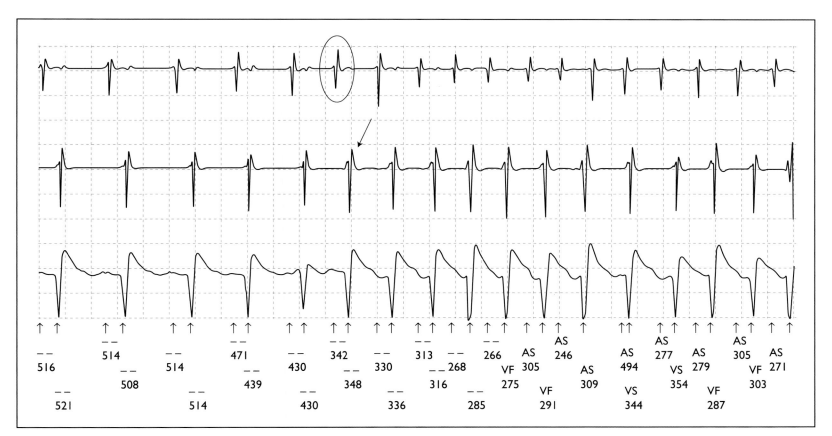

FIGURE 9-46. Inappropriate shock due to an atrial tachycardia. Many patients with heart failure and depressed ventricular function are candidates for implantable cardioverter-defibrillators (ICDs). Atrial tachyarrhythmias are a frequent cause of inappropriate shock in these patients, necessitating the concomitant use of antiarrhythmic drugs to suppress the atrial arrhythmias. The figure depicts intracardiac electrograms for an ICD; shown from *top* to *bottom* are the atrial electrogram, ventricular (near-field) electrogram, ventricular (far-field) electrogram, and device-measured intervals. An atrial flutter that begins with an atrial premature beat (*circled*) leads to a rapid ventricular response (beginning with *arrow*). This is misinterpreted as ventricular fibrillation, leading to shock. Device reprogramming to make use of detection enhancements and medications may be performed to prevent recurrent inappropriate shocks.

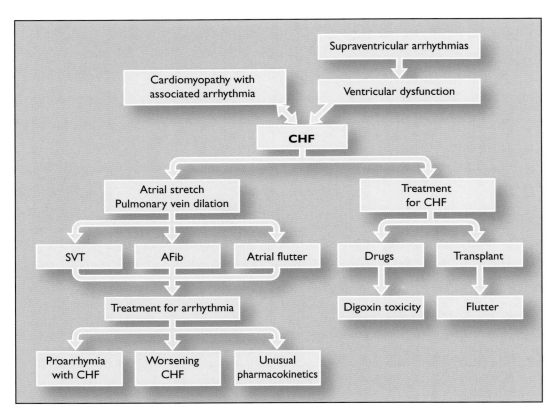

FIGURE 9-47. A stepwise algorithmic approach to the diagnosis and treatment of supraventricular arrhythmia in heart failure. AFib—atrial fibrillation; CHF—congestive heart failure; SVT—supraventricular tachycardia.

REFERENCES

1. Mathew J, Hunsberger S, Fleg J, *et al.*: Incidence, predictive factors, and prognostic significance of supraventricular tachyarrhythmias in congestive heart failure. *Chest* 2000, 118:914–922.

2. Chugh S, Blackshear J, Shen W, *et al.*: Epidemiology and natural history of atrial fibrillation: Clinical implications. *J Am Coll Cardiol* 2001, 37:371–378.

3. Maisel W, Stevenson L: Atrial fibrillation in heart failure: Epidemiology, pathophysiology, and rationale for therapy. *Am J Cardiol* 2003, 91:2D–8D.

4. Ehrlich J, Nattel S, Hohnloser S: Atrial fibrillation and congestive heart failure: Specific considerations at the intersection of two common and important cardiac disease states. *J Cardiovasc Electrophysiol* 2002, 13:399–405.

5. Kalman J, VanHare G, Olgin J, *et al.*: Ablation of 'incisional' reentrant atrial tachycardia complicating surgery for congenital heart disease: Use of entrainment to define a critical isthmus of conduction. *Circulation* 1996, 93:502–512.

6. Pozzoli M, Cioffi G, Traversi E, *et al.*: Predictors of primary atrial fibrillation and concomitant clinical and hemodynamic changes in patients with chronic heart failure: a prospective study in 244 patients with baseline sinus rhythm. *J Am Coll Cardiol* 1998, 32:197–204.

7. Mayr A, Knotzer H, Pajk W, *et al.*: Risk factors associated with new onset tachyarrhythmias after cardiac surgery—a retrospective analysis. *Int J Clin Prac* 2001, 55:108–114.

8. Young J, Gasparini M: Congestive heart failure induced by recipient atrial tachycardia conducted to the donor atrium after orthotopic heart transplantation: complete regression after successful radiofrequency ablation. *Drug Saf* 1999, 20:223–230.

9. Coates WC, Henneman PL, Lewis RJ, Raggi P: Uncommon etiologies of atrial fibrillation. *Acad Emerg Med* 1996, 3:114–119.

10. Vlay SC, Vlay LC, Coyle PK: Combined cardiomyopathy and skeletal myopathy: a variant with atrial fibrillation and ventricular tachycardia. *Pacing Clin Electrophysiol* 2001, 24:1389–1397.

11. Scherf D: Studies on auricular tachycardia caused by aconitine administration. *Proc Exp Biol Med* 1947, 64:233.

12. Haissaguerre M, Jais P, Shah D, *et al.*: Spontaneous initiation of atrial fibrillation by ectopic beats originating in the pulmonary veins. *N Engl J Med* 1998, 339:659–666.

13. Moe G: On the multiploe wavelet hypothesis of atrial fibrillation. *Arch Int Pharmacodyn Ther* 1962, 140:183–188.

14. Kalifa J, Jalife J, Zaitsev A, *et al.*: Intra-atrial pressure increases rate and organization of waves emanating from the superior pulmonary veins during atrial fibrillation. *Circulation* 2003, 158:668–671.

15. Goyal SB, Spodick DH: Electromechanical dysfunction of the left atrium associated with interatrial block. *Am Heart J* 2001, 142:823–827.

16. Anderson RH, Sanchez-Quintana D, Komiya N: Electrophysiological abnormalities of the atrial muscle in patients with paroxysmal atrial fibrillation associated with hyperthyroidism. *Cardiovasc Res* 2002, 54:325–336.

17. Morrison K, Krishnaswamy P, Kazanegra R, *et al.*: Temporal relations of atrial fibrillation and congestive heart failure and their joint influence on mortality: the Framingham Heart Study [see comment]. *Diabetes Care* 2003, 26:2081–2087.

18. Mounsey JP, Kok LC, DiMarco JP, *et al.*: Atrial structure and fibres: morphologic bases of atrial conduction. *J Am Coll Cardiol* 2002, 39:1964–1972.

19. Ernst S, Antz M, Ouyang F, *et al.*: Ostial PV isolation: is there a role for three-dimensional mapping? *Pacing Clin Electrophysiol* 2003, 26:1624–1630.

20. Takase B, Nagata M, Matsui T, *et al.*: Pulmonary vein dimensions and variation of branching pattern in patients with paroxysmal atrial fibrillation using magnetic resonance angiography. *Jpn Heart J* 2004, 45:81–92.

21. Dixen U, Wallevik L, Hansen MS, *et al.*: Prolonged signal-averaged P wave duration as a prognostic marker for morbidity and mortality in patients with congestive heart failure. *Scand Cardiovasc J* 2003, 37:193–198.

22. Mansourati J, Gilard M, Valls-Bertault V, *et al.*: Predictors of primary atrial fibrillation and concomitant clinical and hemodynamic changes in patients with chronic heart failure: a prospective study in 344 patients with baseline sinus rhythm. *Am J Cardiol* 1999, 83:1138–1140.

23. Wang T, Larson M, Levy D, *et al.*: Temporal relations of atrial fibrillation and congestive heart failure and their joint influence on mortality: the Framingham Heart Study. *Circulation* 2003, 107:2920–2925.

24. Nikolic G, Marriott H: Left bundle branch block with right axis deviation: A marker of congestive cardiomyopathy. *J Electrocardiol* 1985, 18:395–404.

25. Goldberger A, Dresselhaus T, Bhargava V: Dilated cardiomyopathy: Utility of the transverse: Frontal plane QRS voltage ratio. *J Electrocardiol* 1985, 18:35–40.

26. Leon A, Greenberg J, Kanuru N, *et al.*: Cardiac resynchronization in patients with congestive heart failure and chronic atrial fibrillation: Effect of upgrading to biventricular pacing after chronic right ventricular pacing. *J Am Coll Cardiol* 2002, 39:1258–1263.

27. Troughton R, Prior D, Pereira J, *et al.*: Plasma B-type natriuretic peptide levels in systolic heart failure: Importance of left ventricular diastolic function and right ventricular systolic function. *J Am Coll Cardiol* 2004, 43:416–422.

28. Mueller C, Scholer A, Laule-Kilian K, *et al.*: Use of B-type natriuretic peptide in the evaluation and management of acute dyspnea. *N Engl J Med* 2004, 350:647–654.

29. Shinagawa K, Li D, Leung TK, Nattel S: Consequences of atrial tachycardia-induced remodeling depend on the preexisting atrial substrate. *Circulation* 2002, 105:251–257.

30. Shinbane JS, Wood MA, Jensen DN, *et al.*: Tachycardia-induced cardiomyopathy: a review of animal models and clinical studies. *J Am Coll Cardiol* 1997, 29:709–715.

31. Landahl S, Hedner T, Hall C, *et al.*: Avoiding drug problems. The safety of drugs for supraventricular tachycardia. *J Intern Med* 1997, 241:269–275.

32. Dries D, Exner D, Gersh B, *et al.*: Atrial fibrillation is associated with an increased risk for mortality and heart failure progression in patients with asymptomatic and symptomatic left ventricular systolic dysfunction: a retrospective analysis of the SOLVD trials. *J Am Coll Cardiol* 1998, 32:695–703.

33. Stein K, Euler D, Mehra R, *et al.*: Do atrial tachyarrhythmias beget ventricular tachyarrhythmias in defibrillator recipients? *J Am Coll Cardiol* 2002, 40:335–340.

34. Wood M, Brown-Mahoney C, Kay G, Ellenbogen K: Clinical outcomes after ablation and pacing therapy for atrial fibrillation: A meta-analysis. *Circulation* 2000, 101:1138–1144.

35. Ozcan C, Jahangir A, Friedman P, *et al.*: Long-term survival after ablation of the atrioventricular node and implantation of a permanent pacemaker in patients with atrial fibrillation. *N Engl J Med* 2001, 344:1043–1051.

36. Ozcan C, Jahangir A, Friedman P, *et al.*: Significant effects of atrioventricular node ablation and pacemaker implantation on left ventricular function and long-term survival in patients with atrial fibrillation and left ventricular dysfunction. *Am J Cardiol* 2003, 92:33–37.

37. Acierno JS Jr, Dai D, Leyne M, *et al.*: Atrial fibrillation. Rhythm versus rate control. *Am J Hum Genet* 2003, 72:1551–1559.

38. Feinberg WM: Anticoagulation for prevention of stroke. *Neurology* 1998, 51:S27–S30.

39. Alaeddini J, Ramee S, Ventura HO, Pedersen OD: Prevalence, prognostic significance, and treatment of atrial fibrillation in congestive heart failure with particular reference to the DIAMOND-CHF study. *Congest Heart Fail* 2003, 9:343–346.

40. Brendorp B, Pedersen OD, Elming H, *et al.*: Can antiarrhythmic drugs save lives in patients with congestive heart failure? *Expert Rev Cardiovasc Ther* 2003, 1:191–202.

41. Naccarelli GV, Hynes J, Wolbrette DL, *et al.*: Maintaining stability of sinus rhythm in atrial fibrillation: antiarrhythmic drugs versus ablation. *Curr Cardiol Rep* 2002, 4:418–425.

42. Elming H, Brendorp B, Pedersen OD, *et al.*: Dofetilide: a new drug to control cardiac arrhythmia. *Expert Opin Pharmacother* 2003, 4:973–985.

43. Pedersen OD, Bagger H, Keller N, *et al.*: Efficacy of dofetilide in the treatment of atrial fibrillation-flutter in patients with reduced left ventricular function: a Danish investigations of arrhythmia and mortality on dofetilide (DIAMOND) substudy. *Circulation* 2001, 104:292–296.

44. Heywood JT: Calcium channel blockers for heart rate control in atrial fibrillation complicated by congestive heart failure. *Can J Cardiol* 1995, 11:823–826.

45. Nolan PE Jr, Nappi J, Pollak PT: Clinical efficacy of amiodarone. *Pharmacotherapy* 1998, 18:127S–137S.

46. DAVID Trial Investigators: Dual-chamber pacing or ventricular backup pacing in patients with an implantable defibrillator: the dual-chamber and VVI implantable defibrillator (DAVID) trial. *JAMA* 2002, 288:3115–3123.

47. Friedman P, Stanton M: Spot welding the gap in atrial flutter ablation. *Circulation* 1999, 99:3206–3208.

48. Pappone C, Rosanio S, Augello G, *et al.*: Mortality, morbidity, and quality of life after circumferential pulmonary vein ablation for atrial fibrillation: outcomes from a controlled nonrandomized long-term study. *J Am Coll Cardiol* 2003, 42:185–197.

VENTRICULAR ARRHYTHMIAS IN ISCHEMIC CARDIOMYOPATHY

Bruce A. Koplan and William G. Stevenson

Ventricular arrhythmias ranging from single premature ventricular beats to sustained ventricular tachycardia and ventricular fibrillation are common in patients with ischemic heart disease. The frequency of ambient ventricular ectopic activity parallels the severity of ventricular dysfunction and heart failure. Ventricular tachycardia (VT) and ventricular fibrillation (VF) are important causes of sudden death. The ability to identify patients at risk for future arrhythmias and sudden death has improved significantly over time. This chapter reviews mechanisms, diagnosis, and therapy of ventricular arrhythmias in patients with ischemic cardiomyopathy. Risk stratification for future sudden death in patients with ischemic cardiomyopathy and prognosis for patients with a prior episode of ventricular arrhythmia are discussed.

Ventricular arrhythmias are characterized by their duration, effect, and electrocardiographic morphology. Sustained arrhythmias require an intervention for termination, such as cardioversion or antiarrhythmic drug administration, or produce severe symptoms, such as syncope. Nonsustained arrhythmias terminate spontaneously without a severe hemodynamic impact. During electrophysiologic studies, induced VTs that last more than 30 seconds are commonly defined as sustained. The QRS morphology is referred to as monomorphic when each QRS complex resembles the preceding and following QRS. Polymorphic VT has a changing QRS complex from beat to beat. Distinction is further complicated by the fact that many patients with ischemic cardiomyopathy have multiple morphologies of monomorphic VT.

The most common forms of sustained ventricular arrhythmia in ischemic cardiomyopathy are polymorphic VT/VF (PMVT/VF), which occurs most commonly in the setting of acute ischemia, and sustained monomorphic VT related to a preexisting myocardial infarct scar. During acute ischemia, the resting membrane potential in ventricular myocytes becomes less negative. Important factors that contribute to this are a rise in extracellular $K+$ concentration and a fall in the extracellular pH [1–3]. Eventually, the peak action potential spike during phase 0 of the monophasic action potential becomes blunted and recovery of cellular excitability becomes slowed, leading to failure of electrical propagation in the ischemic zone. A less negative resting membrane potential along with electrical heterogeneity both transmurally and in the zone of ischemia compared with nearby nonischemic zones provides a substrate for increased excitability and reentry. These features provide a substrate for PMVT/VF. Another common ventricular arrhythmia in ischemic cardiomyopathy is sustained monomorphic VT in the setting of a prior infarct scar. A prior scar leads to heterogeneous conduction with preferential conduction in certain directions around the scar in such a way that the depolarization wave front can reenter areas of the scar. If an appropriate substrate of scar interspersed with excitable tissue is present, the depolarization wave front can reenter isthmuses of excitable tissue within the scar and lead to sustained VT [4].

The nonsustained ventricular arrhythmias seen in ischemic cardiomyopathy may result from the same mechanisms described above for sustained ventricular arrhythmias. Single premature ventricular beats (PVCs) are common in patients with ischemic heart disease and may arise either from afterde-polarizations or reentry. Nonsustained VT (NSVT), either polymorphic or monomorphic, is defined as three or more consecutive ventricular beats. Frequent PVCs and NSVT are associated with future risk of sudden death in patients with a prior infarct [5,6]. Other forms of ventricular arrhythmia, including accelerated idioventricular rhythm, torsades de pointes, and ventricular arrhythmias related to metabolic disarray, are also covered in this chapter.

The recognition of ventricular arrhythmias and the ability to differentiate them from supraventricular arrhythmia are essential. In patients with a wide complex tachycardia, the medical history alone often points to the correct diagnosis. In patients with prior myocardial infarction, wide QRS tachycardia can be assumed to be ventricular in origin with 95% certainty [7]. The surface ECG may be used to differentiate VT from supraventricular tachycardia (SVT). Surface ECG characteristics that differentiate VT from SVT include the presence of electrical concordance in the precordial leads, atrioventricular (AV) dissociation, and onset of the R wave to the nadir of the S wave greater than 100 ms [8]. Additional findings that support VT as the cause of wide complex tachycardia include the presence of fusion and/or capture beats. When the diagnosis remains unclear, characteristics of the bundle branch morphology (which are also covered in this chapter) may also be helpful.

Management of ventricular arrhythmias in patients with ischemic heart disease must be tailored to the particular patient. Acute management involves eliminating, if possible, any active ischemia that may be eliciting an arrhythmia. Algorithms for the acute medical management of ventricular arrhythmias are discussed in this chapter. After the acute management of ventricular arrhythmias has taken place, the next step is to risk stratify patients with ischemic heart disease for future risk of sudden death.

Since the first human recipient of an implantable cardioverter-defibrillator (ICD) in 1980, the ICD has revolutionized the long-term management of ventricular arrhythmias in patients with ischemic cardiomyopathy. Currently, an ICD is the treatment of choice for most patients with a high risk of future ventricular arrhythmias and sudden death. Identification of those individuals (risk stratification) has been studied extensively. One of the most robust and highly used predictors of sudden death in patients with ischemic cardiomyopathy is the baseline ejection fraction. In the absence of a defibrillator, the annual rate of sudden death approaches 5% to 10% in patients with an ejection fraction less than or equal to 30%, and those with preserved functional capacity have an improvement in survival with an ICD [9,10]. Numerous other noninvasive risk factors for sudden cardiac death have been identified, including QRS width, abnormal T wave alternans, abnormal heart rate variability, and QT dispersion [11]. However, the utility of these other noninvasive risk factors in choosing patients for ICD therapy remains unclear. For patients in whom the ejection fraction is moderately reduced (ejection fraction <45%), programmed ventricular stimulation has been demonstrated as a useful tool for risk stratification and selection of patients for ICD therapy [6]. With regard to medical management to reduce future incidence of sudden cardiac death, β-blockers and ACE inhibitors have been demonstrated to be beneficial. Other antiarrhythmic drugs, such as class I or class III antiarrhythmics, have failed to show a mortality reduction, and some of these drugs (class Ia and Ic antiarrhythmics) may even be associated with increased mortality [12].

In patients who already have an ICD but are receiving frequent therapies from their device, antiarrhythmic medications have a role in reducing the frequency of occurrence of arrhythmia [13]. For ICD patients in whom frequent episodes of ventricular arrhythmia cannot be controlled with medication, or those in whom antiarrhythmic medications are contraindicated, catheter ablation has been shown to be effective at reducing the burden of future arrhythmia [4].

The topics mentioned in the preceding paragraphs are described in greater detail later in this chapter. After reviewing the chapter, the reader should have a better understanding of the recognition and management of ventricular arrhythmias related to ischemic heart disease. The reader should also have a better understanding of risk stratification for future sudden death in these patients so that treatment options can be tailored to the future risk of sudden death.

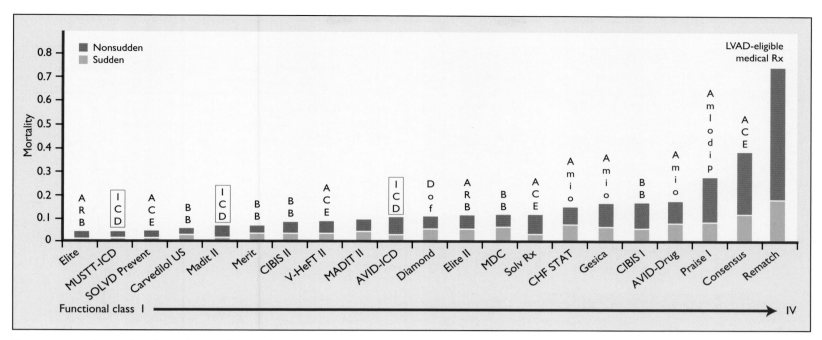

FIGURE 10-1. Annualized incidence of mortality (*total bar height*) and sudden death for selected trials including patients with depressed ventricular function. Annual sudden death risk ranges from less than 2% to more than 10%. As severity of heart failure increases, a greater proportion of deaths are caused by heart failure rather than by sudden death. Therapies assessed in the trials are indicated above the *bars*. ACE—angiotensin-converting enzyme; Amio—amiodarone; Amlodip—amlodipine; ARB—angiotensin receptor blocker; BB—β-blocker; Dof—dofetilide; ICD—implantable cardioverter-defibrillator; LVAD—left ventricular assist device; NYHA—New York Heart Association.

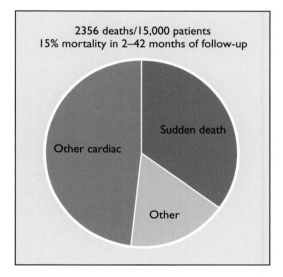

FIGURE 10-2. Meta-analysis of trials of acute myocardial infarction. In patients enrolled in trials of acute myocardial infarction who survived to be discharged from the hospital, 15% died during follow-up ranging from 2 to 42 months; 38% of the deaths were sudden, most likely the result of ventricular arrhythmias. Meta-analysis further indicated that therapy with ACE inhibitors was associated with a 20% reduction in the risk of sudden death [14].

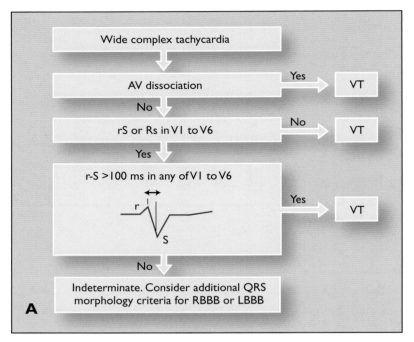

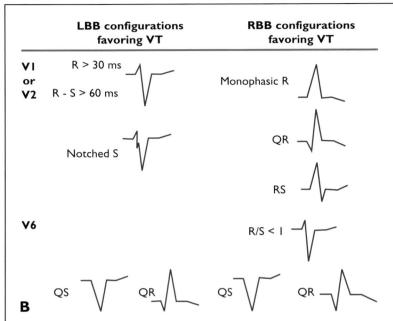

FIGURE 10-3. **A**, An algorithm for distinguishing monomorphic ventricular tachycardia (VT) from supraventricular tachycardia (SVT) with aberrant interventricular conduction. Although such algorithms are useful, errors occur, particularly in patients with advanced ventricular dysfunction. In general, wide QRS tachycardias should be managed presumptively as VT unless proven otherwise. **B**, QRS morphology characteristics that differentiate VT from SVT in a wide QRS tachycardia. Left bundle branch block (LBBB)-type morphologies have a dominant S wave in V_1 or V_2. Notching of the downstroke or a broad R wave favors VT. Right bundle branch block (RBBB) QRS morphologies, shown in the *right column*, have a dominant R wave in V_1 [8]. AV—atrioventricular; rS—greater amplitude of "S" component of QRS complex; Rs—greater amplitude of "R" component of QRS complex.

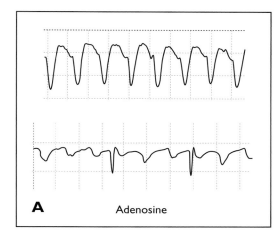

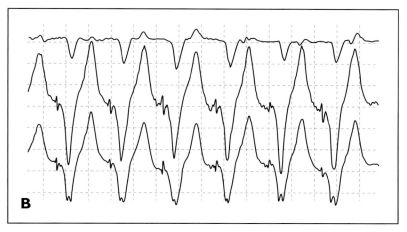

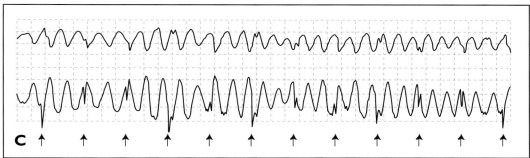

Figure 10-4. Wide complex rhythms that can be mistaken for ventricular tachycardia (VT). **A**, Atrial flutter conducted with one-to-one A-V conduction with aberrancy mimicking VT. Administration of adenosine created transient atrioventricular block, exposing the mechanism of the arrhythmia. Adenosine administration during a wide QRS tachycardia in patients with heart failure may be followed by severe bradyarrhythmias after arrhythmia termination, and may rarely precipitate ventricular fibrillation (VF) [15]. **B**, Wide complex tachycardia due to paced ventricular rhythm during sinus tachycardia in a patient with a DDD pacemaker. The pacing spikes are not evident in the *top tracing*, and this rhythm could be misinterpreted as a slow VT. **C**, Artifact mimicking polymorphic VT/VF that was caused by repetitive motion as the patient brushed his teeth. Absence of symptoms during the arrhythmia, the history, and actual QRS complexes (*arrows*) marching through the rhythm strip at a regular rate establish the diagnosis. Artifacts such as this one may lead to inappropriate testing, including invasive procedures, if not properly recognized [16].

TYPES OF VENTRICULAR TACHYARRHYTHMIAS IN ISCHEMIC CARDIOMYOPATHY

Monomorphic ventricular tachycardia (VT)
   Scar-related reentrant VT
   Bundle branch reentry
Polymorphic VT
   Torsades de pointes associated with QT prolongation
   Acute myocardial ischemia
Ventricular fibrillation
Accelerated idioventricular rhythm
Sinusoidal VT
   Hyperkalemia, ischemia
   Rapid monomorphic VT
Bidirectional VT
   Digoxin toxicity
   Myocarditis

Figure 10-5. Ventricular tachycardia can be classified based on electrocardiogram morphology as indicated. This classification also has utility in suggesting potential causes of the arrhythmia.

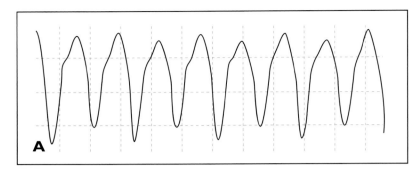

A

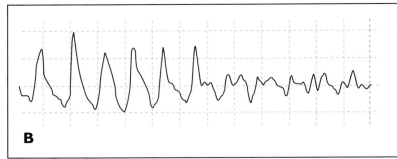

B

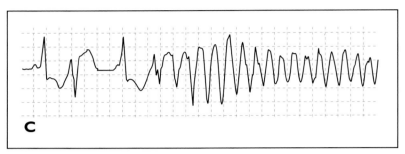

C

FIGURE 10-6. Examples of different electrocardiographic types of ventricular tachycardia (VT) are shown. **A,** Sustained monomorphic ventricular tachycardia. Each QRS is similar to the preceding and following QRS. This form of VT is most often caused by reentry through an area of old infarction (*see* below). **B,** Polymorphic VT degenerating into ventricular fibrillation. This form of tachycardia is commonly associated with active cardiac ischemia, although it may also occur related to prior infarction. **C,** Polymorphic VT torsades de pointes (TDP) (*see* below). Although TDP may be a result of congenital long QT syndromes, acquired forms are more common.

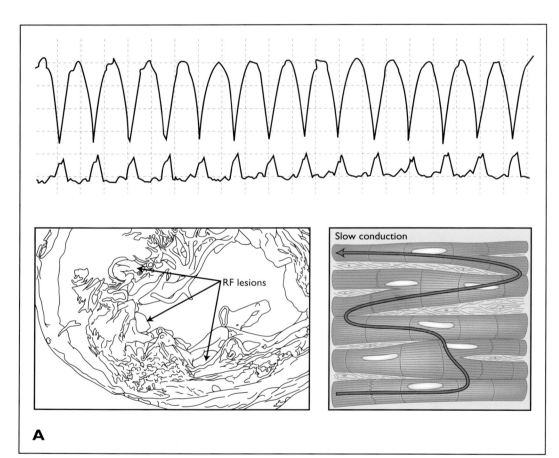

A

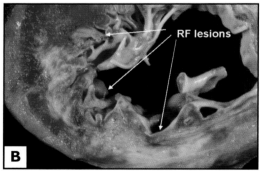

B

FIGURE 10-7. A, Sustained monomorphic ventricular tachycardia (VT) due to reentry through a region of old infarction shown from a two-channel recording. The mechanism is indicated in the schematic at the bottom. The left ventricle is seen in a short-axis view looking toward the mitral valve. Areas of surviving myocyte bundles are present in the inferior wall infarct region bordered by regions of fibrosis, creating channels or isthmuses for conduction through the infarct region. On a macroscopic level, conduction through the isthmus is slow because of a circuitous path for propagation, as illustrated in the schematic shown at the *lower right*. Depolarization of the isthmus does not produce sufficient amplitude electrical activity to be recorded in the surface ECG. The QRS

complex occurs when the circulating wave front reaches the exit of the isthmus, along the infarct border, and propagates across the ventricle. Multiple potential reentry pathways are present in most patients who have had spontaneous VT. The location and size of the circuits vary greatly from patient to patient [17–19].

B, Cross-section from an autopsy specimen of the left ventricle. The patient died of cardiogenic shock and uncontrollable monomorphic VT after failed catheter ablation. An extensive old inferior wall scar is present with dense fibrosis (*gray regions*) mixed with surviving myocytes (*red*). Radiofrequency (RF) catheter ablation lesions are present in the border of the scar (*grey regions with surrounding darker hemorrhagic margins*).

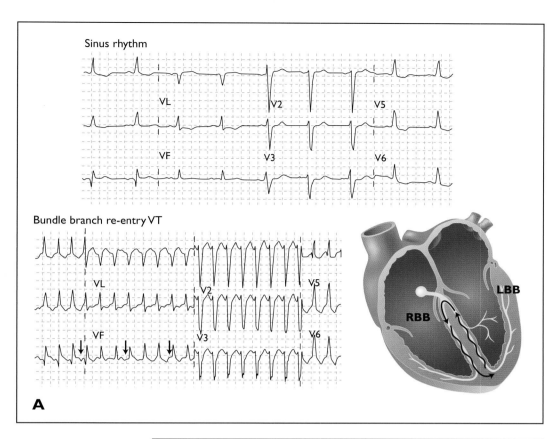

Sinus rhythm

Bundle branch re-entry VT

A

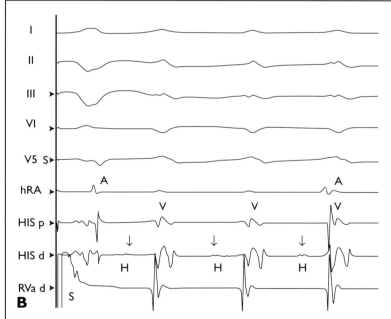

B

FIGURE 10-8. A, Surface electrocardiograms from a patient with old inferior wall myocardial infarction and ventricular tachycardia (VT) due to bundle branch reentry. During sinus rhythm (*top*), interventricular conduction delay is present, consistent with delayed conduction through the Purkinje system. In this case, the tachycardia has a QRS morphology similar to that of sinus rhythm, but atrioventricular (AV) dissociation is present (*arrows* denote p waves). The mechanism is shown in the *panel to the right of the lower figure.* The circulating reentry wave front propagates down the right bundle branch (RBB), producing a QRS that has a left bundle branch block configuration. The wave front continues through the interventricular septum and then travels in retrograde up the left bundle branch (LBB) to complete the circuit. Bundle branch reentry (BBR) causes 5% to 10% of monomorphic VTs that are studied in the electrophysiology laboratory in patients with ischemic cardiomyopathy. BBR may have either a left bundle branch block or right bundle branch block configuration, depending on the direction of revolution through the reentry circuit. It is associated with severe disease in the His-Purkinje system and usually with severe left ventricular dysfunction. Catheter ablation of the right bundle branch is curative, but other, poor residual AV conduction and other scar-related VTs are often present, so implantation of a cardioverter-defibrillator is often warranted [20,21].

B, Surface ECG and intracardiac electrogram example of BBR tachycardia. *The top five tracings* represent simultaneous surface-lead electrograms (standard ECG leads I, II, III, V_1, and V_5) recorded at 200 mm/sec. Simultaneous intracardiac electrograms from the high right atrium (hRA, *fourth from bottom*), proximal His bundle region (HIS p, *third from bottom*), distal His bundle (HIS d, *second from bottom*), and right ventricular apex (Rva d, *bottom electrogram*) are also displayed. BBR is initiated with a premature stimulus (S). Note dissociation between the atrial electrogram (A) and the ventricular electrogram (V) during tachycardia, consistent with VT. A His bundle electrogram (H) precedes each ventricular electrogram, consistent with involvement of this His-Purkinje system in the tachycardia. Radiofrequency ablation of the right bundle branch eliminated this tachycardia.

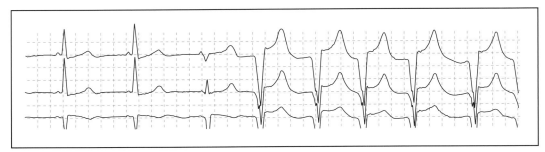

FIGURE 10-9. Accelerated idioventricular rhythm (AIVR). AIVR often occurs in the setting of a slowing of atrial rhythm and may be caused by increased automaticity in Purkinje fibers. It is common during acute myocardial infarction and cardiac

reperfusion, and usually resolves spontaneously. Note the third beat of the rhythm strip, which represents a fusion beat (fusion between sinus rhythm and ventricular rhythm).

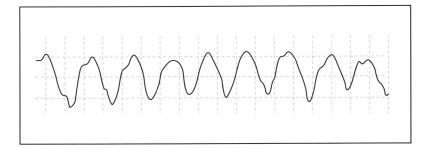

FIGURE 10-10. Sinusoidal ventricular tachycardia due to hyperkalemia. The markedly long QRS duration exceeding 200 ms indicates that conduction through the ventricle is markedly slowed. Hyperkalemia, severe global myocardial ischemia, and anti-arrhythmic drug toxicity (particularly flecainide or propafenone) are potential causes. Immediate therapy should include intravenous calcium gluconate. Sodium bicarbonate administration also rapidly improves conduction. Glucose and insulin administration and measures to reduce serum potassium may then be undertaken [22,23].

RISK FACTORS FOR HYPERKALEMIA IN HEART FAILURE

IMPAIRED RENAL FUNCTION

ACE inhibitors
Angiotensin blockade
β-Blockers
Aldosterone antagonists

HYPERKALEMIA DURING SPIRONOLACTONE THERAPY

RALES pilot trial [25]:
214 patients treated with spironolactone for 12 wk
13% hyperkalemia with spironolactone 25 mg daily
20% hyperkalemia with spironolactone 50 mg daily

RALES—Randomized Aldactone Evaluation Study.

FIGURE 10-11. Risk factors for hyperkalemia in heart failure. Ischemic cardiomyopathy and many heart failure therapies predispose to hyperkalemia. Hyperkalemia suppresses automaticity and slows conduction. Sinusoidal ventricular tachycardia responds to administration of intravenous calcium gluconate and sodium bicarbonate [24,25].

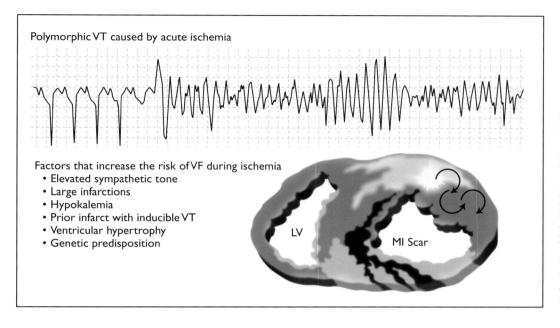

Polymorphic VT caused by acute ischemia

Factors that increase the risk of VF during ischemia
• Elevated sympathetic tone
• Large infarctions
• Hypokalemia
• Prior infarct with inducible VT
• Ventricular hypertrophy
• Genetic predisposition

LV

MI Scar

FIGURE 10-12. Polymorphic ventricular tachycardia (VT) due to acute myocardial infarction (MI). During acute ischemia, potassium leaks from cells into the interstitium, depolarizing adjacent cells and causing ventricular ectopic activity that can reenter through the border region, initiating polymorphic VT that degenerates to ventricular fibrillation (VF). Autopsies in patients with ischemic cardiomyopathy who died suddenly suggest acute ischemia in 54% of sudden death victims, even though symptoms of an ischemic syndrome were usually not clinically appreciated [26]. LV—left ventricle.

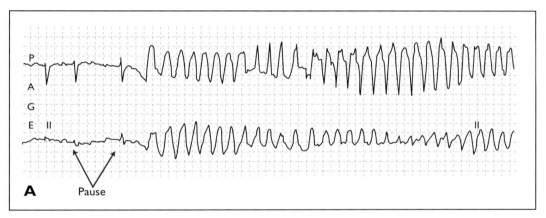

P
A
G
E   II

II

A   Pause

B. CAUSES OF QT PROLONGATION AND TORSADES DE POINTES

Bradycardia	Psychotropic drugs
Electrolytes	Haloperidol
Hypo K, Mg, Ca	Tricyclic antidepressants
Antiarrhythmics	Phenothiazines
Sotalol	Antibiotics
Dofetilide	Erythromycin
Ibutilide	Pentamidine
Quinidine	Trimethoprim-sulfamethoxazole
Procainamide	Other drugs
Disopyramide	Bepridil
Amiodarone (rare)	Probucol

FIGURE 10-13. Polymorphic ventricular tachycardia torsades de pointes (TDP) associated with QT prolongation. **A,** Note the initiation of TDP usually occurs after a long interval (pause) produces further QT prolongation, thus with a long–short sequence. **B,** Although TDP may be associated with congenital long QT syndrome, most cases are caused by another factor that prolongs the QT interval. Diuretic therapy inducing electrolyte abnormalities, and diminished excretion of antiarrhythmic drugs that prolong the QT interval, increase susceptibility of patients with ischemic cardiomyopathy to TDP. In addition, electrophysiologic remodeling of hypertrophy in chronic heart failure is associated with down-regulation of repolarizing potassium currents that may predispose to this arrhythmia [27,28].

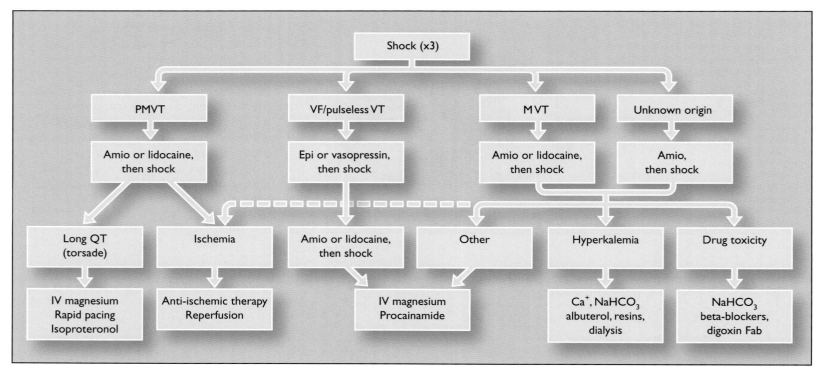

FIGURE 10-14. Acute management of hemodynamically unstable wide complex tachycardia (WCT)/ventricular tachycardia (VT). This algorithm assumes that cardiopulmonary resuscitation is initiated after three unsuccessful shocks and maintained until a pulse is achieved. Amio—amiodarone; Epi—epinephrine; MVT—monomorphic VT; PMVT—polymorphic VT; VF—ventricular fibrillation [29].

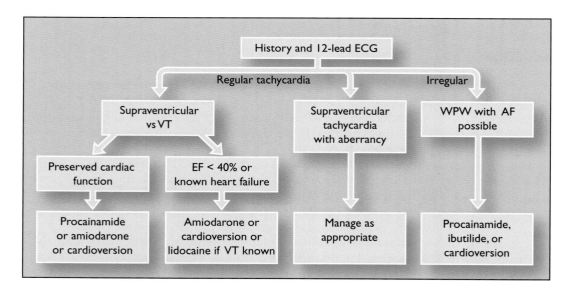

FIGURE 10-15. An approach to stable wide complex tachycardia. AF—atrial fibrillation; EF—ejection fraction; VT—ventricular tachycardia; WPW—Wolff-Parkinson-White.

RISK STRATIFICATION AND LONG-TERM TREATMENT AND PREVENTION OF VENTRICULAR ARRHYTHMIAS IN ISCHEMIC HEART DISEASE

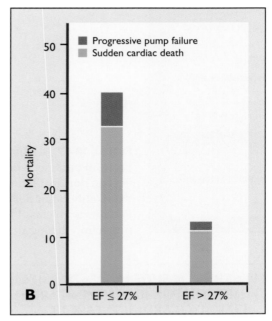

A. SECONDARY PREVENTION TRIALS DEMONSTRATING A MORTALITY BENEFIT FROM ICDS IN ISCHEMIC HEART DISEASE

TRIAL (YEAR)	OUTCOME
AVID (1997)	Resuscitated VF/VT
CIDS (2000)	Resuscitated VF/VT >72 h out from any MI
CASH (2000)	Resuscitated VF/VT >72 h out from any MI

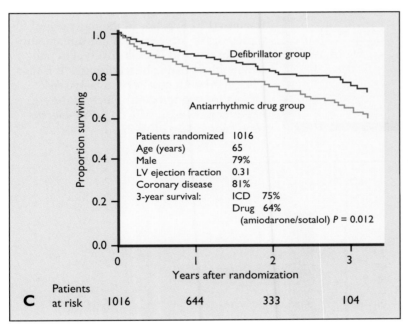

FIGURE 10-16. A, Inclusion criteria from clinical trials demonstrating a mortality benefit from implantable cardioverter-defibrillators (ICDs) in ischemic heart disease. Multiple clinical trials have demonstrated a survival benefit from ICDs for both primary and secondary prevention of sudden cardiac death (SCD) in properly selected patients with ischemic cardiomyopathy [30–33].

B, In patients who have experienced a prior episode of ventricular tachycardia (VT) or ventricular fibrillation (VF), the risk of death either from progressive pump failure or SCD is highly determined by the baseline left ventricular (LV) ejection fraction (EF) [34].

C, Kaplan-Meier survival curve from the Antiarrhythmics Versus Implantable Defibrillators (AVID) trial. Patients resuscitated from VT or VF without a correctable cause, 81% with coronary artery disease, were randomized to ICD versus antiarrhythmic drug. ICDs conferred a significant improvement in mortality. Two smaller trials (Cardiac Arrest Study Hamburg [CASH] and Canadian Implantable Defibrillator Study [CIDS]), although failing to reach statistical significance, displayed similar trends. +EPS—inducible VT at electrophysiology study; MI—myocardial infarction; NSVT—nonsustained VT.

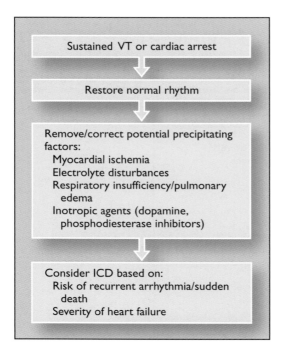

FIGURE 10-17. Arrhythmia management strategy for secondary prevention of arrhythmic death in patients who have survived a sustained episode of ventricular tachycardia or ventricular fibrillation. Therapy is guided by the likely risk of recurrent arrhythmias and the likelihood of deriving a benefit from an implantable cardioverter-defibrillator (ICD). Patients with class IV heart failure are unlikely to benefit unless the ICD provides protection during the wait for cardiac transplantation.

PRIMARY PREVENTION OF SUDDEN DEATH: IMPORTANCE OF VENTRICULAR FUNCTION FOR IDENTIFYING ARRHYTHMIA RISK AFTER MYOCARDIAL INFARCTION

	LVEF <0.40	LVEF >0.40
Infarct survivors, %	22–34	66–78
Sudden death/arrhythmia (annualized incidence), %	3–11	1–2
+ EPS, %	20	6
+ SECG, %	47	24

FIGURE 10-18. Primary prevention of sudden death. The left ventricular ejection fraction (LVEF) is one of the most useful indicators of future risk of life-threatening arrhythmias and overall survival in patients with ischemic heart disease. It is also associated with other noninvasive risk factors for sudden death, such as the signal-averaged ECG (SECG). EPS—electrophysiologic study [35–37].

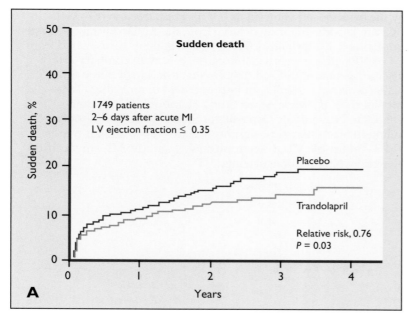

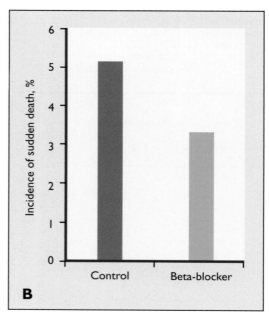

FIGURE 10-19. Agents that reduce the risk of sudden cardiac death. A reduction in sudden cardiac death has been demonstrated through the use of both ACE inhibitors (**A**) and β-blockers (**B**) in patients with ischemic heart disease. Unless contraindicated, these medications should be considered as first-line agents for patients with ischemic heart disease and ventricular dysfunction [38,39]. LV—left ventricular; MI—myocardial infarction.

A. LONG-TERM ANTIARRHYTHMIC DRUG (AAD) THERAPY AFTER MYOCARDIAL INFARCTION: EFFECT ON SUDDEN DEATH AND OVERALL MORTALITY IN THE ABSENCE OF AN IMPLANTABLE CARDIOVERTER-DEFIBRILLATOR

DRUG	MORTALITY	SUDDEN DEATH
Class Ia AADs		
Quinidine	Increased	—
Class Ib AADs		
Lidocaine	Neutral	Neutral
Mexiletine	Neutral	Neutral
Class Ic AADs		
Encainide	Increased	Increased
Moricizine	Increased	—
Flecainide	Increased	Increased
β-Blockers	Decreased	Decreased
Class III AADs		
Amiodarone	Neutral	Decreased
d,l-Sotalol	Neutral	Neutral
d-Sotalol	Increased	—
Dofetilide	Neutral	Neutral
Calcium channel blockers	Neutral	—

B. AMIODARONE FOR PRIMARY PREVENTION OF SUDDEN DEATH: META-ANALYSIS OF POST–MYOCARDIAL INFARCTION AND HEART FAILURE TRIALS

THE GOOD

13% Reduction in total mortality

29% Reduction in sudden death

Predictors of benefit

Initial heart rate >90 bpm (GESICA); additive benefit to β-adrenergic blockers (EMIAT/CAMIAT)

THE BAD

Amiodarone discontinued in 41% of patients by 2 y

Placebo discontinued in 27% of patients

Risk of pulmonary toxicity: 1%/y

CAMIAT—Canadian Amiodarone Myocardial Infarction Arrhythmia Trial (Pilot); EMIAT—European Myocardial Infarction Amiodarone Trial; GESICA—Randomized Trial of Low-Dose Amiodarone in Severe Congestive Heart Failure.

C. AMIODARONE TOXICITIES

EFFECT	% AFFECTED
Bradycardia	2.4
Hypothyroidism	7
Hyperthyroidism	1.4
Neuropathy	0.5
Pulmonary effects	1.6
Liver effects	1.0

FIGURE 10-20. Antiarrhythmic drug (AAD) therapy for the prevention of sudden death and overall mortality. **A**, Aside from β-blocker therapy, antiarrhythmic drugs other than amiodarone fail to reduce mortality, and many have increased mortality in patients with depressed ventricular function and coronary artery disease. Proarrhythmia (such as torsades de pointes) and other toxicities may be the cause [12,35,40–43]. **B**, Amiodarone therapy has been evaluated in patients surviving myocardial infarction who had markers of increased risk for sudden death (depressed ventricular function and/or ambient ventricular ectopy). The trials were generally neutral or suggested a small benefit. Meta-analysis suggests a beneficial effect on mortality and sudden death, but with substantial toxicities. Implantable cardioverter-defibrillators are clearly superior to amiodarone in efficacy for prevention of sudden death [44]. **C**, Some of the more common toxicities of amiodarone along with their rate of occurrence [45–47].

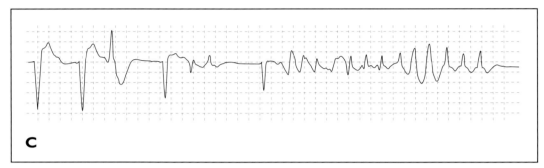

A. PRIMARY PREVENTION OF SUDDEN DEATH WITH IMPLANTABLE CARDIOVERTER-DEFIBRILLATORS IN ISCHEMIC HEART DISEASE

STUDY (YEAR)	TARGET POPULATION
MADIT-II (2002)	EF ≤30%, >1 mo from any MI, >3 mo from revascularization
MADIT (1996)	EF ≤35%, NSVT, +EPS, >3 wk from any MI, >3 mo from any revascularization
MUSTT (1999)	EF ≤40%, NSVT ≥4 d after any MI or revascularization, +EPS

EF—ejection fraction; EPS—electrophysiologic study; MADIT—Multicenter Automatic Defibrillator Implantation Trial; MI—myocardial infarction; MUSTT—Multicenter Unsustained Tachycardia Trial; NSVT—nonsustained ventricular tachycardia.

B

C

FIGURE 10-21. Survival benefit of implantable cardioverter-defibrillators (ICDs). **A**, Inclusion criteria of trials of ICDs in ischemic heart disease. Multiple clinical trials have demonstrated a survival benefit from ICDs for both primary and secondary prevention of sudden cardiac death in properly selected patients with ischemic cardiomyopathy [6,10,48]. **B**, Nonsustained ventricular tachycardia (NSVT) is observed in more than 60% of patients with chronic heart failure. It is a marker of disease severity and increased mortality from sudden and nonsudden death. Suppression of NSVT does

not reduce sudden death. Approximately one-third of patients with NSVT and left ventricular ejection fraction <0.40 have inducible ventricular tachycardia (VT) at electrophysiologic testing. The Multicenter Unsustained Tachycardia Trial (MUSTT) supports implantation of an ICD to reduce mortality in these patients. **C**, Nonsustained polymorphic VT is relatively unusual and should raise concern for myocardial ischemia and causes of torsades de pointes. In MUSTT, the majority of VTs were less than 10 beats in duration and slower than 180 bpm [6].

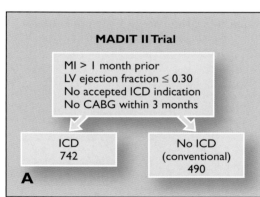

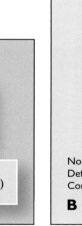

MADIT II Trial

MI > 1 month prior
LV ejection fraction ≤ 0.30
No accepted ICD indication
No CABG within 3 months

ICD
742

No ICD
(conventional)
490

A

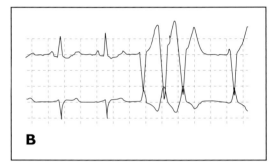

Mean follow-up = 20 mo

	Mortality
ICD	14.2%
No ICD	19.8%

Defibrillator

Conventional

No. at Risk					
Defibrillator	742	503(0.91)	274(0.84)	110(0.78)	9
Conventional	490	329(0.90)	170(0.78)	65(0.69)	3

B

FIGURE 10-22. Survival of patients with ischemic heart cardiomyopathy and left ventricular (LV) ejection fraction of 30% or less from the Multicenter Automatic Defibrillator Implantation Trial (MADIT)-II. **A**, Inclusion criteria and trial design of MADIT-II.

B, Survival curves from MADIT-II. Implantable cardioverter-defibrillator (ICD; *dotted line*) versus conventional medical therapy (*solid line*) for primary prevention. CABG—coronary artery bypass graft; MI—myocardial infarction; SCD—sudden cardiac death.

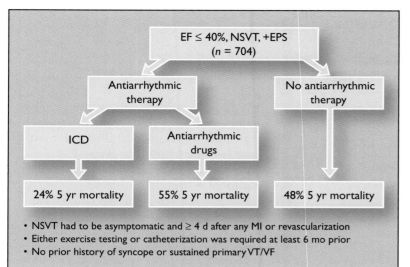

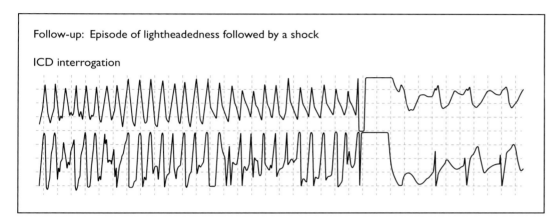

24% 5 yr mortality   55% 5 yr mortality   48% 5 yr mortality

- NSVT had to be asymptomatic and ≥ 4 d after any MI or revascularization
- Either exercise testing or catheterization was required at least 6 mo prior
- No prior history of syncope or sustained primary VT/VF

FIGURE 10-23. Electrophysiologic-guided study (EPS) of implantable cardioverter-defibrillators (ICDs). In patients with ischemic cardiomyopathy and less severe reduction of ejection fraction (EF ≤40%), ICDs have been demonstrated to confer a mortality benefit when the decision is guided by electrophysiologic study [6]. MI—myocardial infarction; NSVT—nonsustained ventricular tachycardia; VT/VF—ventricular tachycardia/ventricular fibrillation.

Follow-up: Episode of lightheadedness followed by a shock

ICD interrogation

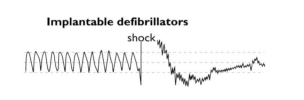

FIGURE 10-24. Intracardiac recording from a patient who received an appropriate therapy from an implantable cardioverter-defibrillator (ICD) for ventricular fibrillation that may have otherwise resulted in sudden death.

Implantable defibrillators

Indications:

Secondary prevention:
- Resuscitated from VT/VF without a clear correctable secondary cause
Primary prevention:
- Prior MI + LVEF ≤ 0.30 + QRS > 120 ms
- Prior MI EF < 0.40 + NSVT + inducible VT

FIGURE 10-25. Indications for implantable cardioverter-defibrillators (ICDs) in patients with ischemic cardiomyopathy. Information derived from clinical trials has led to these indications for ICDs in patients with ischemic cardiomyopathy. EF—ejection fraction; LVEF—left ventricular EF; MI—myocardial infarction; NSVT—nonsustained ventricular tachycardia; VT—ventricular tachycardia. (*Adapted from* American Heart Association. *Consensus Statement on Indications for Implantable Devices.*)

INDICATIONS FOR AN IMPLANTABLE CARDIOVERTER-DEFIBRILLATOR IN PATIENTS WITH ISCHEMIC HEART DISEASE

CLASS I

VF/VT arrest not due to a reversible cause

Spontaneous sustained VT in association with structural heart disease

Syncope of undetermined origin and inducible VT at EPS

NSVT, prior MI, LV dysfunction, and inducible VF/VT at EPS not suppressible by a class I antiarrhythmic drug

CLASS IIA

Patents with LVEF ≤30%, at least 1 mo post MI and 3 mo post coronary artery revascularization surgery

CLASS IIB

Cardiac arrest presumed to be caused by VF when EPS is precluded by other medical conditions

Severe symptoms attributable to sustained ventricular tachyarrhythmias while awaiting cardiac transplantation

Syncope with advanced structural heart disease in which thorough invasive and noninvasive investigation has failed to define a cause

CLASS III

Ventricular tachyarrhythmias due to a transient or reversible disorder (*eg*, acute MI, electrolyte imbalance, drugs, or trauma) when correction of the disorder is considered feasible and likely to substantially reduce the risk of recurrent arrhythmia

Significant psychiatric illnesses that may be aggravated by device implantation or may preclude systematic follow-up

Terminal illnesses with projected life expectancy of 6 mo

NYHA class IV drug-refractory congestive heart failure in patients who are not candidates for cardiac transplantation

Figure 10-26. Indications for implantable defibrillators in patients with ischemic heart disease. Class I: conditions for which there is evidence and/or general agreement that a given procedure or treatment is useful and effective. Class II: conditions for which there is conflicting evidence and/or a divergence of opinion about the usefulness/efficacy of a procedure or treatment; class IIa: weight of evidence/opinion is in favor of usefulness/efficacy; class IIb: usefulness/efficacy is less well established by evidence/opinion. Class III: conditions for which there is evidence and/or general agreement that the procedure/treatment is not useful/effective and in some cases may be harmful. EPS—electrophysiologic study; MI—myocardial infarction; NSVT—nonsustained ventricular tachycardia; VF—ventricular fibrillation; VT—ventricular tachycardia. LV—left ventricle; LVEF—left ventricular ejection fraction; NSVT—nonsustained ventricular tachycardia; NYHA—New York Heart Association. (*Modified from* American Heart Association. *Scientific Statement.* 1998 [update 2002].)

PATIENTS WHO SHOULD NOT RECEIVE AN IMPLANTABLE CARDIOVERTER-DEFIBRILLATOR (ICD)

Patients who, regardless of arrhythmia risk, should not receive an ICD include those who:

Are bedridden with class IV symptoms

Are awaiting transplantation in the hospital

Have incessant VT or active ischemia (an ICD may be warranted after these issues are controlled)

Figure 10-27. Patients who should not receive an implantable cardioverter-defibrillator (ICD). The decision to implant an ICD must be tailored to the patient. Regardless of the future risk of arrhythmia, some patients with severe medical comorbidities may not be appropriate candidates. In addition, certain active medical conditions, such as ongoing cardiac ischemia or incessant ventricular tachycardia (VT) should be controlled prior to device implantation.

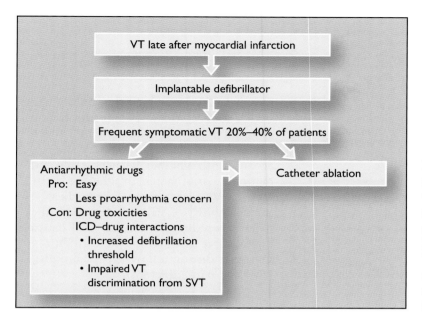

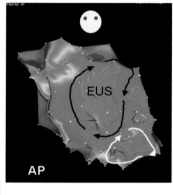

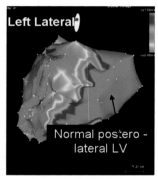

FIGURE 10-28. Implantable cardioverter-defibrillators (ICDs) as first-line therapy. ICDs are first-line therapy for patients with ventricular tachycardia (VT) or ventricular fibrillation (VF) that is not clearly the result of a correctable secondary cause, such as acute myocardial infarction. Of those who develop VT, more than 70% experience a recurrence of the arrhythmia during follow-up. Those with VF have a lower risk of recurrence, but the risk still exceeds 30%. Those with frequent symptomatic recurrences require further therapy to reduce episodes [49]. SVT—supraventricular VT.

FIGURE 10-29. Catheter ablation of recurrent ventricular tachycardia (VT). Catheter ablation of recurrent VT requires identification of the regions contained in the large infarcts that support reentry. Catheter mapping during VT is often not possible when VT produces hemodynamic instability. **A**, Ablation has been facilitated by use of "voltage maps" of the ventricles. The maps are acquired by moving a mapping catheter point by point around the left ventricle. The amplitude of the electrograms at each point are indicated by color codes. Normal amplitude regions (>1.5 millivolts) are purple; amplitude diminishes as colors proceed to blue, green, yellow, and red. Gray areas are electrically unexcitable scar (EUS) that has a pacing threshold greater than 10 milliamperes. This type of plot clearly defines the location of the anterior wall infarction in this patient and exposes potential channels of excitable myocytes that may support reentry. Pacing in these regions may further help locate regions of slow conduction and exit sites from reentry circuits. Radiofrequency (RF) ablation lesions are then placed during stable sinus rhythm through selected target regions. This approach markedly reduces VT recurrences and the resulting implantable cardioverter-defibrillator therapies in the majority of patients, regardless of the presence of multiple morphologies of VT and unstable VT [50–52].

B, Simultaneously recorded surface electrogram tracings recorded during RF ablation of VT (ablation artifact seen in *bottom tracing*). VT is present with the first nine QRS complexes. RF energy was applied in a critical isthmus region as defined by voltage mapping during sinus rhythm (*see* panel A), and the tachycardia terminates during the RF application and sinus rhythm ensues (last three QRS complexes).

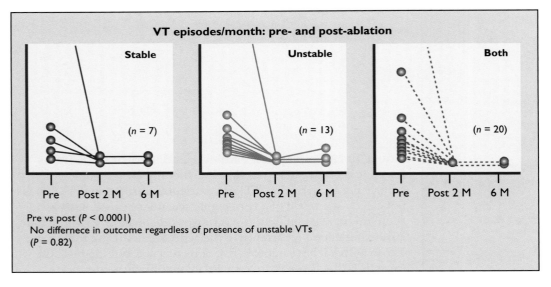

FIGURE 10-30. Reduction in monthly ventricular tachycardia (VT) episodes for 1 month prior to ablation and at 2 and 6 months after ablation for patients according to whether VT was stable and mappable or unstable, or whether both types of VT were present. Regardless of the stability of VT, catheter ablation markedly reduced episodes of VT causing implantable cardioverter-defibrillator therapies during follow-up at 2 months (2M) and 6 months (6M).

REFERENCES

1. Harris A, Bisteni A, Russell RA, *et al.*: Excitatory factors in ventricular tachycardia resulting from myocardial ischemia; potassium a major excitant. *Science* 1954, 199:200–203.

2. Coronel R, Fiolet JW, Wilms-Schopman JG, *et al.*: Distribution of extracellular potassium and electrophysiologic changes during two-stage coronary ligation in the isolated, perfused canine heart. *Circulation* 1989, 80:165–177.

3. Pogwizd SM, Corr PB: Mechanisms underlying the development of ventricular fibrillation during early myocardial ischemia. *Circ Res* 1990, 66:672–695.

4. Soejima K, Stevenson WG: Catheter ablation of ventricular tachycardia in patients with ischemic heart disease. *Curr Cardiol Rep* 2003, 5:364–368.

5. Maggioni AP, Zuanetti G, Franzosi MG, *et al.*: Prevalence and prognostic significance of ventricular arrhythmias after acute myocardial infarction in the fibrinolytic era. GISSI-2 results [see comment]. *Circulation* 1993, 87:312–322.

6. Buxton AE, Lee KL, Fisher JD, *et al.*: A randomized study of the prevention of sudden death in patients with coronary artery disease. Multicenter Unsustained Tachycardia Trial Investigators. *N Engl J Med* 1999, 341:1882–1890.

7. Tchou P, Young P, Mahmud R, *et al.*: Useful clinical criteria for the diagnosis of ventricular tachycardia. *Am J Med* 1988, 84:53–56.

8. Brugada P, Brugada J, Mont L, *et al.*: A new approach to the differential diagnosis of a regular tachycardia with a wide QRS complex [see comment]. *Circulation* 1991, 83:1649–1659.

9. Greenberg H, Case RB, Moss AJ, *et al.*: Analysis of mortality events in the Multicenter Automatic Defibrillator Implantation Trial (MADIT-II). *J Am Coll Cardiol* 2004, 43:1459–1465.

10. Moss AJ, Zareba W, Hall WJ, *et al.*: Prophylactic implantation of a defibrillator in patients with myocardial infarction and reduced ejection fraction. *N Engl J Med* 2002, 346:877–883.

11. Stevenson WG, Epstein LM: Predicting sudden death risk for heart failure patients in the implantable cardioverter-defibrillator age [comment]. *Circulation* 2003, 107:514–516.

12. Epstein AE, Hallstrom AP, Rogers WJ, *et al.*: Mortality following ventricular arrhythmia suppression by encainide, flecainide, and moricizine after myocardial infarction. The original design concept of the Cardiac Arrhythmia Suppression Trial (CAST). *JAMA* 1993, 270:2451–2455.

13. Pacifico A, Hohnloser SH, Williams JH, *et al.*: Prevention of implantable-defibrillator shocks by treatment with sotalol. d,l-Sotalol Implantable Cardioverter-Defibrillator Study Group [see comment]. *N Engl J Med* 1999, 340:1855–1862.

14. Domanski MJ, Exner DV, Borkowf CB, *et al.*: Effect of angiotensin converting enzyme inhibition on sudden cardiac death in patients following acute myocardial infarction. A meta-analysis of randomized clinical trials. *J Am Coll Cardiol* 1999, 33:598–604.

15. Pelleg A, Pennock RS, Kutalek SP: Proarrhythmic effects of adenosine: one decade of clinical data. *Am J Ther* 2002, 9:141–147.

16. Knight BP, Pelosi F, Michaud GF, *et al.*: Clinical consequences of electrocardiographic artifact mimicking ventricular tachycardia. *N Engl J Med* 1999, 341:1270–1274.

17. de Bakker JM, Coronel R, Tasseron S, *et al.*: Ventricular tachycardia in the infarcted, Langendorff-perfused human heart: role of the arrangement of surviving cardiac fibers [see comment]. *J Am Coll Cardiol* 1990, 15:1594–1607.

18. de Bakker JM, van Capelle FJ, Janse MJ, *et al.*: Slow conduction in the infarcted human heart. 'Zigzag' course of activation. *Circulation* 1993, 88:915–926.

19. Stevenson WG, Friedman PL, Sager PT, *et al.*: Exploring post-infarction reentrant ventricular tachycardia with entrainment mapping. *J Am Coll Cardiol* 1997, 29:1180–1189.

20. Blanck Z, Dhala A, Deshpande S, *et al.*: Bundle branch reentrant ventricular tachycardia: cumulative experience in 48 patients [see comment]. *J Cardiovasc Electrophysiol* 1993, 4:253–262.

21. Lopera G, Stevenson WG, Soejima K, *et al.*: Identification and ablation of three types of ventricular tachycardia involving the His-Purkinje system in patients with heart disease. *J Cardiovasc Electrophysiol* 2004, 15:52–58.

22. Luu M, Stevenson WG, Stevenson LW, *et al.*: Diverse mechanisms of unexpected cardiac arrest in advanced heart failure. *Circulation* 1989, 80:1675–1680.

23. Kittleson M, Hurwitz S, Shah MR, *et al.*: Development of circulatory-renal limitations to angiotensin-converting enzyme inhibitors identifies patients with severe heart failure and early mortality. *J Am Coll Cardiol* 2003, 41:2029–2035.

24. Bozkurt B, Agoston I, Knowlton AA: Complications of inappropriate use of spironolactone in heart failure: when an old medicine spirals out of new guidelines. *J Am Coll Cardiol* 2003, 41:211–214.

25. Pitt B, Chang P, Grossman W, *et al.*: Rationale, background, and design of the randomized angiotensin receptor antagonist—angiotensin-converting enzyme inhibitor study (RAAS). *Am J Cardiol* 1996, 78:1129–1131.

26. Uretsky BF, Thygesen K, Armstrong PW, *et al.*: Acute coronary findings at autopsy in heart failure patients with sudden death: results from the assessment of treatment with lisinopril and survival (ATLAS) trial [see comment]. *Circulation* 2000, 102:611–616.

27. Middlekauff HR, Stevenson WG, Saxon LA, Stevenson LW: Amiodarone and torsades de pointes in patients with advanced heart failure. *Am J Cardiol* 1995, 76:499–502.

28. Tomaselli GF, Rose J: Molecular aspects of arrhythmias associated with cardiomyopathies. *Curr Opin Cardiol* 2000, 15:202–208.

29. Guidelines 2000 for Cardiopulmonary Resuscitation and Emergency Cardiovascular Care: Part 6: advanced cardiovascular life support: section 6: pharmacology II: agents to optimize cardiac output and blood pressure. The American Heart Association in collaboration with the International Liaison Committee on Resuscitation. *Circulation* 2000, 102(8 Suppl):I129–I35.

30. The Antiarrhythmics Versus Implantable Defibrillators (AVID) Investigators: A comparison of antiarrhythmic-drug therapy with implantable defibrillators in patients resuscitated from near-fatal ventricular arrhythmias. *N Engl J Med* 1997, 337:1576–1584.

31. Connolly SJ, Gent M, Roberts RS, *et al.*: Canadian Implantable Defibrillator Study (CIDS): a randomized trial of the implantable cardioverter defibrillator against amiodarone. *Circulation* 2000, 101:1297–1302.

32. Kuck KH, Cappato R, Siebels J, Ruppel R: Randomized comparison of antiarrhythmic drug therapy with implantable defibrillators in patients resuscitated from cardiac arrest: the Cardiac Arrest Study Hamburg (CASH). *Circulation* 2000, 102:748–754.

33. Connolly SJ, Hallstrom AP, Cappato R, *et al.*: Meta-analysis of the implantable cardioverter defibrillator secondary prevention trials. AVID, CASH and CIDS studies. Antiarrhythmics vs Implantable Defibrillator study. Cardiac Arrest Study Hamburg. Canadian Implantable Defibrillator Study. *Eur Heart J* 2000, 21:2071–2078.

34. Szabo BM, Crijns HJ, Wiesfeld AC, *et al.*: Predictors of mortality in patients with sustained ventricular tachycardias or ventricular fibrillation and depressed left ventricular function: importance of beta-blockade. *Am Heart J* 1995, 130:281–286.

35. Exner DV, Reiffel JA, Epstein AE, *et al.*: Beta-blocker use and survival in patients with ventricular fibrillation or symptomatic ventricular tachycardia: the Antiarrhythmics Versus Implantable Defibrillators (AVID) trial. *J Am Coll Cardiol* 1999, 34:325–333.

36. Pedretti R, Etro MD, Laporta A, *et al.*: Prediction of late arrhythmic events after acute myocardial infarction from combined use of noninvasive prognostic variables and inducibility of sustained monomorphic ventricular tachycardia. *Am J Cardiol* 1993, 71:1131–1141.

37. Copie X, Hnatkova K, Blankoff I, *et al.*: Risk of mortality after myocardial infarction: value of heart rate, its variability and left ventricular ejection fraction [in French]. *Arch Mal Coeur Vaiss* 1996, 89:865–871.

38. Kober L, Torp-Pedersen C, Carlsen JE, *et al.*: A clinical trial of the angiotensin-converting-enzyme inhibitor trandolapril in patients with left ventricular dysfunction after myocardial infarction. Trandolapril Cardiac Evaluation (TRACE) Study Group [see comment]. *N Engl J Med* 1995, 333:1670–1676.

39. Hjalmarson A: Effects of beta blockade on sudden cardiac death during acute myocardial infarction and the postinfarction period. *Am J Cardiol* 1997, 80:35J–39J.

40. Waldo AL, Camm AJ, deRuyter H, *et al.*: Effect of d-sotalol on mortality in patients with left ventricular dysfunction after recent and remote myocardial infarction. The SWORD Investigators. Survival With Oral d-Sotalol [see comment]. *Lancet* 1996, 348:7–12. [Erratum appears in *Lancet* 1996, 348:416.]

41. Kober L, Bloch Thomsen PE, Moller M, *et al.*: Effect of dofetilide in patients with recent myocardial infarction and left-ventricular dysfunction: a randomised trial. *Lancet* 2000, 356:2052–2058.

42. Reimold SC, Chalmers TC, Berlin JA, Antman EM: Assessment of the efficacy and safety of antiarrhythmic therapy for chronic atrial fibrillation: observations on the role of trial design and implications of drug-related mortality. *Am Heart J* 1992, 124:924–932.

43. Greene H: Randomized antiarrhythmic drug therapy in survivors of cardiac arrest (The CASCADE study). *Am J Cardiol* 1993, 72:280–287.

44. Anonymous. Effect of prophylactic amiodarone on mortality after acute myocardial infarction and in congestive heart failure: meta-analysis of individual data from 6500 patients in randomised trials. Amiodarone Trials Meta-Analysis Investigators [see comment]. *Lancet* 1997, 350:1417–1424.

45. Weinberg BA, Miles WM, Klein LS, *et al.*: Five-year follow-up of 589 patients treated with amiodarone. *Am Heart J* 1993, 125:109–120.

46. Dusman RE, Stanton MS, Miles WM, *et al.*: Clinical features of amiodarone-induced pulmonary toxicity. *Circulation* 1990, 82:51–59.

47. Ott MC, Khoor A, Leventhal JP, *et al.*: Pulmonary toxicity in patients receiving low-dose amiodarone. *Chest* 2003, 123:646–651.

48. Moss AJ, Hall WJ, Cannom DS, *et al.*: Improved survival with an implanted defibrillator in patients with coronary disease at high risk for ventricular arrhythmia. *N Engl J Med* 1996, 335:1933–1940.

49. Raitt MH, Klein RC, Wyse DG, *et al.*: Comparison of arrhythmia recurrence in patients presenting with ventricular fibrillation versus ventricular tachycardia in the Antiarrhythmics Versus Implantable Defibrillators (AVID) trial. *Am J Cardiol* 2003, 91:812–816.

50. Soejima K, Suzuki M, Maisel WH, *et al.*: Catheter ablation in patients with multiple and unstable ventricular tachycardias after myocardial infarction: short ablation lines guided by reentry circuit isthmuses and sinus rhythm mapping. *Circulation* 2001, 104:664–669.

51. Soejima K, Stevenson WG, Maisel WH, *et al.*: Electrically unexcitable scar mapping based on pacing threshold for identification of the reentry circuit isthmus: feasibility for guiding ventricular tachycardia ablation. *Circulation* 2002, 106:1678–1683.

52. Marchlinski FE, Callans DJ, Gottlieb CD, Zado E: Linear ablation lesions for control of unmappable ventricular tachycardia in patients with ischemic and nonischemic cardiomyopathy. *Circulation* 2000, 101:1288–1296.

VENTRICULAR ARRHYTHMIAS IN NONISCHEMIC DILATED CARDIOMYOPATHY

Kalyanam Shivkumar, Miguel Valderrabano, and Jagat Narula

Nonischemic dilated cardiomyopathies (NIDCM) comprise a heterogeneous set of diseases typically characterized by systolic dysfunction of the left ventricle or both ventricles. Myocardial dysfunction in this syndrome may be secondary to hypertensive, diabetic, familial, autoimmune, and metabolic causes. The major cause of morbidity and mortality (often sudden cardiac death) is related to disorders of cardiac rhythm. Although several in-hospital studies have implicated bradyarrhythmias and asystole as underlying mechanisms for death, ventricular tachyarrhythmias substantially contribute to mortality in these patients. Arrhythmogenesis in these patients may result from functional or structural abnormalities and may be initiated by reentrant or triggered mechanisms. Although, ischemic cardiomyopathy is the typical setting in which a structural substrate for reentry has been defined, patients with nonischemic cardiomyopathy may also harbor areas of low voltage/scars that provide the substrate for reentry.

The priority for management of nonischemic cardiomyopathy is to reduce the risk of sudden cardiac death. Although several earlier studies had shown promise in utilizing autonomic tests to define the risk for sudden death, recent studies have failed to confirm the predictive value of autonomic function tests. Medical therapies that are utilized for the management of heart failure (especially β-blockers) have a profound effect on reducing the risk of sudden death, but the use of implantable cardioverter-defibrillators (ICDs) offers the major intervention strategy to prevent sudden death in these patients. Most studies of ICDs have included patients with both ischemic and nonischemic cardiomyopathy. However, recent studies, such as Defibrillators in Nonischemic Cardiomyopathy Treatment Evaluation (DEFINITE), have focused exclusively on patients with nonischemic cardiomyopathy. One of the largest trials comparing amiodarone and ICD in heart failure, the Sudden Cardiac Death in Heart Failure Trial (SCD-HeFT), included a large proportion of patients with NIDCM. This trial has shown a significant improvement in survival in patients who received an ICD.

MOLECULAR IONIC CHANGES IN HEART FAILURE THAT MAY CONTRIBUTE TO ARRHYTHMOGENESIS

MYOCARDIAL PROTEINS	CHANGES DURING HF
Calcium channel	Most studies report a reduction
Na-Ca exchanger	Up-regulation
Ca pump of SR	Down-regulation
Phospholamban	Down-regulation
I_{to}	Reduction
$I_{K,S}$	Reduction
I_{K1}	Reduction
Late I_{Na}	Increased

FIGURE 11-1. Molecular ionic changes in heart failure that may contribute to arrhythmogenesis. It is well known that the rate of sudden cardiac death is inversely related to the left ventricular ejection fraction (LVEF). This is especially true when the LVEF is below 30% to 35%, the point at which mortality is increased by more than threefold. About 50% of deaths among heart failure (HF) patients are caused by ventricular arrhythmias. Unlike ischemic cardiomyopathy, these arrhythmias are often triggered by activity caused by after-depolarizations. Reentry also plays a role in nonischemic dilated cardiomyopathy (NIDCM). Scar tissue and scattered fibrosis may occur in such patients, creating potential reentrant circuits. Besides human studies from explanted hearts following orthotopic heart transplantation, many HF animal models have been established for mechanistic studies. As shown in the table, recent studies have demonstrated that cardiac action potential (AP) duration is prolonged in HF because of alteration of outward potassium, inward calcium, and late sodium currents. These changes are believed to be heterogeneous among different types of ventricular myocytes, leading to transmural heterogeneity of repolarization and therefore QT interval dispersion [1–4]. Increased sympathetic nerve sprouting in explanted hearts of cardiomyopathic patients with a history of clinical tachyarrhythmias has been reported [5] and represents an intriguing additional piece of the puzzle in the pathogenesis of ventricular arrhythmias in these patients.

Changes in ionic current density in individual myocytes during HF have long been implicated in the arrhythmogenesis in NIDCM (*see* Fig. 11-2). Recent experiments on cardiac tissue "wedge preparations" obtained from dogs with pacing-induced HF confirmed that AP duration is not only prolonged but also heterogeneous from epicardium to endocardium. Optical mapping studies [1] have shown that the prolongation of AP duration of the M cells, located in the middle layer of myocardium, accounts for increases in the QT interval in HF animals and subsequently may cause a significant increase in the spatial gradient of repolarization across the ventricular wall. As stated earlier, the prolonged AP would serve as substrate for delayed afterdepolarization. At the same time, a significant increase of spatial gradient of repolarization would cause the development of functional block, leading to reentrant ventricular tachycardia (VT), and increased susceptibility of reentry breakup, causing polymorphic VT. These findings suggest that a restoration of AP duration and reduction of transmural QT dispersion may be key factors in the development of antiarrhythmics and pharmacologic management of HF patients. I_{to}—transient outward potassium current; $I_{K,s}$—slow component of delayed rectifier potassium channel; I_{K1}—inward rectifier potassium channel; I_{Na}—late component of inward sodium current; SR—sarcoplasmic reticulum.

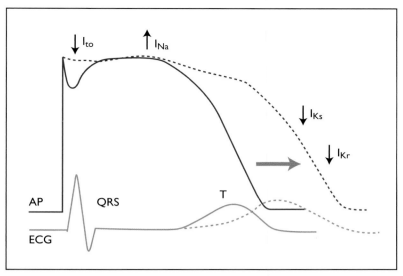

FIGURE 11-2. Alterations in ionic regulation leading to changes in cardiac excitability: action potential (AP) and ECG changes in heart failure. The characteristic finding in heart failure is the prolongation of the AP duration. Cardiac AP is generated by the extremely well-orchestrated function of different ion channels in the sarcolemma. The illustration shows a stylized AP and the underlying ionic currents responsible for the changes in membrane potential. The AP itself is a plot of membrane potential over time by the balance between inward and outward currents. Generally, the direction of the current is determined by the flow of positive ions, such as sodium (Na), calcium (Ca), and potassium (K). The inward current is defined as positive ions moving from the extracellular space into the intracellular space, and the outward current as positive ions moving in the reverse direction. When there is net inward current, the membrane potential becomes positive or depolarized, *ie*, it is less negative compared with the resting membrane potential. The converse is true when there is net outward current or the membrane potential becomes negative again or repolarized, *ie*, close to the resting membrane potential. At times, the membrane potential becomes more negative than the resting potential; this is referred to as "hyperpolarization." At any given point along the AP trace, there are both inward and outward currents that are operative, and the AP itself is governed by the balance between the currents. Phase 0 of the AP is the result of a rapid influx of Na via the voltage-gated Na channels in response to a depolarizing stimulus. This is followed by phase 1 as a result of the activation of an inward Ca current (via L-type Ca channels) and an early outward K current, called the transient outward current (I_{to}). Phase 2 of the AP is largely the result of the persistent activation of the inward Ca currents. Repolarization involves a concerted activation of several K currents. The major repolarizing currents in ventricular myocytes are I_{Kr} (rapid component of the delayed rectifier current) and I_{Ks} (slow component of the delayed rectifier current). The molecular bases of these currents have been determined with the cloning and expression of the corresponding ion channels. Prolongation of cardiac AP duration is critical to the triggered activity because of alteration of outward K, inward Ca, and late Na currents. These changes are believed to be heterogeneous among different types of ventricular myocytes, leading to transmural heterogeneity of repolarization and therefore QT interval dispersion. Such changes may eventually lead to development of functional block and may result in reentrant ventricular tachycardia (VT) and increased susceptibility of reentry breakup, causing polymorphic VT. I_{Na}—late component of inward sodium current.

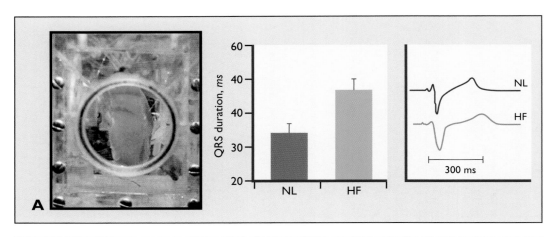

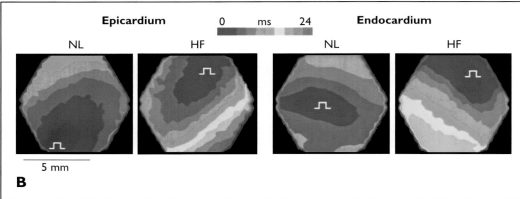

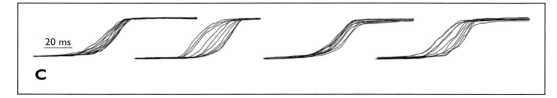

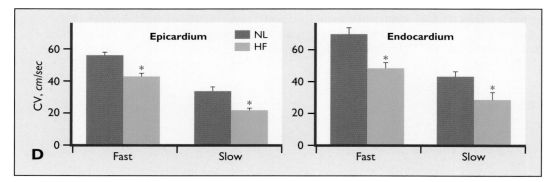

FIGURE 11-3. Experimental evidence of exaggerated transmural electrophysiologic heterogeneity. Experiments utilizing "wedge preparations" from a pacing-induced canine heart failure (HF) model confirm that action potential (AP) duration is not only prolonged but also heterogeneous from epicardium to endocardium. Optical mapping studies [1] show that the prolongation of AP duration of the M cells, which make up most of the middle layer of myocardium, accounts for the increase of QT interval in HF animals and subsequently causes a significant increase in the spatial gradient of repolarization across the ventricular wall. As stated earlier, the prolonged AP would serve as substrate for delayed afterdepolarization. In the meantime, a significant increase in the spatial gradient of repolarization would cause the development of functional block, leading to reentrant ventricular tachycardia (VT) and increased susceptibility of reentry breakup, causing polymorphic VT. **A,** Data obtained from a canine wedge preparation in a custom-designed imaging chamber. This preparation is mounted with the cut transmural surface facing the optical window. The duration of the QRS complex of the volume-conducted ECG was prolonged significantly in HF wedges. **B,** Depolarization isochronal maps of the epicardial and endocardial surfaces of representative canine wedge preparations from normal (NL) and failing (HF) ventricles paced from the sites (indicated by the *square wave*) demonstrate propagation of the electrical wave front. **C,** Representative AP upstrokes from sites along the slow axis of propagation in each layer that denotes slowing of impulse propagation in HF. **D,** Summary bar plots of left ventricular epicardial and endocardial conduction velocities (CV) along the fast and slow axes of propagation. Fast and slow components of CV are significantly reduced in wedges from failing hearts. *Asterisks* denote $P < 0.05$. (*Adapted from* Akar *et al*. [6].)

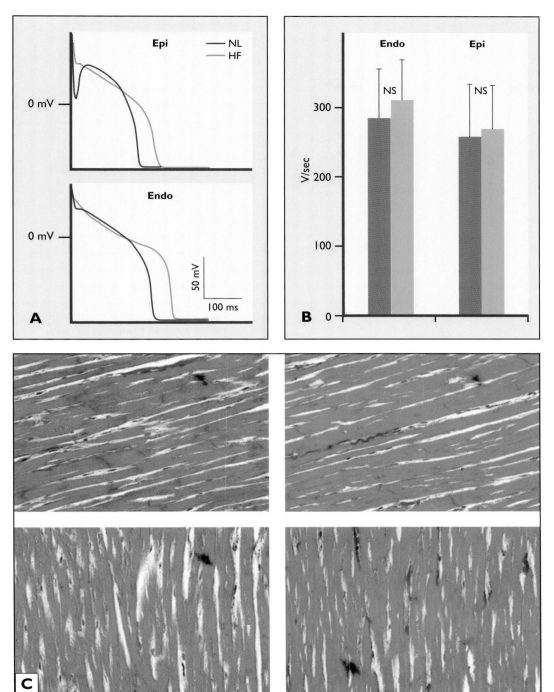

Figure 11-4. Epicardial (EPI) and endo-cardial (ENDO) tissue in normal (NL) and failing (HF) hearts. **A,** Representative action potentials recorded using the patch clamp technique in current-clamp mode in isolated epicardial and endocardial myo-cytes from a normal and failing left vent-ricle [6]. **B,** Bar plot of the average action potential upstroke velocity in epicardial and endocardial cells of normal and failing hearts. **C,** Masson trichrome stains of epicardial and endocardial tissue slices from a normal and a failing heart. NS—not significant.

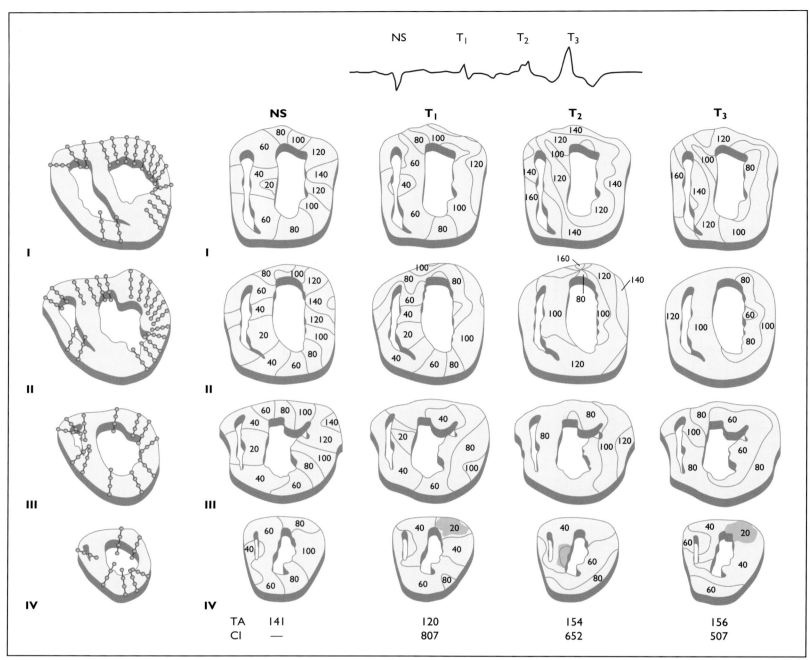

FIGURE 11-5. Focal ventricular tachycardia in nonischemic dilated cardiomyopathy (NIDCM): triggered activity or automaticity—mapping and histologic correlations (similar to Fig. 11-3). The figure shows three-dimensional activation sequences of sinus beat and subsequent spontaneous three-beat ventricular tachycardia (VT) from a patient with NIDCM. The *left* side of the figure shows the location of plunge electrodes placed in explanted hearts. The location of the electrodes in the right ventricle, septum, and interventricular septum are shown. The numbers correspond to activation times; 39 plunge-needle electrodes were placed in the left and right ventricles and interventricular septum. Electrodes were evenly distributed. Interelectrode distance averaged 0.5 to 1.5 cm between endocardial sites, 1 to 3 cm between epicardial sites, and 2.5 to 8 mm between sites of focal initiation and immediately adjacent sites. Each electrode contained four bipolar pairs separated by 2.5 mm, with an inter-bipolar distance of 500 µm. Electrograms were recorded from 156 intramural sites. There is termination of the preceding sinus beat (NS) in the midlateral left ventricle in level II. T_1 arose from an apical subendocardial site by a focal mechanism, as judged by the absence of intervening electrical activity for 665 ms from the termination of NS to the initiation of T_1 (colored *blue*). Beats T_2 and T_3 also arose by a focal mechanism from apical subendocardial sites (colored *blue*), with T_3 initiating at the same site as T_1. Each beat terminated in the basal posterolateral left ventricle, with no evidence of reentry Calibration bar = 300 ms. *Panels I to IV* are serial sections of the heart, from the base to the apex. T_1 to T_3 represent the beats of VT. The numbers represent activation times. The sequence of activation shows reentry across the myocardial wall occurring during this short run of non-sustained VT. (*Adapted from* Pogwizd *et al.* [7].)

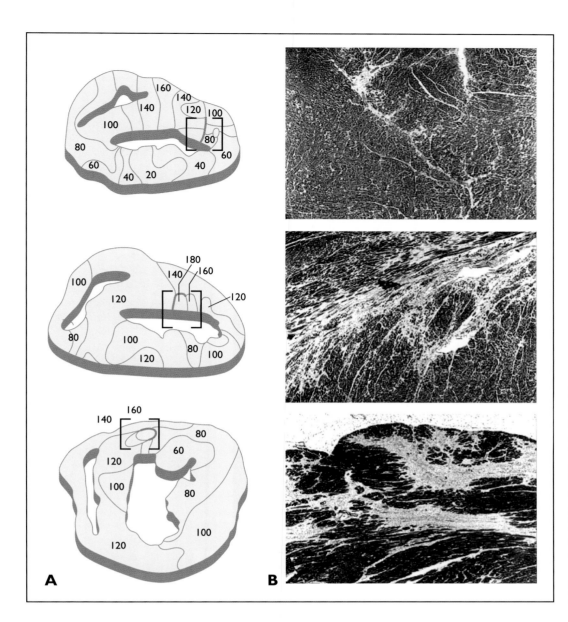

FIGURE 11-6. Histologic characterization of the site of conduction block reveals exaggerated fibrosis in myocardial slices. **A**, Rows 1 through 3 are sections from activation maps, with *thick lines* denoting sites of conduction block (enclosed in *brackets*). **B**, Corresponding photomicrographs of trichrome-stained sections of myocardium in vicinity of block (denoted by *brackets* at left). Sections in rows 1 through 3 demonstrate extensive nontransmural interstitial and replacement fibrosis at subendocardial (rows 1 and 2) and midmyocardial (row 3) sites of conduction block. (*Adapted from* Pogwizd *et al.* [7].)

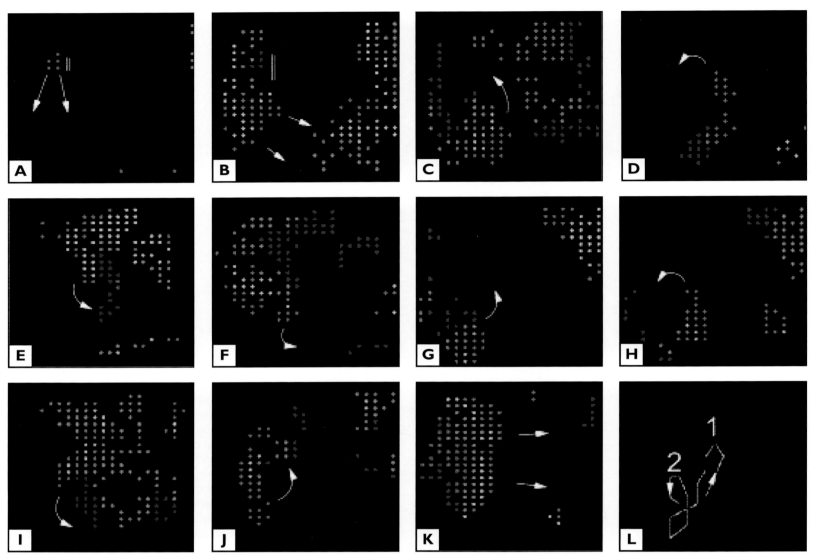

FIGURE 11-7. Experimental evidence for reentrant tachycardia in nonischemic dilated cardiomyopathy (NIDCM). The panels show plaque electrode mapping of reentrant wave fronts in an explanted heart with NIDCM. Reentry is initiated by epicardial breakthrough with a line of conduction block parallel to the epicardial fiber orientation. **A–K,** Selected frames from the dynamic display of the activation patterns during ventricular tachycardia. **L,** Trajectory of the tip of the reentrant wave fronts, demonstrating the meandering nature of the core. *Numbers 1 and 2* indicate the first and second cycles of reentry. The time of each frame is shown in *parentheses* above the panels. The beginning of the data acquisition was taken as time zero. The *double-headed arrow* at the right lower border of the figure displays myocardial fiber orientation. (*Adapted from* Wu *et al.* [8].)

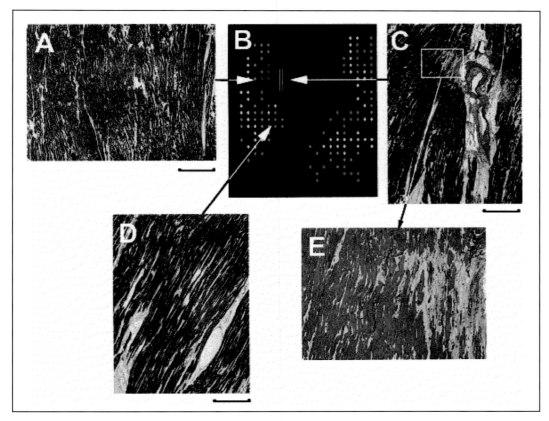

FIGURE 11-8. Plaque electrode mapping of reentrant wave fronts in the explanted heart (same heart as in Fig. 11-7). Histologic findings correspond to activations shown in Figure 11-3. **A, C–E,** Sections of the left ventricular myocardium parallel to the epicardium in heart number 1. With trichrome stain, small veins with perivascular fibrosis (*blue*) are clearly seen in **C** (*arrows*). The magnified view (**E**) also shows interstitial and replacement fibrosis. (Magnification × 100.) The areas of fibrosis in **C** and **E** correspond to the line of conduction block in **B** (same frame as Fig. 11-7B). However, in the areas without conduction block, histologic examination showed either normal tissue (**A**) or only mild fibrosis (**D**). (Calibration lines 1 mm.) (*Adapted from* Wu *et al.* [8].)

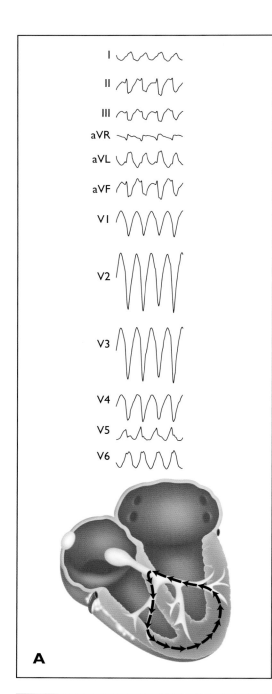

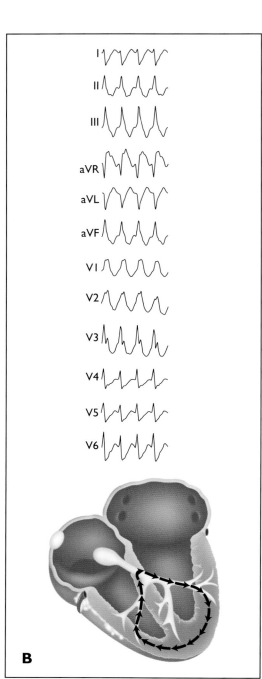

Figure 11-9. Bundle branch reentrant ventricular tachycardia (VT). **A** and **B**, Reentry within the conduction system. Bundle branch reentry presents with an electrocardiographic morphology of typical right or left bundle branch block. Bundle branch reentry can be successfully managed utilizing catheter ablation. When the right bundle is activated in the antegrade direction, it gives rise to an electrocardiographic pattern consistent with typical left bundle branch block (**A**). When the left bundle is activated in the antegrade direction, it gives rise to an electrocardiographic appearance of right bundle branch block (**B**). **C**, Intramyocardial reentry. The ECG shows an apical septal VT (with negative precordial concordance).

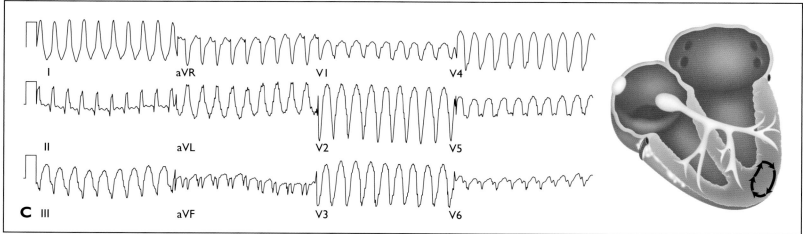

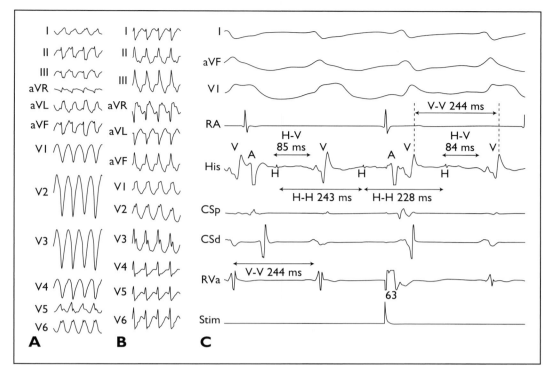

FIGURE 11-10. Intracardiac tracings of bundle branch reentry. **A** and **B**, Wide complex tachycardias from the same patient shown in Figure 11-9A and B, with alternating left and right bundle branch block patterns. **C**, Intracardiac recordings of right bundle branch block ventricular tachycardia advancement by premature ventricular stimulation. A single premature ventricular beat is introduced that captures the His bundle retrogradely (HH interval is shortened from 244 ms to 228 ms), and the subsequent ventricular activation is advanced with unchanged HV interval. CSd—carotid sinus denervation; CSp—carotid sinus pressure; RA—right atrium; RVa—right ventricular apex; Stim—stimulus. (*Adapted from* Valderrabano and Gallik [9].)

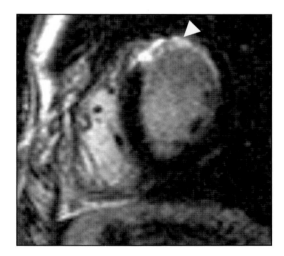

FIGURE 11-11. In vivo demonstration of myocardial scars or structural substrates for reentry in nonischemic dilated cardiomyopathy (NIDCM). The figure shows a contrast-enhanced MRI of a patient with dilated cardiomyopathy and a coronary arteriogram that demonstrated nonsignificant stenotic lesions. There is significant scarring in the ventricle (areas of increased contrast enhancement: *arrowhead*). In a study of 28 patients with NIDCM, 21% were found to have hyperenhancement on contrast-enhanced MRI [6]. Therefore, a subset of patients with dilated cardiomyopathy may still have well-defined myocardial scars. It is likely that such scars can provide an anatomic substrate that can sustain macroreentrant tachycardias. (*Courtesy of* David Bello, MD; UCI College of Medicine, Irvine CA).

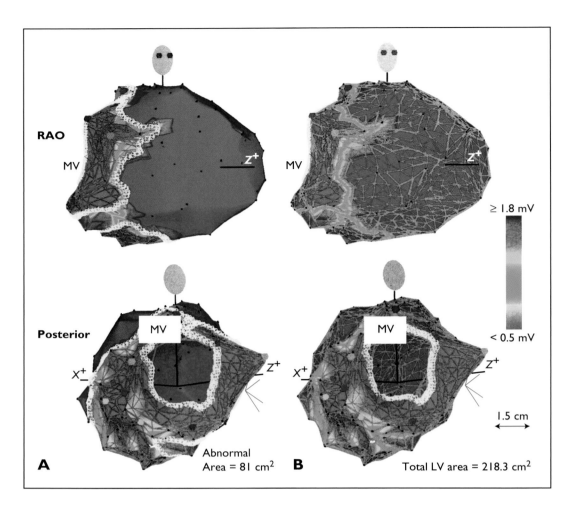

FIGURE 11-12. Myocardial scar as substrate for reentry. Three-dimensional voltage maps of the left ventricular (LV) endocardium in nonischemic dilated cardiomyopathy were constructed using electroanatomic mapping and displayed in right anterior oblique (RAO) and posterior projections. Purple areas represent normal endocardium (1.8 mV) with dense scar depicted as red (<0.5 mV). Border zone (0.5 to 1.8 mV) is defined as areas with the color gradient between red and purple. Endocardial surface area was estimated by using a computer algorithm. **A,** The extent of abnormal endocardium was estimated by measuring contiguous areas of abnormal electrogram recordings, represented by the nonpurple area. The area was first outlined and then divided into multiple, nonoverlapping triangular segments. **B,** The overall extent of abnormal endocardium (<1.8 mV) can be determined as the sum of all abnormal segments. The basal electrogram abnormalities in this figure have been known to provide the substrate for ventricular tachycardias. (*Adapted from* Hsia *et al.* [10].)

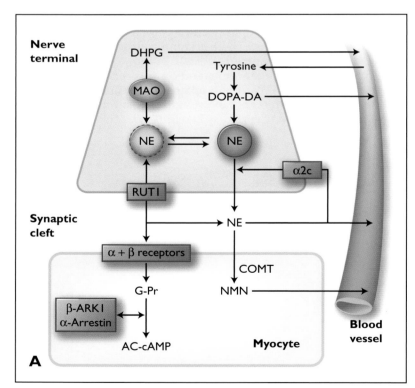

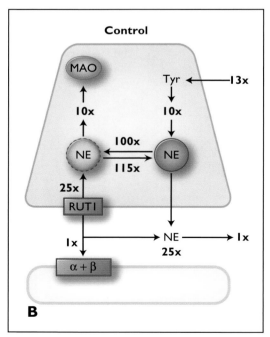

FIGURE 11-13. Predisposition to disease progression and arrhythmogenesis. The exaggerated adrenergic state in heart failure may contribute to arrhythmogenesis; the role of parasympathetic influences is still being debated. **A,** Synthesis, storage, release, and reuptake of norepinephrine (NE) in a cardiac synaptic terminal. Tyrosine (Tyr) is transported actively into the axoplasm to be converted to dihydroxyphenylalanine (DOPA) by tyrosine hydroxylase and subsequently to dopamine (DA) by cytoplasmic enzymes.

Continued on next page

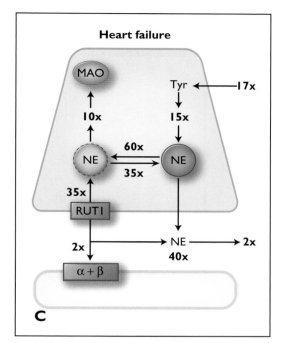

C

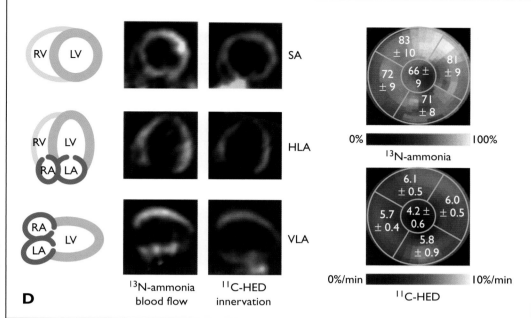

D

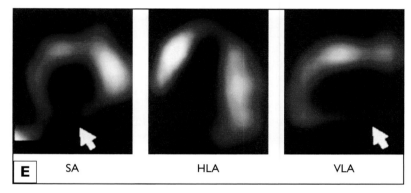

E

FIGURE 11-13. *(Continued)* **B** and **C**, The processes of synthesis, vesicular-axoplasmic exchange, metabolism, release, neuronal and extraneuronal uptake, spillover, and turnover of NE for sympathetic nerves of the normal (**B**) and failing (**C**) human heart at rest. Both NE release and uptake are increased in the failing heart; the efficiency of the NE uptake is reduced such that cardiac spillover of NE is increased disproportionately more than neuronal uptake. As such, cardiac NE stores are 50% lower in heart failure. Numbers with each arrow represent the rates of each process in a hundredth of actual picomoles per minute value (100 pg or 1x is the normal amount of NE spilled into the circulation, and representation as 1/100 of values allows easier understanding of the relative changes in the NE cascade). A noninvasive assessment of inefficiency of reuptake mechanisms is clinically feasible by performing MIBG (iobenguane) scans. **D**, Role of neuronal imaging in cardiomyopathy. PET images were obtained in a patient with dilated cardiomyopathy and reduced left ventricular (LV) function following the injection of ^{13}N-ammonia and 40 minutes after the injection of C-11 hydroxyephedrine (^{11}C-HED). The tomographic slices are displayed in short-axis (SA), horizontal long-axis (HLA), and vertical long-axis (VLA) views. There is relatively homogeneous distribution of ^{13}N-ammonia, indicating integrity of myocardial perfusion. However, there is markedly reduced retention of ^{11}C-HED, indicating partial denervation of the LV in this patient with dilated cardiomyopathy. The retention index is reduced to 6% (normal values > 12%). The area of denervation is most evident in the distal anterior wall and apical area of the LV,

confirming reports that injury of the autonomic nervous system is a heterogeneous process in patients with congestive heart failure. This PET example confirms several reports, which have shown reduced ^{123}I-metaiodobenzylguanidine (^{123}I-mIBG) retention in the myocardium of patients with congestive heart failure. The SPECT ^{123}I-mIBG retention, however, can only be assessed semiquantitatively by placing regions of interest over the mediastinum and the myocardium and calculating a relative retention ratio. A ratio over 2 is considered normal. Patients with denervation display a reduced ratio of tracer retention. Values below 1.2 identify patients at high risk for subsequent cardiovascular complications. There are data indicating the prognostic value of ^{11}C-HED in patients with congestive heart failure confirming the ^{123}I-mIBG observations. The advantage of PET is that it provides an absolute quantification of ^{11}C-HED tracer retention in the myocardium of patients with heart failure. LA—left atrium; RA—right atrium; RV—right ventricle. **E**, Neuronal imaging and cardiac arrhythmias. ^{123}I-metaiodobenzylguanidine (^{123}I-mIBG) SPECT images were obtained in a 54-year-old man with idiopathic right ventricular outflow tract tachycardia. The tomographic slices are displayed in short-axis (SA), horizontal long-axis (HLA), and vertical long-axis (VLA) views. ^{123}I-mIBG images acquired 4 hours following injection show a marked ^{123}I-mIBG retention defect in the midventricular and basal inferior walls (*arrows*), suggesting regional sympathetic denervation. Unfortunately, the right ventricle cannot be imaged by radionuclide techniques due to thin myocardial walls. (**B** and **C** *adapted from* Narula and Sarkar [11].)

ROLE OF EP TESTING IN NIDCM PATIENTS WITH SYMPTOMS SUGGESTIVE OF ARRHYTHMIA (PALPITATIONS, SYNCOPE, NEAR-SYNCOPE)

Assessment of sinus node function

Assessment of conduction system

Atrioventricular node conduction

Infranodal conduction (of relevance to heart block as well as a substrate for bundle branch reentry)

Tachycardia inducibility

Supraventricular tachycardias

Bundle branch reentry

Intramyocardial reentry

FIGURE 11-14. Role of electrophysiologic (EP) testing in nonischemic dilated cardiomyopathy (NIDCM) patients with symptoms suggestive of arrhythmia (palpitations, syncope, near-syncope). Ventricular arrhythmias are not uncommon in patients with NIDCM. The Cardiomyopathy Trial (CAT) showed that up to 53% of these patients have unsustained ventricular tachycardia VT on Holter monitoring [12]. Initially thought to be of prognostic relevance, its value has been questioned recently by the results of the Sudden Cardiac Death in Heart Failure Trial (SCD-HeFT) and the Marburg Cardiomyopathy Study [13]. The clinical spectrum of arrhythmia in these patients varies from asymptomatic premature ventricular contractions to palpitations, syncope, and even sudden death. This broad range of presentation is particularly distressing to the clinician asked to evaluate such patients. EP testing should be utilized as a diagnostic tool in the approach to patients with nonischemic cardiomyopathy and symptoms suggestive of arrhythmia. Of particular significance is the inducibility of bundle-branch reentry, which tends to be rapid and very symptomatic and can be cured by radiofrequency ablation (*see* Fig. 11-9). It should be noted, however, that EP testing (tachycardia inducibility) in the absence of symptoms or a clear clinical correlation has very limited value as a prognostic tool in these patients [14]. Apart from the EP study, commonly used tests for risk stratification in NIDCM have included ECG parameters with variable predictive values. QRS duration appears to be the strongest predictor of risk of sudden cardiac death. On the other hand, QT dispersion, QT dynamics, and microvolt T-wave alternans are of limited value.

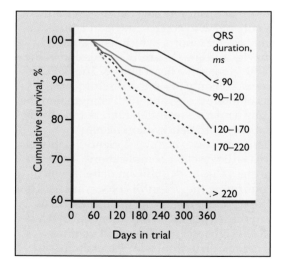

FIGURE 11-15. Utility of QRS duration as a marker for risk. The Vesnarinone Survival Trial (VEST) demonstrated QRS duration to be an independent predictor of mortality. Patients with QRS duration greater than 200 ms had a fivefold greater mortality risk than those with QRS duration less than 90 ms. Resting ECG is a powerful, accessible, and inexpensive marker of prognosis in patients with dilated cardiomyopathy and congestive heart failure. The mechanism of QRS prolongation in heart failure has been a subject of intense investigation, and it appears that the mechanism could be related to proximal conduction delays and actual slowing of propagation at the level of the His-Purkinje muscle junction. An example of left bundle conduction delay is shown in Figure 11-16. (*Adapted from* Gottipaty *et al.* [15].)

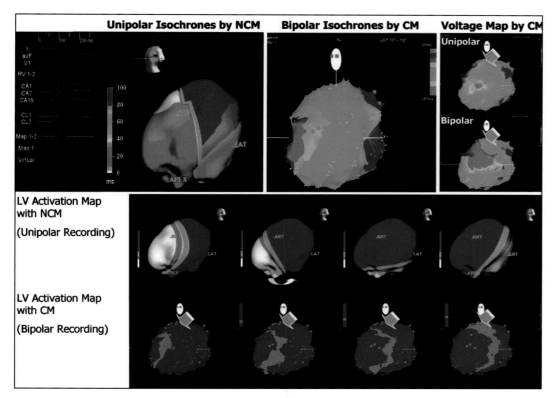

FIGURE 11-16. Characterization of left ventricular (LV) activation in patients with heart failure and left bundle branch block: surface ECG, intracardiac recordings of unipolar (map 1) contact (CM), and corresponding noncontact (NCM, virtual) electrograms. Epicardial unipolar recording was acquired with a 16-pole microcatheter inserted into an anterior vein (CA1 most distal, CA7 centered between, and CA15 most proximal) and an eight-pole microcatheter inserted into a lateral vein (CL1 most distal and CL7 most proximal). A line of block crossed over the anterior vein, creating activation delay between CA1 through 7 and CA15, with the latter aligned in time to CL1 and CL7. The unipolar isochronal map shows a line of block, and the bipolar isochronal map (*top middle*) shows an increased density of isochronal lines without evidence of a line of block. The unipolar voltage map (*top right*) shows fragmented electrograms of normal voltage (range, 2 to 6 mV) in the anterior region (*arrow*). In contrast, the bipolar voltage map shows low-voltage double potentials (*dots*) in the same region. Unipolar isopotential activation sequence (*middle*) shows a U-shaped activation front that rotated around the apex and activated the lateral wall late; the bipolar propagation map (*bottom*) shows a longer activation time in the anterior region (*arrows*). (*Adapted from* Auricchio *et al.* [16].)

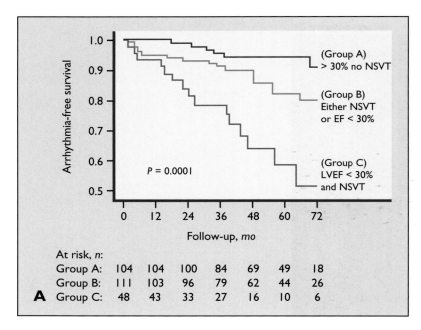

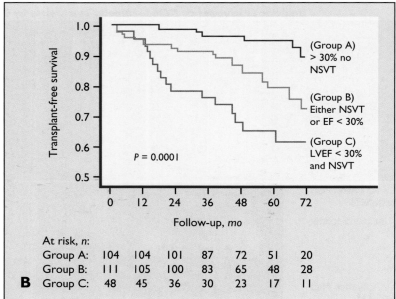

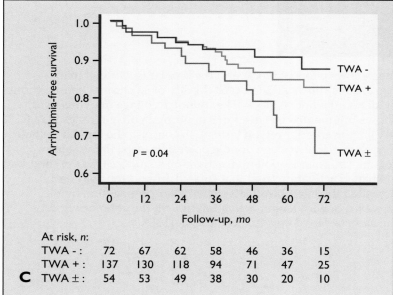

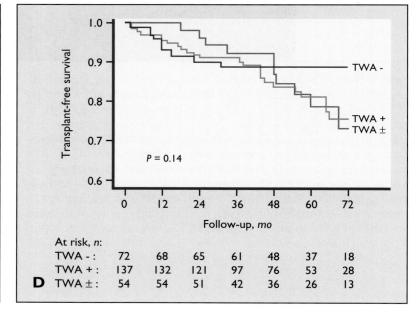

FIGURE 11-17. Risk stratification in nonischemic dilated cardiomyopathy (NIDCM). Several studies have sought to stratify the risk of sudden cardiac death in patients with NIDCM utilizing noninvasive markers of autonomic function, such as T-wave alternans (TWA), baroreflex sensitivity (BRS), and heart rate variability (HRV). There have been nonuniform findings reported in the literature. The most recent data are from the Marburg dilated cardiomyopathy trial [13], which included 343 patients with dilated cardiomyopathy with idiopathic dilated cardiomyopathy who underwent Holter ECG, QTc dispersion, HRV, BRS, and microvolt TWA testing. On multivariate analysis, only left ventricular ejection fraction (LVEF) was a significant arrhythmia risk predictor. Specifically, there was an increase in relative risk by 2.3 per 10% reduction in ejection fraction. Nonsustained ventricular tachycardia (NSVT) showed a trend toward increased mortality in this group of patients. Similarly, the use of β-blockers also demonstrated a trend toward increased arrhythmic events. **A** and **B**, Survival with and without NSVT. **C** and **D**, Survival by TWA classification. Arrhythmia-free survival was best in patients with higher LVEF and no evidence of NSVT. (*Adapted from* Grimm *et al.* [13].)

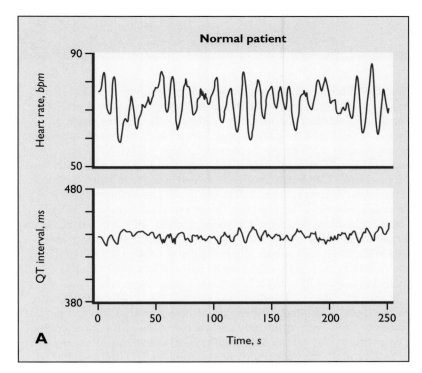

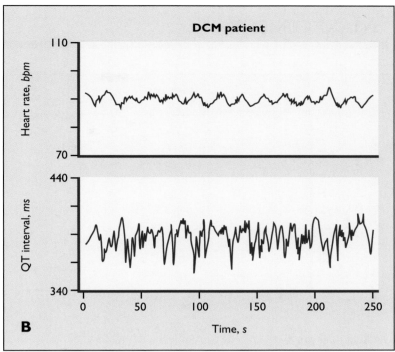

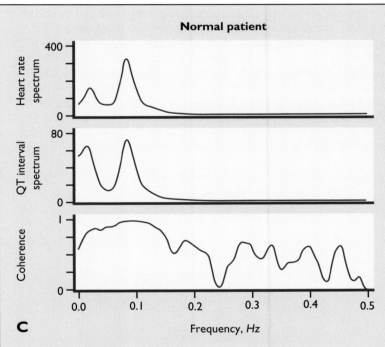

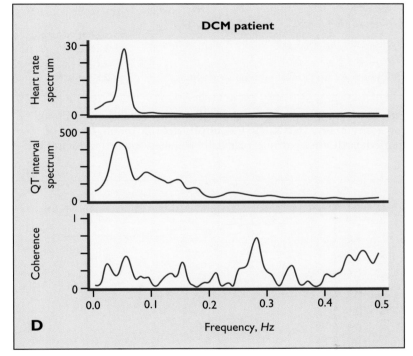

FIGURE 11-18. QT interval dynamics in nonischemic dilated cardiomyopathy (DCM). Beat-to-beat variability in QT intervals was studied in 83 patients with ischemic and nonischemic cardiomyopathy [2]. This study demonstrated that QT interval variability did not depend on ejection fraction or spatial distribution of QT at baseline; however, New York Heart Association functional class was a good predictor. In normal subjects (**A**), heart rate variability may be large, with very little fluctuation in QT variability; however, the converse is noted in the patient with DCM (**B**). Power and coherence spectra for heart rate and QT interval from a normal patient (**C**)—the same patient as in **A**—and from a patient with DCM (**D**)—the same patient as in **B**. The data show that QT variability changes are nonlinear compared with that of heart rate. (*Adapted from* Berger *et al.* [2].)

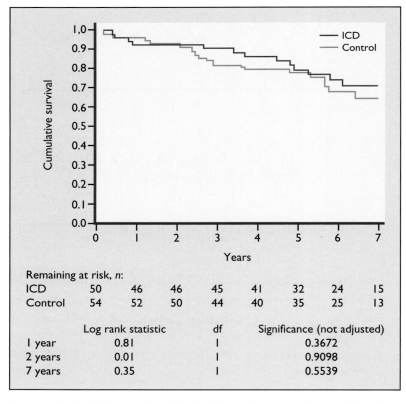

	Log rank statistic	df	Significance (not adjusted)
1 year	0.81	1	0.3672
2 years	0.01	1	0.9098
7 years	0.35	1	0.5539

FIGURE 11-19. Pilot study of defibrillators in nonischemic dilated cardiomyopathy (NIDCM). Electrophysiologic management of dilated cardiomyopathy is primarily directed toward reducing the

risk of sudden death. The most effective therapies to reduce the risk of sudden cardiac death in this setting are implantable cardioverter-defibrillators (ICDs). Most of the studies have included both ischemic and nonischemic cardiomyopathy patients. Some studies, such as the Cardiomyopathy Trial (CAT), Amiodarone Versus Implantable Defibrillator in Patients with Nonischemic Cardiomyopathy and Asymptomatic Nonsustained Ventricular Tachycardia (AMIOVIRT), and Defibrillators in Nonischemic Cardiomyopathy Treatment Evaluation (DEFINITE), were exclusively preformed in patients with NIDCM. Studies such as the Comparison of Medical Therapy, Resynchronization, and Defibrillation Therapies in Heart Failure (COMPANION) trial and the Sudden Cardiac Death in Heart Failure Trial (SCD-HeFT) included almost 50% NIDCM patients.

In the pilot study of defibrillators in NIDCM [12], patients with recent onset of dilated cardiomyopathy (6 months) and an ejection fraction <30% were randomly assigned to either an ICD or control. The primary end point of the trial was all-cause mortality at 1 year of follow-up. Fifty patients were assigned to ICD therapy and 54 to control treatment. The trial was terminated after the inclusion of 104 patients because the all-cause mortality rate at 1 year did not reach the expected 30% in the control group. After a mean follow-up of 5.5 2.2 years, 30 deaths had occurred (13 in the ICD group and 17 in the control group). Cumulative survival was not significantly different between the two groups (93% and 80% in the control group versus 92% and 86% in the ICD group after 2 and 4 years, respectively). There were only four deaths in the ICD group and two deaths in the control arm of the trial in the first year. It was reported that even if the target of 1348 patients was included, the trial would have been underpowered.

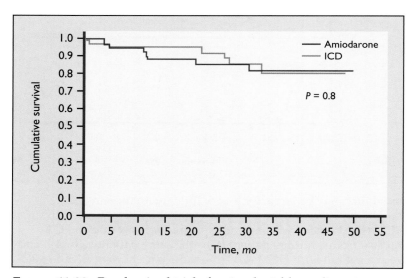

FIGURE 11-20. Randomized trial of an implantable cardioverter-defibrillator (ICD) versus amiodarone in patients with dilated cardiomyopathy. The purpose of the Amiodarone Versus Implantable Defibrillator in Patients with Nonischemic Cardiomyopathy and Asymptomatic Nonsustained Ventricular Tachycardia (AMIOVIRT) study, a multicenter randomized trial, was to compare total mortality during therapy with amiodarone or an ICD in patients with nonischemic dilated cardiomyopathy (NIDCM) and nonsustained ventricular tachycardia (NSVT) [17]. In this trial, 103 patients with NIDCM, a left ventricular ejection fraction of 35%, and asymptomatic

NSVT were randomized to receive either an ICD or amiodarone. This trial was discontinued early because of the inability to demonstrate statistical significance, which was likely based on prospectively defined criteria. Patients surviving at 1 year (90% vs 96%) and 3 years (88% vs 87%) in the amiodarone and ICD groups, respectively, were not statistically different ($P = 0.8$). Quality of life was also similar in both arms ($P = $ not significant). There was a trend with amiodarone, as compared with the ICD, toward improved arrhythmia-free survival ($P = 0.1$) and lower cost during the first year of therapy. (*Adapted from* Strickberger *et al.* [17].)

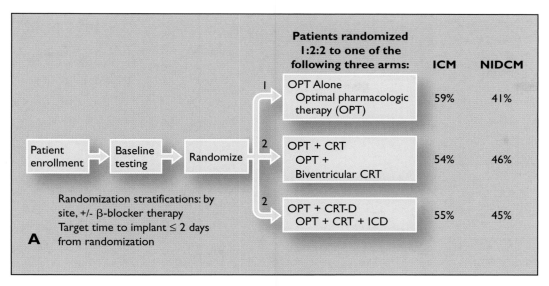

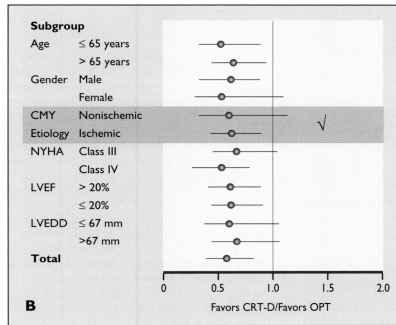

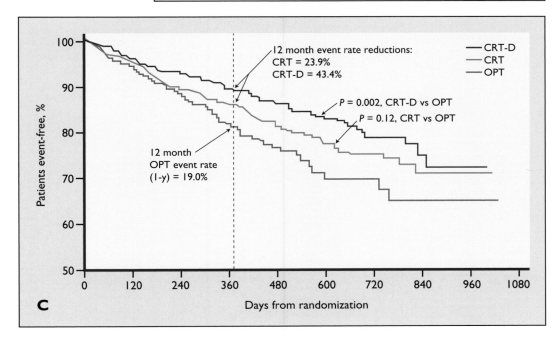

FIGURE 11-21. Defibrillators (with cardiac resynchronization capability) compared with cardiac resynchronization or pharmacotherapy alone. **A**, In the Comparison of Medical Therapy, Resynchronization, and Defibrillation Therapies in Heart Failure (COMPANION) trial, a total of 1520 patients who had advanced heart failure (New York Heart Association [NYHA] class III or IV) due to ischemic or non-ischemic cardiomyopathies (CMY) and a QRS interval of at least 120 ms were randomly assigned in a 1:2:2 ratio to receive optimal pharmacologic therapy (OPT; diuretics, angiotensin-converting enzyme inhibitors, β-blockers, and spironolactone) alone or in combination with cardiac resynchronization therapy with either a pacemaker (CRT) or a pacemaker-defibrillator (CRT-D) [18]. **B**, The primary composite end point was the time to death from or hospitalization for any cause. As compared with OPT alone, CRT decreased the risk of the primary end point (hazard ratio, 0.81; *P* = 0.014) as did CRT-D (hazard ratio, 0.80; *P* = 0.01). **C**, The risk of the combined end point of death from or hospitalization for heart failure was reduced by 34% in the CRT group (*P* < 0.002) and by 40% in the CRT-D group (*P* < 0.001 for the comparison with the OPT group). A pacemaker reduced the risk of the secondary end point of death from any cause by 24% (*P* = 0.059). There was a 36% reduction in death from any cause in the CRT-D group (*P* = 0.003). Among patients with non-ischemic dilated cardiomyopathy (NIDCM), CRT-D was associated with a significantly lower risk of death from any cause, as compared with OPT (hazard ratio, 0.50; 95% CI, 0.29 to 0.88; *P* = 0.015). ICM—ischemic cardiomyopathy; LVEDD—left ventricular end-diastolic dimension; LVEF—left ventricular ejection fraction.

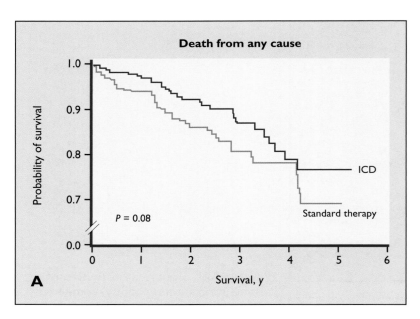

A

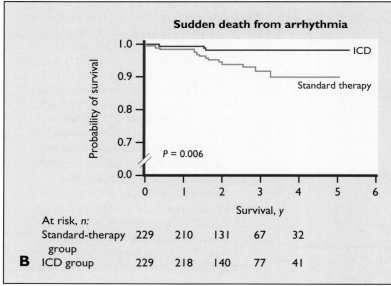

B

FIGURE 11-22. Randomized trial of defibrillators in nonischemic dilated cardiomyopathy (NIDCM). The Defibrillators in Non-ischemic Cardiomyopathy Treatment Evaluation (DEFINITE) enrolled 458 patients with NIDCM, a left ventricular ejection fraction (LVEF) of less than 36%, and premature ventricular complexes (PVCs) or nonsustained ventricular tachycardia (NSVT) [19]. A total of 229 patients were randomly assigned to receive standard medical therapy and 229 to receive standard medical therapy plus a single-chamber implantable cardioverter-defibrillator (ICD). In this trial, 458 patients with NIDCM, LVEF <36%, and PVCs or NSVT were randomized to standard therapy or standard therapy with ICD. **A,** At follow-up (29 ± 14.4 months), fewer patients died in the ICD group than in the standard-therapy group (28 vs 40), but the difference was not significant (P = 0.08). **B,** Sudden death from arrhythmia was lower in the ICD group compared with the standard-therapy group. This trial, in contrast to the Sudden Cardiac Death in Heart Failure Trial (SCD-HeFT; *see* Fig. 11-23), enrolled only nonischemic cardiomyopathy patients.

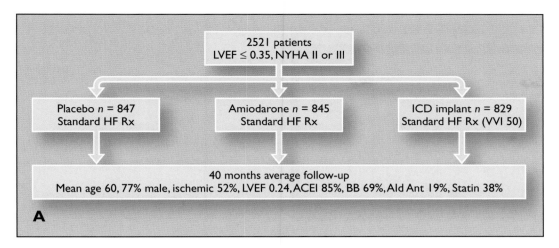

A

2521 patients
LVEF ≤ 0.35, NYHA II or III

Placebo n = 847
Standard HF Rx

Amiodarone n = 845
Standard HF Rx

ICD implant n = 829
Standard HF Rx (VVI 50)

40 months average follow-up
Mean age 60, 77% male, ischemic 52%, LVEF 0.24, ACEI 85%, BB 69%, Ald Ant 19%, Statin 38%

B

	HR	97.5% CI	P
Amiodarone vs placebo	1.06	0.86–1.30	0.53
ICD vs placebo	0.77	0.62–0.96	0.007

— Amiodarone
— ICD therapy
— Placebo

Mortality / Months of follow-up

C

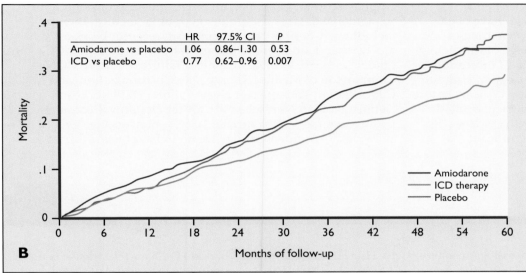

Patient group		N	HR	97.5% CI
All patients		1692	1.06	0.86, 1.30
NYHA class	Class II	1195	0.85	0.65, 1.11
	Class III	497	1.44	1.05, 1.97
CHF etiology	Ischemic	879	1.05	0.81, 1.36
	Nonischemic	813	1.07	0.76, 1.51

0.5 1 2 4

D

Patient group		N	HR	97.5% CI
All patients		1676	0.77	0.62, 0.96
NYHA class	Class II	1160	0.54	0.40, 0.74
	Class III	516	1.16	0.84, 1.61
CHF etiology	Ischemic	884	0.79	0.60, 1.04
	Nonischemic	792	0.73	0.50, 1.04

0.25 0.5 1 2

Figure 11-23. The Sudden Cardiac Death-Heart Failure Trial (SCD-HeFT). In SCD-HeFT, only patients with New York Heart Association (NYHA) class II or III heart failure (HF), either ischemic or non-ischemic cardiomyopathy, and a left ventricular ejection fraction (LVEF) of 35% or less were eligible for enrollment [20]. **A**, Trial design. There were 2521 patients enrolled in 148 centers in North America and New Zealand. Patients were randomized to best medical therapy, best medical therapy plus amiodarone, or best medical therapy plus the insertion of an implantable cardioverter-defibrillator (ICD). The median age of the 2521 patients was 60 years, 23% were female, the average duration of heart failure was 24 months, and the mean LVEF was 25%. Seventy percent of patients were in NYHA class II, and the remainder were in class III. Fifty-two percent of patients had ischemic heart disease, and the mean QRS duration was 112 ms. The baseline use of ACE inhibitors (ACEI) was 85%, 96% if angiotensin receptor blockers were included. β-Blockers (BB) were prescribed in 69% of patients at baseline, and this improved to 78% at last follow-up identification. **B**, Survival. The primary outcome of the trial demonstrated that ICD implantation reduces all-cause mortality 23% when compared with placebo, whereas amiodarone did not improve mortality. The 3-year rates of all-cause mortality for the ICD, amiodarone, and placebo were 17.1%, 24.0%, and 22.3%, respectively; 5-year all-cause mortality was 28.9%, 34.1%, and 35.8%, respectively. **C** and **D**, The relative risk of mortality with amiodarone relative to placebo over the 5 years of the study was 1.06 (97.5% CI, 0.86 to 1.30). Subgroup analysis did not show any favorable interaction between patients treated with β-blockers and randomization to amiodarone. This trial demonstrates that in heart failure, LVEF less than or equal to 35%, and NYHA class II or III heart failure symptoms, amiodarone offers absolutely no survival advantage. Shown are the relative numbers of patients with ischemic and nonischemic cardiomyopathy in comparing the three groups. Ald Ant—aldosterone antagonist; CHF—congestive heart failure; HR—hazard ratio. (*Adapted from* Cleland *et al.* [20].)

ALGORITHM FOR ICD IMPLANTATION IN PATIENTS WITH NIDCM

CLINICAL CHARACTERISTIC	EF	QRS WIDTH	RECOMMENDATION	EVIDENCE
VT, VF arrest	Any, %	Any	ICD	ACC/AHA guidelines [21]
Class III or IV CHF	30–35	≥ 120 ms	Bi-V ICD	COMPANION [18]
NSVT	<35	Any	ICD	DEFINITE [19]
LV dysfunction	<35	Any	ICD	SCD-HeFT
Syncope	<35	Any	ICD	Fonarow et al. [22]
				Knight et al. [23]

FIGURE 11-24. Algorithm for implantable cardioverter-defibrillator (ICD) implantation in patients with nonischemic dilated cardiomyopathy (NIDCM). Patients who have been resuscitated from ventricular tachycardia (VT)/ventricular fibrillation (VF) arrest meet the American College of Cardiology (ACC)/American Heart Association (AHA) class I indication for implantation of ICDs. Patients who have low ejection fraction (EF) and QRS prolongation with class III or class IV heart failure symptoms benefit from implantation of a biventricular (Bi-V) ICD. In summary, all patients with NIDCM with evidence of serious arrhythmias, QRS prolongation, and significant symptoms of heart failure should be offered an ICD. It must be emphasized that patients with NIDCM being considered for implantable devices should be on optimal medical therapy including ACE inhibitors/angiotensin receptor blockers, β-blockers, and aldosterone antagonists, according the ACC/AHA guidelines. CHF—congestive heart failure; COMPANION—Comparison of Medical Therapy, Resynchronization, and Defibrillation Therapies in Heart Failure; DEFINITE—Defibrillators in Nonischemic Cardiomyopathy Treatment Evaluation; LV—left ventricle; NSVT—nonsustained VT; SCD-HeFT—Sudden Cardiac Death in Heart Failure Trial.

REFERENCES

1. Akar FG, Rosenbaum DS: Transmural electrophysiological heterogeneities underlying arrhythmogenesis in heart failure. *Circ Res* 2003, 93:638–645.

2. Berger RD, Kasper EK, Baughman KL, *et al.*: Beat-to-beat QT interval variability: novel evidence for repolarization lability in ischemic and nonischemic dilated cardiomyopathy. *Circulation* 1997, 96:1557–1565.

3. Janse MJ. Electrophysiological changes in heart failure and their relationship to arrhythmogenesis. *Cardiovasc Res* 2004, 61:208–217.

4. Kaab S, Nuss HB, Chiamvimonvat N, *et al.*: Ionic mechanism of action potential prolongation in ventricular myocytes from dogs with pacing-induced heart failure. *Circ Res* 1996, 78:262–273.

5. Cao JM, Fishbein MC, Han JB, *et al.*: Relationship between regional cardiac hyperinnervation and ventricular arrhythmia. *Circulation* 2000, 101:1960–1969.

6. Akar FG, Spragg DD, Tunin RS, *et al.*: Mechanisms underlying conduction slowing and arrhythmogenesis in nonischemic dilated cardiomyopathy. *Circ Res* 2004, 95:717–725.

7. Pogwizd SM, McKenzie JP, Cain ME: Mechanisms underlying spontaneous and induced ventricular arrhythmias in patients with idiopathic dilated cardiomyopathy. *Circulation* 1998, 98:2404–2414.

8. Wu TJ, Ong JJ, Hwang C, *et al.* Characteristics of wave fronts during ventricular fibrillation in human hearts with dilated cardiomyopathy: role of increased fibrosis in the generation of reentry. *J Am Coll Cardiol* 1998, 32:187–196.

9. Valderrabano M, Gallik D: A tachycardia with changing bundle branch block patterns: what is the mechanism? *Pacing Clin Electrophysiol* 2004, 27:394–396.

10. Hsia HH, Callans DJ, Marchlinski FE: Characterization of endocardial electrophysiological substrate in patients with nonischemic cardiomyopathy and monomorphic ventricular tachycardia. *Circulation* 2003, 108:704–710.

11. Narula J, Sarkar K: A conceptual paradox of MIBG uptake in heart failure: retention with incontinence! *J Nucl Cardiol* 2003, 10:700–704.

12. Bansch D, Antz M, Boczor S, *et al.*: Primary prevention of sudden cardiac death in idiopathic dilated cardiomyopathy: the Cardiomyopathy Trial (CAT). *Circulation* 2002, 105:1453–1458.

13. Grimm W, Christ M, Bach J, *et al.*: Noninvasive arrhythmia risk stratification in idiopathic dilated cardiomyopathy: results of the Marburg Cardiomyopathy Study. *Circulation* 2003, 108:2883–2891.

14. Grimm W, Hoffmann J, Menz V, *et al.*: Programmed ventricular stimulation for arrhythmia risk prediction in patients with idiopathic dilated cardiomyopathy and nonsustained ventricular tachycardia. *J Am Coll Cardiol* 1998, 32:739–745.

15. Gottipaty V, Krelis S, Lu F, *et al.* The resting electrocardiogram provides a sensitive and inexpensive marker of prognosis in patients with chronic congestive heart failure [abstract]. *J Am Coll Cardiol* 1999, 33:145A.

16. Auricchio A, Fantoni C, Regoli F, *et al.*: Characterization of left ventricular activation in patients with heart failure and left bundle branch block. *Circulation* 2004,109:1133–1139.

17. Strickberger SA, Hummel JD, Bartlett TG, *et al.*: Amiodarone versus implantable cardioverter-defibrillator: randomized trial in patients with nonischemic dilated cardiomyopathy and asymptomatic nonsustained ventricular tachycardia—AMIOVIRT. *J Am Coll Cardiol* 2003, 41:1707–1712.

18. Bristow MR, Saxon LA, Boehmer J, *et al.*: Cardiac-resynchron-ization therapy with or without an implantable defibrillator in advanced chronic heart failure. *N Engl J Med* 2004, 350:2140–2150.

19. Kadish A, Dyer A, Daubert JP, *et al.*: Prophylactic defibrillator implantation in patients with nonischemic dilated cardiomyopathy. *N Engl J Med* 2004, 350:2151–2158.

20. Cleland JG, Ghosh J, Freemantle N, *et al.*: Clinical trials update and cumulative meta-analyses from the American College of Cardiology: WATCH, SCD-HeFT, DINAMIT, CASINO, INSPIRE, STRATUS-US, RIO-Lipids and cardiac resynchronisation therapy in heart failure. *Eur J Heart Fail* 2004, 6:501–508.

21. Gregoratos G, Abrams J, Epstein AE, *et al.*: ACC/AHA/NASPE 2002 guideline update for implantation of cardiac pacemakers and antiarrhythmia devices: summary article: a report of the American College of Cardiology/American Heart Association Task Force on Practice Guidelines (ACC/AHA/NASPE Committee to Update the 1998 Pacemaker Guidelines). *Circulation* 2002, 106:2145–2161.

22. Fonarow GC, Feliciano Z, Boyle NG, *et al.*: Improved survival in patients with nonischemic advanced heart failure and syncope treated with an implantable cardioverter-defibrillator. *Am J Cardiol* 2000, 85:981–985.

23. Knight BP, Goyal R, Pelosi F, *et al.*: Outcome of patients with nonischemic dilated cardiomyopathy and unexplained syncope treated with an implantable defibrillator. *J Am Coll Cardiol* 1999, 33:1964–1970.

NOVEL IMPLANTABLE NONPACING DEVICES IN HEART FAILURE

David A. Cesario, Dwight W. Reynolds, and Charles D. Swerdlow

Changes in intravascular volume and ventricular systolic and/or diastolic performance that precede symptomatic exacerbations of heart failure are associated with elevations of cardiac filling pressures. Optimal day-to-day management of patients with chronic heart failure requires accurate assessment of these fluid status parameters. Because patients with chronic heart failure adapt to chronic increases in intravascular volume and filling pressures, traditional clinical assessment may not detect an exacerbation until it is severe. Percutaneous, invasive measurements of filling pressures by right heart catheterization provides diagnostic, therapeutic, and prognostic information in the treatment of heart failure [1]. Repeated right heart catheterizations may help tailor therapy [2], but they are expensive, inconvenient for patients, and associated with significant risks. Furthermore, percutaneous invasive monitoring assesses patients only while they are resting and supine. Optimally, monitoring would be performed continuously to assess the hemodynamic effects of the activities of daily living, to evaluate changes in therapy, to provide real-time early warning of exacerbations, and to identify their proximate causes. Continuous monitoring of heart failure using implantable devices is technically feasible. The first generation of implantable heart-failure monitors is currently undergoing clinical trials, and a new generation is under development.

Various other novel monitoring devices currently under investigation include the intrathoracic impedance sensor, which provides an indirect measure of lung and cardiac fluid content, and thus intravascular volume. Intracardiac electrograms are routinely available in cardiac resynchronization pacemakers and implantable cardioverter-defibrillators. They may provide information relevant to the monitoring of heart failure patients, including commonly used parameters (*eg*, heart-rate variability or ventricular rate during atrial fibrillation) and new parameters (*eg*, ST segment deviation as a measure of ischemia). In some patients, such data may identify reversible, proximate causes of heart failure exacerbations, such as arrhythmias or ischemia.

Furthermore, potential new therapies such as cardiac contractility modulation may allow direct inotropic modulation in heart failure patients by nonexcitatory stimuli delivered through implantable devices. Similarly, implantable devices are being developed that may modulate sympathetic and parasympathetic stimulation of myocardial architecture to induce inotropic or bradycardic effects, respectively. Although many of these devices are in their infancy, the ultimate goal in the treatment of heart failure patients is to cohesively integrate the data obtained from these implantable monitors into novel treatment regimens. Such devices will provide an ultimate interface between the electrophysiology and heart failure disciplines.

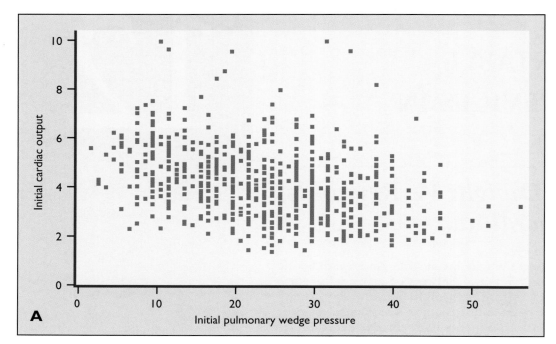

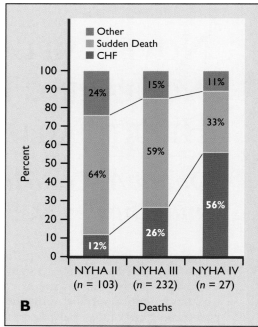

FIGURE 12-1. Need for improved monitoring. **A**, There is a marked variability in the initial hemodynamic profiles (cardiac output and pulmonary wedge pressure) of patients with heart failure. This figure depicts the wide spectrum of initial hemodynamic values seen in a sample of 700 patients referred for possible heart transplantation. This plot illustrates that many of these patients had normal pulmonary capillary wedge pressures, and some had cardiac outputs as high as 8 to 10 L/min. Further, the hemodynamic profile cannot always be predicted by the patient history and a physical exam [3,4]. These data demonstrate the importance of tailoring heart failure treatment to each individual patient and suggest a potential need for improved monitoring devices for heart failure patients. (*Adapted from* Stevenson [5].)

B, The severity of heart failure alters the mode of death. Cardiac arrhythmias are common in heart failure patients and their frequency is related to the severity of cardiac dysfunction. Greater than 40% of the total mortality in heart failure patients is due to sudden cardiac death. Sudden cardiac death predominates in patients with mild-to-moderate heart failure; pump failure and other causes of death are less common in these patients. However, as the severity of heart failure increases, death from pump failure becomes more pronounced [6,7]. CHF—congestive heart failure; NYHA—New York Heart Association. (*Adapted from* Englestein [7].)

A. PROPERTIES OF SENSORS USED FOR IMPLANTABLE MONITORS

Relationship between sensed parameter and clinical condition

Power source and power consumption

Method of data transmission (including lead vs leadless)

Frequency of data acquisition

Requirement for special sensor and/or lead

User interface: complexity and ease of use

Reliability

Stability of measurements

Ease of calibration

B. PARAMETERS MEASURED BY OR FOR IMPLANTABLE MONITORS

Hemodynamic monitors

Types of implantable pressure transducers

Locations of pressure sensors

   Right ventricle (Chronicle*)

   Left atrium (HeartPod†)

   Right ventricle (CardioMEMS‡)

   Pulmonary artery (Remon§)

Physiologic monitoring

Lung water (transthoracic impedance)

Sensors used for rate-responsive pacing

Thoracic impedance

Peak endocardial acceleration

Core body temperature

Mixed venous oxygen

Parameters derived from pacemaker of ICD electrograms

Heart rate variability

Atrial and ventricular rate ICD

Atrial fibrillation: prevalence and ventricular

ST segments

Ischemia monitor

---

*Medtronics, Inc., Minneapolis, MN.
†Savacor, Inc., Los Angeles, CA.
‡CardioMEMS, Atlanta, GA.
§Remon Medical Technologies Ltd., Caesarea, Israel.

FIGURE 12-2. Recently, a number of implantable devices have been developed in an attempt to better assess the clinical status of ambulatory heart failure patients, and ultimately to aid the physician in optimizing the outpatient treatment regimens of these patients. The first generation of heart failure monitoring devices employs various technologies to monitor classic hemodynamic variables. Currently both right ventricular and left atrial hemodynamic monitoring systems are undergoing clinical evaluation.

A, The properties of the sensor largely define the capabilities and limitations of any implanted monitoring system. For any sensor, the relationship between the sensed parameter and the clinical condition of interest is critical. This relationship is particularly important in heart failure, because it is a complex clinical syndrome not defined by a single clinical variable. Pressure has been the mainstay of clinical, invasive monitoring of heart failure because of the 1) close relationship between left atrial pressure and pulmonary edema, 2) ease of measuring pulmonary capillary wedge pressure as a surrogate for left atrial pressure, and 3) limitations of fluid-filled catheters for measuring other parameters. Pressure is the most commonly measured parameter by implantable sensors, and implantable monitoring devices have been proposed based on pressure measured in the left atrium,

pulmonary artery, or right ventricle. However, heart failure sensors may measure a variety of other parameters such as those listed in **B**.

Properties of the power source are also important determinants of the capabilities of an implantable monitor. Monitors with implantable power sources can measure and store data at programmable intervals and alert the patient automatically, but their service life is limited by battery capacity and a lead is usually required to connect the extracardiac power supply to the intracardiac sensor. Externally powered monitors may not require leads and may be smaller in size, because they are not limited by implantable batteries. Additionally, the absence of implantable batteries may give external monitors an increased service life. However, external devices can perform measurements only when the patient is in proximity to the power source; but because all data analysis is performed externally, their electronics can be upgraded more easily and at less cost.

Most monitors require implantation of a special sensor and/or lead, but some measurements can be made using standard pacemaker leads. Other factors to consider include complexity of the user interface, sensor reliability, stability of measurements, and ease of calibration. ICD—implantable cardioverter-defibrillator.

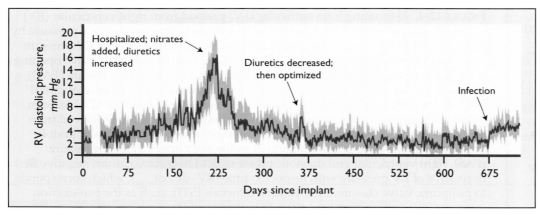

Figure 12-6. Long-term trend plot of right ventricular (RV) diastolic pressure that has been recorded by a chronically implanted, RV hemodynamic monitor (Chronicle Model 9520, Medtronic, Inc., Minneapolis, MN) from a patient with heart failure. Both average values and variations are shown. These data were transmitted via standard telephone lines, electronically stored, and displayed for review by clinicians. Pressure increases correspond to hospitalization for heart failure, reduction in diuretic dose, and possibly to infection. The RV implantable hemodynamic monitor provides similar graphical displays of estimated pulmonary artery diastolic pressures (a surrogate for left ventricular preload heart rates), RV systolic pressure, and activity levels.

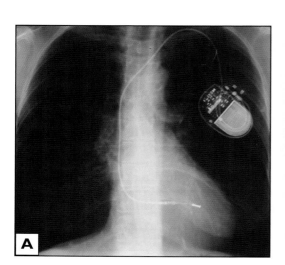

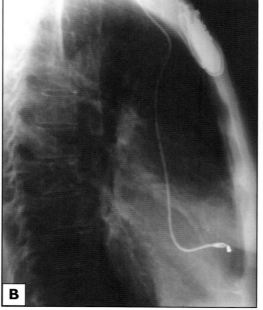

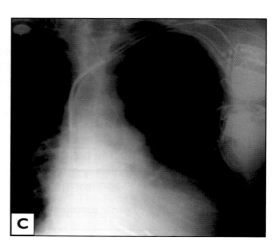

Figure 12-7. Posteroanterior (**A**) and lateral (**B**) chest radiographs of a patient previously implanted with a left prepectoral implantable hemodynamic monitor (IHM) (Chronicle Model 9520 and Model 4328A lead, Medtronic, Inc., Minneapolis, MN). The lead, implanted in the extrathoracic subclavian vein using a percutaneous introducer, courses down the left subclavian and innominate veins and the superior vena cava into the right atrium, across the tricuspid valve, and into the right ventricle. The tined tip of the lead, a unipolar electrode, is passively fixed in trabeculations in the mid-interventricular septal area. The pressure measuring capsule resides approximately 3-cm proximal to the tip of the lead in the right ventricle. Care is taken at implant to assure that passive fixation (to avoid subsequent lead dislodgement) and the pressure waveforms are unaffected by the tricuspid valve or other motion artifact.

C, A portable anteroposterior chest radiograph of a patient implanted with both an IHM (Chronicle Model 9520, Medtronic, Inc.) and a dual chamber implantable cardioverter-defibrillator (ICD), demonstrating implantation of all three leads via the extrathoracic left subclavian vein with separate left prepectoral pockets for the two devices. This approach has been used to avoid putting left and right subclavian/innominate veins at risk of occlusion as well as to facilitate incorporation of these multiple leads into a future, single device combining dual chamber ICD and IHM capabilities. At implantation, care must be taken to assure there is no pressure measurement artifact caused by cardiac motion (tricuspid valve and myocardium), or by inadvertent contact between the leads involving the pressure recording capsule. The tip of the right ventricular IHM lead is placed preferentially into a nonapical (usually septal) location to avoid pressure capsule malfunctions that have occurred with right ventricular apical placement. These malfunctions have been associated with thrombofibrotic covering. The formation of this covering is reportedly facilitated by low blood flow velocities in the right ventricular apex.

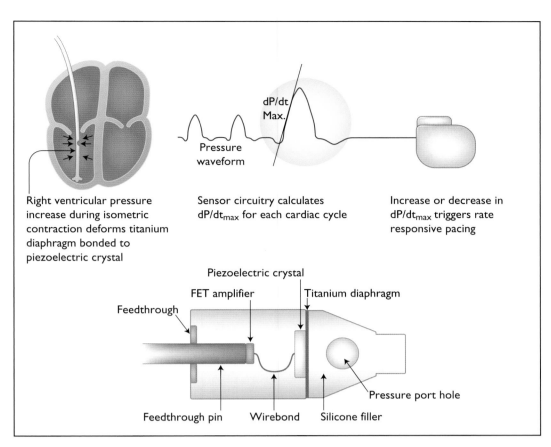

Right ventricular pressure increase during isometric contraction deforms titanium diaphragm bonded to piezoelectric crystal

Sensor circuitry calculates dP/dt_{max} for each cardiac cycle

Increase or decrease in dP/dt_{max} triggers rate responsive pacing

dP/dt Max.

Pressure waveform

Piezoelectric crystal

FET amplifier

Titanium diaphragm

Feedthrough

Pressure port hole

Feedthrough pin   Wirebond   Silicone filler

FIGURE 12-8. An alternative implantable pressure sensor based on electrical currents generated by a piezoelectric crystal has been used for rate-responsive pacing. Pressure changes deform a titanium diaphragm bonded to the crystal. The resulting electrical signal is amplified to produce pressure waveforms and differentiated to determine dP/dt_{max}. To date, no piezoelectric pressure sensor has been developed for clinical use.

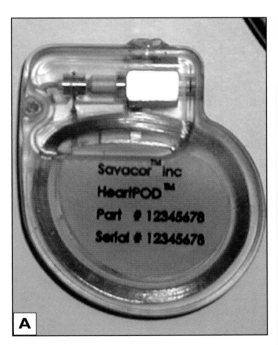

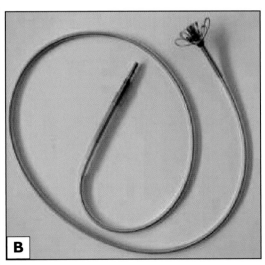

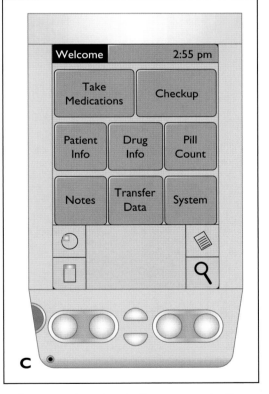

FIGURE 12-9. Implantable left atrial pressure monitor. A left atrial pressure monitor under development (HeartPOD, Savacor, Inc., Los Angeles, CA) is implanted either in a pacemaker-like operation using transseptal catheterization or at cardiac surgery. The system includes a sensor module and lead (**A**) that measure left atrial pressure, core temperature, and the intracardiac electrogram; a communications coil in a polymeric housing (**B**); and a patient advisory module (**C**) made up of a modified, hand-held "palm-type" computer, software, and radiofrequency transmitter/receiver. The lead, similar to a pacemaker lead, connects the sensor housing to the communications coil module, which is typically implanted subcutaneously in the infraclavicular region. The hand-held computer serves as the patient's interface with the implanted monitor. It provides external power to the implant that is transmitted via the communications coil to the sensor, and it acquires real-time physiologic signals using radiofrequency telemetry. The implanted unit performs measurements only when the coil is in radiofrequency communication with a patient advisory module (*see* Fig. 12-26).

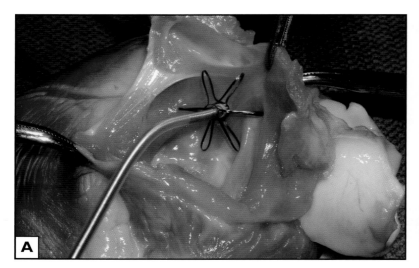

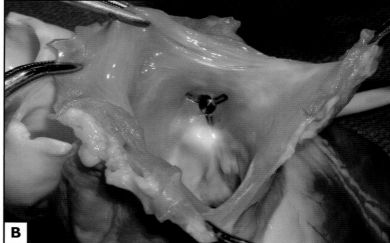

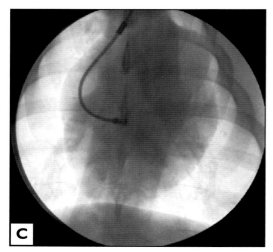

FIGURE 12-10. The 3 mm-diameter sensor housing of the HeartPOD (Savacor, Inc., Los Angeles, CA) left atrial pressure monitor is deployed via transseptal catheterization in a manner similar to larger devices used for closure of atrial septal defects. It is fixed to the interatrial septum by foldable nitinol retention struts, similar to those used to fixate closure devices. **A** and **B**, The right and left atrial sides of the unit, respectively, at the time of implantation in a pig. The sensor is completely covered with neoendocardium within 3 weeks. **C**, Radiograph of the monitor in situ in a pig.

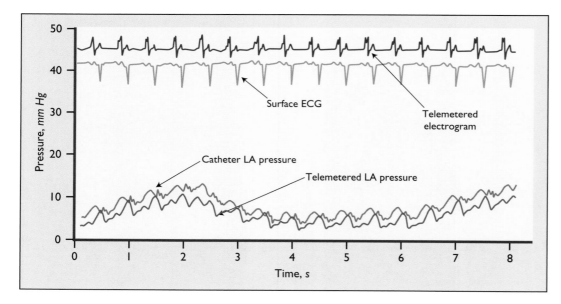

FIGURE 12-11. The sensor system measures left atrial (LA) pressure, core body temperature, and the intracardiac electrogram. Temperature recordings may permit identification of changes in pressure caused by intercurrent infections. Electrograms permit diagnosis of arrhythmias and correlation of atrial and ventricular electrograms with pressure waveforms. Real-time telemetered LA electrogram and surface electrocardiogram (ECG) are shown at the *top*. The LA electrogram has a large atrial component and small ventricular component. At the *bottom*, telemetered LA pressure correlates closely with pressure measured using a fluid-filled catheter/electronic pressure transducer in the left atrium. Signals are from a 4-month old pig implant and have not been corrected for transducer drift.

Initial implantable heart failure monitoring devices assessed standard hemodynamic variables; however, more recent monitors are able to assess novel variables. These newer monitors are attempting to assess variables like lung water as a measure of volume overload, and endocardial acceleration as a measure of contractile state, arrhythmia burden, and myocardial ischemia. The goal of these devices is to assess additional factors in an attempt to provide the clinician with a better overall clinical assessment of the heart failure patient and ultimately aid in the adjustment of the treatment regimen.

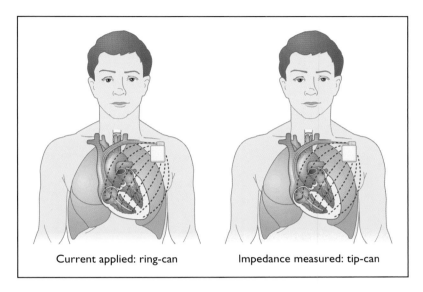

Current applied: ring-can   Impedance measured: tip-can

FIGURE 12-12. Assessment of volume overload by the lung water concept. There is an inverse relationship between thoracic electrical impedance and lung water content [11]. Thoracic impedance is measured by applying a high frequency, low-amplitude current between two electrodes and measuring impedance between the same or a different pair of electrodes. Transthoracic impedance has been used noninvasively to measure heart failure with mixed results [12]. In pacemakers, the respiratory change in intrathoracic impedance has been used as a sensor for rate-responsive pacing [13]. This technology provides highly reliable measurements that are stable over time. Recently, it has been adapted to use measured lung water as an implantable monitor to predict exacerbations of heart failure [14]. Current is applied between an electrode on a pacing or defibrillation lead in the right ventricle and the casing (can) of a pectoral pulse generator. The advantage of this method of monitoring heart failure is that it can be applied using standard pacing or defibrillation electrodes. No special transducer, sensor, or lead is required.

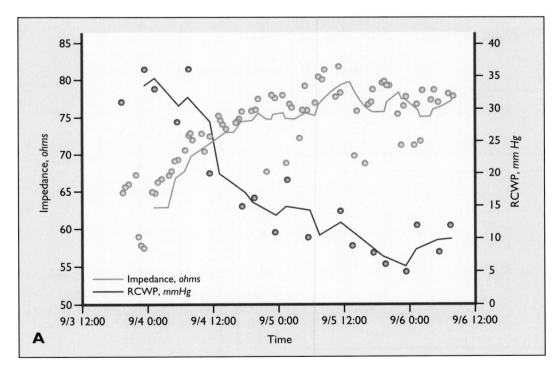

A

FIGURE 12-13. Lung water: single-patient validation. **A,** The temporal relationship between intrathoracic impedance and invasively measured pulmonary capillary wedge pressure (PCWP) in a patient hospitalized for an exacerbation of heart failure. The Y-axis shows impedance (*left*) and PCWP (*right*). Over 6 days of monitoring, PCWP falls from 35 mm to 10 mm and impedance increases from 62 Ω to 78 Ω.

Continued on next page

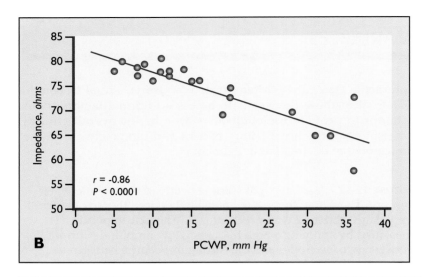

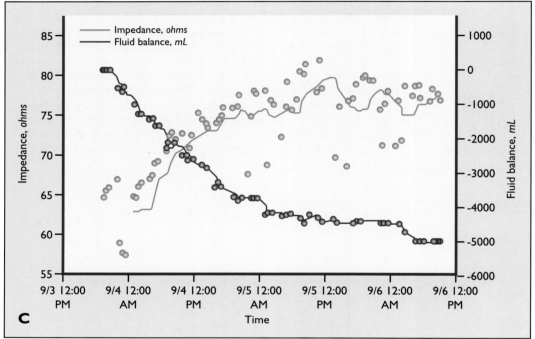

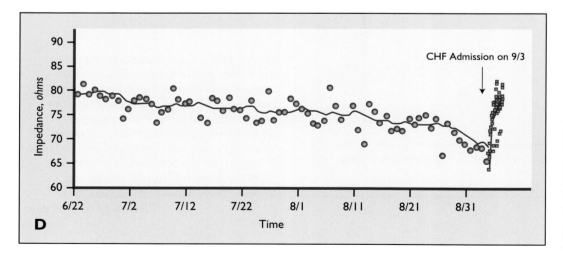

Figure 12-13. *(Continued)* **B,** The regression plot of intrathoracic impedance versus PCWP in the same patient. **C,** The inverse temporal relationship between impedance and fluid balance in the same patient. **D,** Intrathoracic impedance reduction prior to hospitalization for heart failure in the same patient. Impedance declines by 25% over 2 weeks prior to hospitalization.

Continued on next page

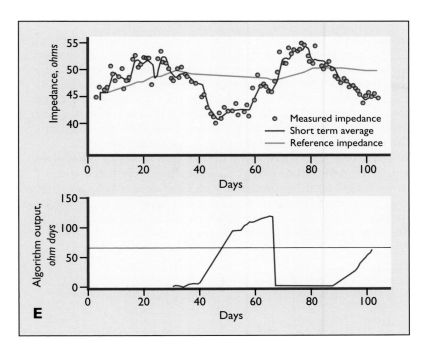

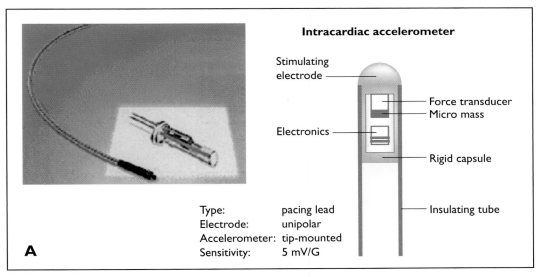

FIGURE 12-13. *(Continued)* **E,** An algorithm for predicting heart failure hospitalization based on intrathoracic impedance data has been developed using data from a clinical trial of 33 patients. The algorithm compares the cumulative difference between a short-term average of impedance data and reference impedance. The algorithm provides advance warning (median 2 weeks) for 70% to 80% of hospitalizations with about one false-positive warning per year [14]. CHF—congestive heart failure.

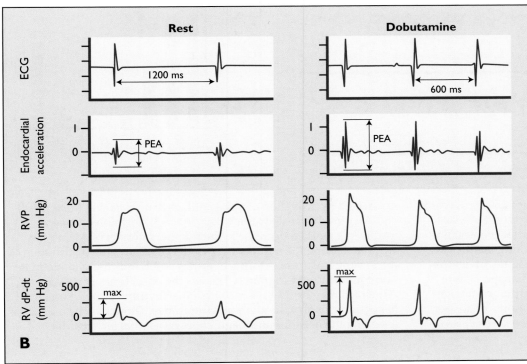

FIGURE 12-14. Evaluation of contractile state by endocardial acceleration. In addition to intra-thoracic impedance, several types of sensors originally developed for rate-responsive pacing may also be used for monitoring heart failure. An advantage of these sensors is their established reliability in implanted devices. Accelerometers may be used to measure myocardial acceleration. During the iso-volumic contraction, peak endocardial acceleration (PEA), a sensitive indicator of contractile function, may be used as a surrogate for maximum dpP/dt [15,16]. **A,** An accelerometer (Sorin Biomedica, Saluggia, Italy) on a right ventricular lead. **B,** Surface electrocardiogram (ECG), the signal generated by the accelerometer representing endocardial acceleration, and right ventricular pressure (RVP) at rest and during dobutamine infusion. This signal is being investigated as a sensor for heart failure. A potential limitation relates to variation in correlation between local right ventricular contractile state and global measures of heart failure.

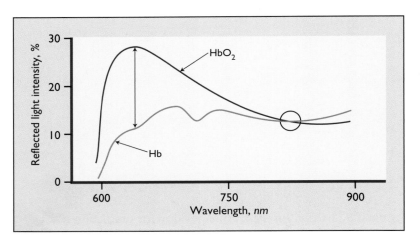

FIGURE 12-15. Surrogate indicators of cardiac output by assessment of mixed venous oxygen. The inverse relationship between mixed venous oxygen concentration and cardiac output has long been used as a gold standard measurement of cardiac output in cardiac catheterization. Implantable oxygen sensors are based on optical reflectivity. The differential reflectivity of oxy-hemoglobin (HgbO$_2$) and deoxy-hemoglobin (Hgb) depends on wavelength. The maximum differential reflectivity is near 660 nm (red). Reflectivity is insensitive to the ratio of oxy- to deoxy-hemoglobin near 805 nm (infrared). Oxygen sensors thus include red and infrared light emitting diodes as well as an optical detector. Tissue in growth degraded function of early implantable oxygen sensors. To date, oxygen sensors have not been used successfully in chronically implanted clinical monitors.

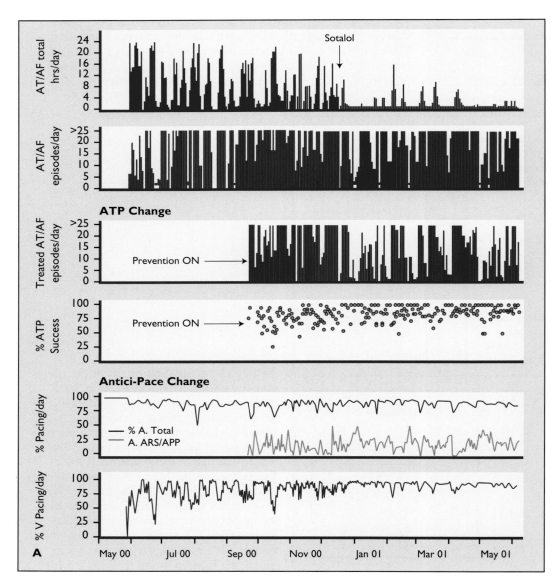

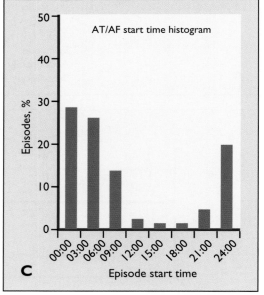

Ventricular response (in AF)		
	# Beats	
<80 bpm	0	(0%)
80–100 bpm	3	(0%)
100–120 bpm	124	(4%)
120–140 bpm	175	(6%)
140–160 bpm	344	(12%)
160–180 bmp	912	(33%)
180–200 bpm	880	(32%)
>200 bpm	319	(12%)

FIGURE 12-16. Diagnostic information from implantable cardioverter defibrillators (ICDs). Atrial fibrillation (AF) may exacerbate heart failure because of loss of atrial transport, inappropriate ventricular rates, or irregularity of ventricular rhythm. Monitoring features of present atrial ICDs or other atrial arrhythmia management devices may provide valuable information regarding the management of heart failure. These data from an atrial antitachycardia pacemaker provide an example. **A**, Shows that the number of hours of AF per day (*top panel*) and number of episodes per day (*second panel*) is unaffected by activation of atrial antitachycardia pacing (*third panel*) and AF prevention algorithms (*fourth panel*). Addition of sotalol results in a marked decrease in the number of hours of AF per day without altering the number of episodes. **B**, Shows the distribution of mean ventricular rates during episodes of AF, indicating inadequate rate control. The histogram (**C**) shows the onset times of episodes of AF, which may be useful in dosing antiarrhythmic drugs. Similar histograms display duration of AF episodes. These may be useful for assessing the need for anticoagulation. AT—atrial tachycardia.

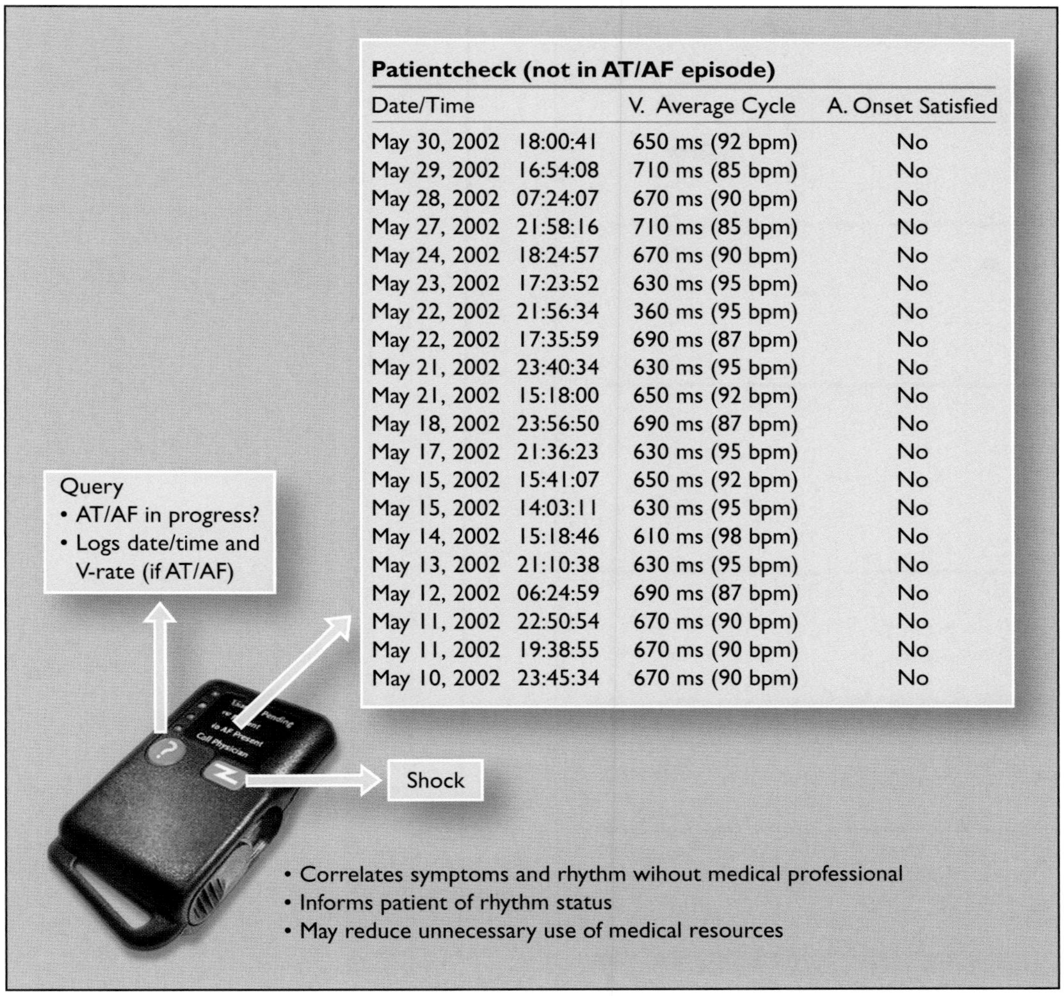

Patientcheck (not in AT/AF episode)

Date/Time		V. Average Cycle	A. Onset Satisfied
May 30, 2002	18:00:41	650 ms (92 bpm)	No
May 29, 2002	16:54:08	710 ms (85 bpm)	No
May 28, 2002	07:24:07	670 ms (90 bpm)	No
May 27, 2002	21:58:16	710 ms (85 bpm)	No
May 24, 2002	18:24:57	670 ms (90 bpm)	No
May 23, 2002	17:23:52	630 ms (95 bpm)	No
May 22, 2002	21:56:34	360 ms (95 bpm)	No
May 22, 2002	17:35:59	690 ms (87 bpm)	No
May 21, 2002	23:40:34	630 ms (95 bpm)	No
May 21, 2002	15:18:00	650 ms (92 bpm)	No
May 18, 2002	23:56:50	690 ms (87 bpm)	No
May 17, 2002	21:36:23	630 ms (95 bpm)	No
May 15, 2002	15:41:07	650 ms (92 bpm)	No
May 15, 2002	14:03:11	630 ms (95 bpm)	No
May 14, 2002	15:18:46	610 ms (98 bpm)	No
May 13, 2002	21:10:38	630 ms (95 bpm)	No
May 12, 2002	06:24:59	690 ms (87 bpm)	No
May 11, 2002	22:50:54	670 ms (90 bpm)	No
May 11, 2002	19:38:55	670 ms (90 bpm)	No
May 10, 2002	23:45:34	670 ms (90 bpm)	No

Query
- AT/AF in progress?
- Logs date/time and V-rate (if AT/AF)

Shock

- Correlates symptoms and rhythm wihout medical professional
- Informs patient of rhythm status
- May reduce unnecessary use of medical resources

FIGURE 12-17. Patient assistant for atrial implantable cardioverter defibrillator (ICD). The patient assistant for atrial ICDs permits determination of rhythm status and permits patients to deliver patient-activated shocks, a model for patient-delivered therapy based on implantable monitors. The data log at *top right* shows interrogations performed daily or twice daily by a patient in whom anticoagulation was contraindicated. AF—atrial fibrillation; AT—atrial tachycardia.

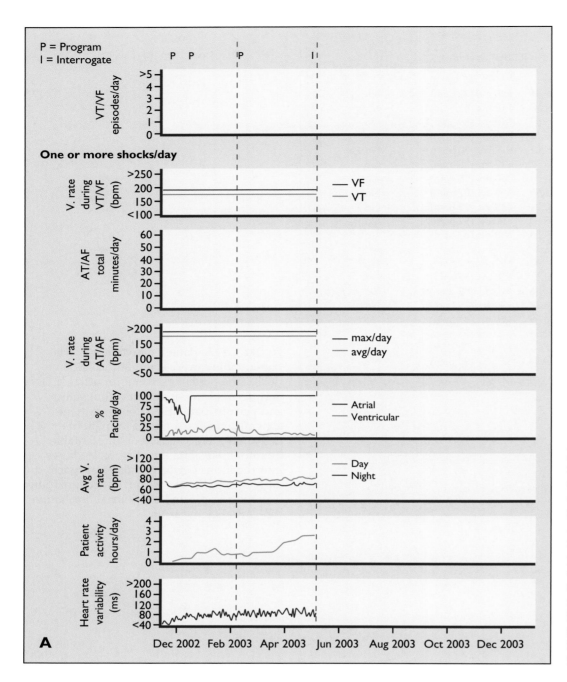

FIGURE 12-18. Diagnostics from a cardiac resynchronization implantable cardioverter-defibrillator (ICD). Present cardiac resynchronization ICDs provide limited diagnostic data for heart failure management. **A**, The fraction of ventricular paced beats fell after hospital discharge due to an inappropriately high value of the sensed atrioventricular delay. Shortening of this delay at the second programming session (*P*) resulted in 100% ventricular pacing. An increase in activity level occurred several months later, but the relationship between improved cardiac resynchronization therapy and patient activity is uncertain.

Continued on next page

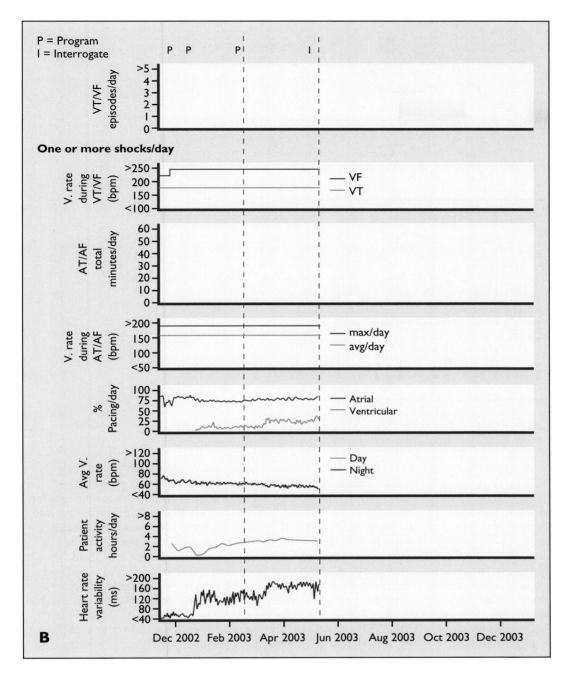

FIGURE 12-18. *(Continued)* **B,** An exacerbation of heart failure in December was associated with decreasing activity per day, reaching a low at the end of the month when the patient was hospitalized. Heart rate variability increases at the time of in-hospital treatment for heart failure. The percent of atrial pacing also increases during hospitalization as resting tachycardia resolves.

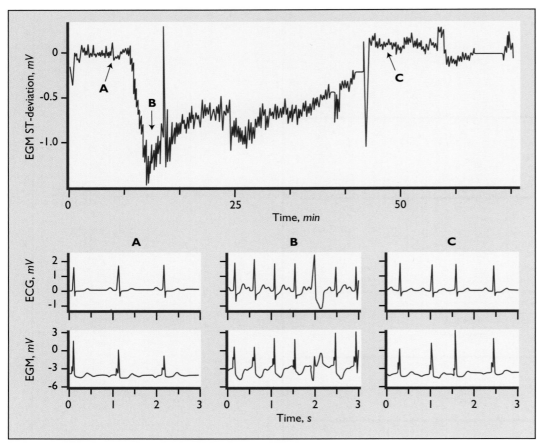

FIGURE 12-19. Ischemia monitoring. Ischemia is an important cause of morbidity and mortality in patients with heart failure. An implantable ischemia monitor is under development as an adjunct to pacemakers or implantable cardioverter defibrillators (ICDs) [17]. It is based on ST-segment deviation measured from intracardiac electrograms (EGM). Standard high-pass filters used in pacemakers and ICDs render these devices insensitive to ST-segment shifts. Thus, an implantable ischemia monitor must either use unfiltered EGMs or unfilter the EGM signal in software using a deconvolution algorithm. Power consumption required for continuous monitoring is an additional problem for implementing an implantable ischemia monitor. Presently, ICDs record high-resolution EGMs and employ microprocessor-intensive rhythm analysis algorithms only when triggered by tachycardia. Ischemia monitoring of patient-triggered events or of antecedents to tachycardias could be implemented with limited effect on power consumption. If implantable monitors were required to meet the same signal quality standards as the surface electrocardiogram (ECG) for ischemia monitoring, power consumption would increase substantially because of requirements for continuous recording of high resolution EGMs (high sampling rate, number of bits required per sample, and bandwidth) and because of the greater duty cycle for the implanted microprocessor.

The figure shows ST segment deviation during a treadmill exercise test recorded from between the right ventricular coil and the can or housing of an ICD. The signal was telemetered and recorded by a specially designed Holter monitor and then passed through a deconvolution algorithm to reduce the high-pass filter from 2.5 Hz to 0.5 Hz. The *top panel* shows the time course of ST segment deviations on the intracardiac EGM. The *lower two panels* show the surface ECG and corresponding intracardiac EGM at three different times corresponding to (**A**) baseline, (**B**) ischemia, and (**C**) recovery.

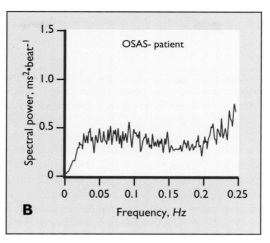
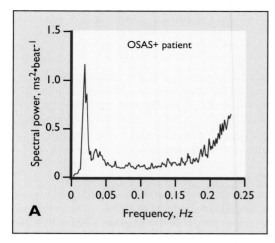

FIGURE 12-20. Heart rate fluctuations in obstructive sleep apnea (OSA). New indications for implantable monitors in patients with cardiovascular disease are constantly on the horizon. OSA has been receiving increased attention as a potentially treatable risk factor for cardiovascular disease [18,19]. OSA has been associated with several characteristic heart rhythm disturbances and recent investigational efforts have focused on monitoring heart rate variability as a surrogate for changes in autonomic tone in this disorder [20,21].

This figure depicts spectral analysis of the interbeat interval increment in obstructive sleep apnea syndrome (OSAS+) (**A**) and normal control patients (OSAS-) (**B**). A spike of very low frequency oscillations occurs in the vast majority of patients with OSA [22].

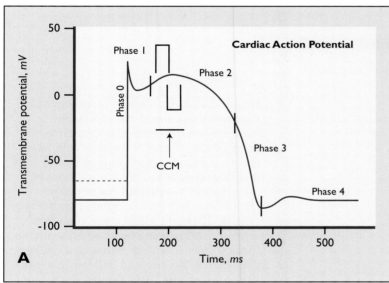
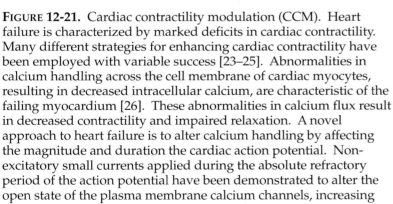
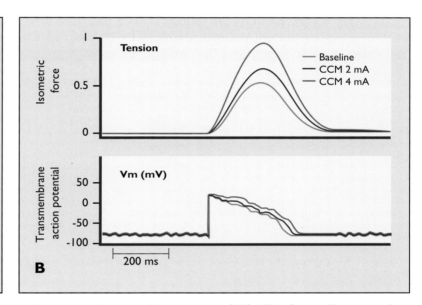

FIGURE 12-21. Cardiac contractility modulation (CCM). Heart failure is characterized by marked deficits in cardiac contractility. Many different strategies for enhancing cardiac contractility have been employed with variable success [23–25]. Abnormalities in calcium handling across the cell membrane of cardiac myocytes, resulting in decreased intracellular calcium, are characteristic of the failing myocardium [26]. These abnormalities in calcium flux result in decreased contractility and impaired relaxation. A novel approach to heart failure is to alter calcium handling by affecting the magnitude and duration the cardiac action potential. Non-excitatory small currents applied during the absolute refractory period of the action potential have been demonstrated to alter the open state of the plasma membrane calcium channels, increasing calcium entry into cardiac myocytes [27]. This figure illustrates the effects of square-wave current pulses applied during the action potential plateau in isolated rabbit papillary muscle. In this method of CCM, nonexcitatory pulses are delivered immediately before the peak of developed tension. Steady state intracellular recordings demonstrate action potential duration, and isometric force (tension) correlates with the amplitude of CCM pulses. **A**, A characteristic cardiac action potential. The *bar* represents the period for CCM delivery. In **B**, the *top curve* depicts steady-state isometric force recordings at baseline and during CCM delivery at two different amplitude settings (2 mA and 4 mA). The *lower curve* shows accompanying increases in action potential duration at the same CCM settings [28]. (*Adapted from* Augello *et al.* [28].)

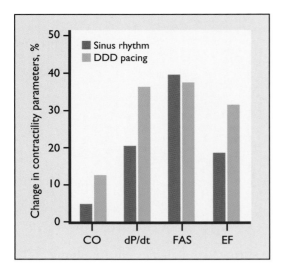

FIGURE 12-22. Cardiac contractility modulation (CCM) improves systolic performance. This figure depicts a series of bar graphs illustrating the average percent change in various systolic parameters from an acute animal model of heart failure during the application of CCM signals relative to baseline. Application of the CCM signal (for a period of 10 minutes) did not alter intrinsic heart rate, but increased peak systolic pressure and pulse pressure. Increases in cardiac output (CO), peak dP/dt, fractional shortening (FAS), and ejection fraction (EF) were noted with the application of CCM during sinus rhythm and dual chamber (DDD) pacing. The average percent increases in these parameters, over baseline measurements, are depicted in the bar graph during sinus rhythm and DDD pacing. Echocardiographic measurements demonstrated that CCM elicited a local improvement in left ventricular function with increased wall thickening noted specifically in areas adjacent to the CCM lead [29]. A preliminary human study has reported that CCM is feasible in patients with heart failure [30]. (*Adapted from* Sabbah *et al.* [29].)

INTEGRATION INTO CLINICAL CARE

INTEGRATION OF IMPLANTABLE MONITORING INTO CLINICAL CARE OF HEART FAILURE PATIENTS

Adjust therapy dynamically based on present value of monitored parameters (tailored therapy)
Evaluate patient tolerance of daily activities objectively
  Exercise tolerance
  Stress
Identify precipitants of heart failure exacerbation
  Arrhythmias
  Ischemia
  Sleep apnea
Improve care during hospitalization for heart failure
  Reduce need for invasive monitoring
  Permit earlier discharge with accurate outpatient monitoring
Improve management by generalists and less-experienced health care providers
Identify new prognostic indices

FIGURE 12-23. Integration of implantable monitors into clinical care. The table suggests possible roles of implantable monitors in the care of patients with heart failure. Given the open-loop nature of early monitoring systems, reliable methods of transmitting meaningful, "actionable" clinical information in a timely manner are crucial. To be of clinical value, data from implantable monitors must be presented to cardiologists, internists, nurse practitioners, physician assistants, and patients in a form that is meaningful to each, and at a time and place where they can act on the information.

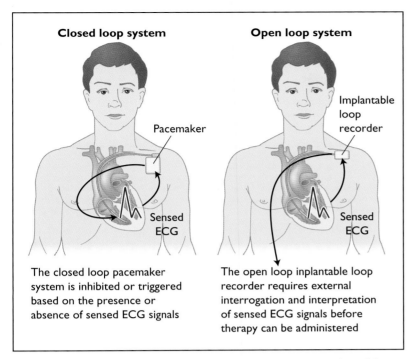

FIGURE 12-24. Open versus closed loop paradigms. Implantable monitors can be integrated into clinical care using either open-loop or closed-loop paradigms. Pacemakers, the prototypical implanted cardiac electronic devices, function as closed-loop systems. The presence or absence of an intracardiac electrogram is sensed. The pacemaker's algorithm then determines whether to deliver therapy (a pacing pulse), and when to deliver it. Some heart failure therapies may be amenable to closed-loop systems. These include cardiac resynchronization therapy, investigational inotropic electrical therapies, and drug delivery using implantable drug pumps. However, the mainstay of present therapy for heart failure remains drugs administered from external reservoirs. For this reason, first generation heart failure monitoring devices are implemented as open-loop systems, such as the implantable loop recorder shown in the figure. The therapy arm of open-loop systems may require real time involvement of either the patient alone or of both a health care provider and the patient.

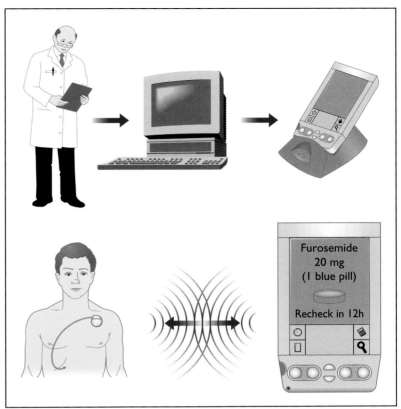

FIGURE 12-25. Open-loop system involving patient and health care provider. The internet-based network for monitoring, Chronicle (Medtronic, Inc., Minneapolis, MN) implantable hemodynamic monitor, involves the patient and the health care provider in the therapy arm. The patient places a hand receiver over the implantable monitor. Telemetered data stored in the implanted monitor are received and stored in the patient's external home monitor. The remote monitor functions as a modem, transmitting data via any phone line to a secure central server where the data are processed. Data are then displayed in appropriate formats on web sites for the patient, the patient's physicians, or other health care providers. Health care providers can then use these data to monitor the patient and alter therapy. This system is now being evaluated in a randomized, clinical trial to determine if it can reduce hospitalizations for heart failure. In one arm of the study, physicians can use data from the implantable monitor to manage patients. In the other arm, the same physicians are blinded to implantable monitor data. In the present version undergoing clinical study, the home monitor does not provide information about clinical status directly to the patient.

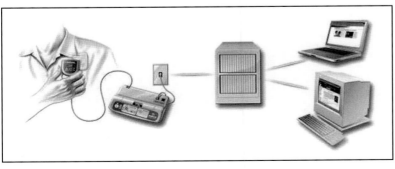

FIGURE 12-26. Open-loop system providing dynamic instructions to the patient. An example of such a system is based on the hand-

held patient advisory module intended for use in conjunction with a left atrial pressure monitor (HeartPOD, Savacor, Inc., Los Angeles, CA). During an office visit, the physician user enters patient-specific conditional instructions such as medication doses into a computer and transmits it to the patient advisory module. The patient uses the advisory module to download real-time pressure signals. The advisory module performs real-time analysis of the telemetered data and displays the patient's preprogrammed instructions based on values of the measured data. If integrated into an information network, the system could be modified so that the advisory module transmits monitoring data to the health care provider. The health care provider could then transmit modified patient instructions to the advisory module.

References

1. Luchsinger PC, Seipp HW Jr, Patel DJ: Relationship of pulmonary artery-wedge pressure to left atrial pressure in man. *Circ Res* 1962, 11:315–318.

2. O'Quin R, Marini JJ: Pulmonary artery occlusion pressure: clinical physiology, measurement, and interpretation. *Am Rev Respir Dis* 1983, 128:319–326.

3. Stevenson LW, Perloff JK: The limited reliability of physical signs for estimating hemodynamics in chronic heart failure. *JAMA* 1989, 261:884–888.

4. Badgett RG, Lucey CR, Mulrow CD: Can the clinical examination diagnose left-sided heart failure in adults? *JAMA* 1997, 277:1712–1719.

5. Stevenson LW: Therapy tailored for symptomatic heart failure. *Heart Fail* 1995, 11:87–107.

6. Effect of metoprolol CR/XL in chronic heart failure: Metoprolol CR/XL Randomised Intervention Trial in Congestive Heart Failure (MERIT-HF). *Lancet* 1999, 353:2001–2007.

7. Engelstein ED: Prevention and management of chronic heart failure with electrical therapy. *Am J Cardiol* 2003, 91:62F–73F.

8. Reynolds DW, Bartelt N, Taepke R, Bennett TD: Measurement of pulmonary artery diastolic pressure from the right ventricle. *J Am Coll Cardiol* 1995, 25:1176–1182.

9. Ohlsson A, Bennett T, Nordlander R, *et al.*: Monitoring of pulmonary arterial diastolic pressure through a right ventricular pressure transducer. *J Card Fail* 1995, 1:161–168.

10. Magalski A, Adamson P, Gadler F, *et al.*: Continuous ambulatory right heart pressure measurements with an implantable hemodynamic monitor: a multicenter, 12-month follow-up study of patients with chronic heart failure. *J Card Fail* 2002, 8:63–70.

11. Grimbert F, Jacquot C, Bossat F, *et al.*: Pulmonary water and thoracic impedance. Evaluation of a measurement technic. *Ann Anesthesiol Fr* 1975, 16(Spec No 2-3):157–163.

12. Gilbert J, Lazio L: Managing congestive heart failure with thoracic electrical bioimpedance. *AACN Clin Issues* 1999, 10:400–405.

13. Lau CP, Ward DE, Camm AJ: Single-chamber cardiac pacing with two forms of respiration-controlled rate-responsive pacemaker. *Chest* 1989, 95:352–358.

14. Stadler RW, Wang L, Yu CM, *et al.*: Automated detection of decreases in intrathoracic impedance to predict congestive heart failure admissions [abstract]. *Pacing Clin Electrophysiol* 2003, 26:932.

15. Bongiorni MG, Soldati E, Arena G, *et al.*: Is local myocardial contractility related to endocardial acceleration signals detected by a transvenous pacing lead? *Pacing Clin Electrophysiol* 1996, 19:1682–1688.

16. Bombardini T, Gaggini G, Marcelli E, *et al.*: Peak endocardial acceleration reflects heart contractility also in atrial fibrillation. *Pacing Clin Electrophysiol* 2000, 23:1381–1385.

17. Stadler RW, Lu SN, Nelson SD, Stylos L: A real-time ST-segment monitoring algorithm for implantable devices. *J Electrocardiol* 2001, 34(suppl)119–126.

18. Peppard PE, Young T, Palta M, Skatrud J: Prospective study of the association between sleep-disordered breathing and hypertension. *N Engl J Med* 2000, 342:1378–1384.

19. Shahar E, Whitney CW, Redline S, *et al.*: Sleep-disordered breathing and cardiovascular disease: cross-sectional results of the Sleep Heart Health Study. *Am J Respir Crit Care Med* 2001, 163:19–25.

20. Guilleminault C, Connolly SJ, Winkle RA: Cardiac arrhythmia and conduction disturbances during sleep in 400 patients with sleep apnea syndrome. *Am J Cardiol* 1983, 52:490–494.

21. Shiomi T, Guilleminault C, Sasanabe R, *et al.*: Augmented very low frequency component of heart rate variability during obstructive sleep apnea. *Sleep* 1996, 19:370–377.

22. Roche F, Duverney D, Court-Fortune I, *et al.*: Cardiac interbeat interval increment for the identification of obstructive sleep apnea. *Pacing Clin Electrophysiol* 2002, 25:1192–1199.

23. Erlemeier HH, Kupper W, Bleifeld W: Intermittent infusion of dobutamine in the therapy of severe congestive heart failure—long-term effects and lack of tolerance. *Cardiovasc Drugs Ther* 1992, 6:391–398.

24. Chatterjee K: Phosphodiesterase inhibitors: alterations in systemic and coronary hemodynamics. *Basic Res Cardiol* 1989, 84(suppl 1):213–224.

25. Tisdale JE, Patel R, Webb CR, *et al.*: Electrophysiologic and pro-arrhythmic effects of intravenous inotropic agents. *Prog Cardiovasc Dis* 1995, 38:167–180.

26. McMurray J, Pfeffer MA: New therapeutic options in congestive heart failure: Part II. *Circulation* 2002, 105:2223–2228.

27. Wood EH, Heppner RL, Weidmann S: Inotropic effects of electric currents. I. Positive and negative effects of constant electric currents or current pulses applied during cardiac action potentials. II. Hypotheses: calcium movements, excitation-contraction coupling and inotropic effects. *Circ Res* 1969, 24:409–445.

28. Augello G, Santinelli V, Vicedomini G, *et al.*: Cardiac contractility modulation by non-excitatory electrical currents. The new frontier for electrical therapy of heart failure. *Ital Heart J* 2004, 5 (suppl 6):68S–75S.

29. Sabbah HN, Haddad W, Mika Y, *et al.*: Cardiac contractility modulation with the impulse dynamics signal: studies in dogs with chronic heart failure. *Heart Fail Rev* 2001, 6:45–53.

30. Pappone C, Augello G, Rosanio S, *et al.*: First human chronic experience with cardiac contractility modulation by nonexcitatory electrical currents for treating systolic heart failure: mid-term safety and efficacy results from a multicenter study. *J Cardiovasc Electrophysiol* 2004, 15:418–427.